Sports and Exercise Medicine: Muscle Injuries

Sports and Exercise Medicine: Muscle Injuries

Edited by **Pablo De Souza**

hayle
medical

New York

Published by Hayle Medical,
30 West, 37th Street, Suite 612,
New York, NY 10018, USA
www.haylemedical.com

Sports and Exercise Medicine: Muscle Injuries
Edited by Pablo De Souza

International Standard Book Number: 978-1-63241-357-4 (Hardback)

Printed in the United States of America.

Contents

Preface

This insightful book on common injuries in the domain of sports medicine provides updated information to readers. A very common pathology in sports and a leading cause of sport activity suspension is muscle tear. This book is aimed at presenting a review on the current knowledge available on muscle tears in athletes, specifically regarding the biology of muscle healing, both traditional and modern surgical treatments as well as preventive measures. This book will be a valuable resource for sports medicine practitioners including physicians, physiotherapists and fitness coaches.

Various studies have approached the subject by analyzing it with a single perspective, but the present book provides diverse methodologies and techniques to address this field. This book contains theories and applications needed for understanding the subject from different perspectives. The aim is to keep the readers informed about the progress in the field; therefore, the contributions were carefully examined to compile novel researches by specialists from across the globe.

Indeed, the job of the editor is the most crucial and challenging in compiling all chapters into a single book. In the end, I would extend my sincere thanks to the chapter authors for their profound work. I am also thankful for the support provided by my family and colleagues during the compilation of this book.

Editor

General Aspect

Nutritional Interventions as Potential Strategy to Minimize Exercise-Induced Muscle Injuries in Sports

Giuseppe D'Antona

Additional information is available at the end of the chapter

1. Introduction

Muscle injury has been related to resistance exercise and prolonged endurance exercise paradigms both leading to significant local mechanical constraints followed by focal disorders such as sarcolemmal damage and leakage of intracellular proteins, oedema, myofibrillar disorganization and microtrauma-triggered inflammation. These unfavorable events lead to variable soreness, swelling, loss in muscle strength and function with reduced range of motion.

To date strategies finalized to minimize exercise-induced muscle injury are scarce and often not adequately supported by research studies.

Based on the notion that dietary supplementations may exert a variety of beneficial effects on the skeletal muscle, in the last 20 years there has been a great deal of interest in nutritional strategies aiming to attenuate signs and symptoms of exercise induced muscle injuries. Anyhow a large number of variables influences the muscular outcome of nutritional supplements, strongly depending on nutrient type, genotype, age, and regulation of nutrient sensing pathways.

Overall there is a paucity of studies on the topic, partly related to the high number of supplements to be considered and their combined use. In general nutrients as vitamins (as vitamin C), N-acetyl-cysteine, L-carnitine, creatine, and branched chain amino acids (BCAA) may exert a potential beneficial role but the underlying cellular mechanism, the optimal dosage and the duration of the pretreatment/treatment period are currently unknown.

This chapter addresses the current knowledge on the potential use of nutritional supplements in preventing and/or minimizing muscle injuries due to resistance or endurance exercise training.

"If the soreness then, be caused by the same conditions which produce fatigue, namely the presence of diffusible waste products of activity we should expect to find, as we do find, that it takes the course described above, passing away within few hours of the work itself" [1]

In 1900 Theodore Hugh first described that exercise induced muscle injury is not a fatigue phenomenon but the consequence of mechanical overload followed by structural and functional muscular changes [1].

Cycles of repetitive eccentric and concentric contractions represent a fundamental source of mechanical stress for active skeletal muscle and vulnerability of skeletal muscle fibers appears to be particularly evident in unaccustomed individuals. In fact conditioning of the muscle through prior similar activity may minimize damage appearance (so called "repeated bout effect") [2]. Overall the process appears as a fundamental step for the arising of exercise-induced plastic response as it is followed by muscle remodeling and adaptation [3]. However muscle damage may delay muscle recovery from exercise and performance thus reducing the athletes compliance to exercise programmes.

The direct consequence of mechanical stress on active skeletal muscle fibers is the appearance of soreness (delayed onset muscle soreness, DOMS), stiffness and reduced force production. This is particularly the case as a consequence of strenuous physical work involving heavy resistance exercise including eccentric (i.e. lengthening) actions [4-6]. In these conditions force loss appears immediately post-exercise whereas soreness becomes evident within 24-48 hours after and, as the force impairment, may last several days depending of the extent of damage [7]. At the microscopic and submicroscopic level fibers damage, which preferentially involves fast twitch fibers [8], is already evident within minutes from the mechanical insult [9] displays throughout individual fibers (i.e. focal injury), and includes plasma membrane disruption accompanied by the loss of muscle proteins in the serum (i.e. creatine kinase (CK), myoglobin, lactate dehydrogenase (LDH), aldolase, troponin), myofibrillar disorders as streaming and broadening of the Z-lines, loss of sarcomeres register, the appearance of regions of overextended sarcomeres, regional disorganization of the myofilaments, subsarcolemmal lipofuscin granules accumulation, alterations of the proteoglycan components, increased interstitial space, and capillary damage [10-15]. Interestingly dramatic changes in the organization of the membrane systems involved in excitation-contraction coupling have been also found following eccentric contractions [16]. The most commonly identified alterations include disorders of the T tubule, changes in the direction and spatial orientation of the triads, and the appearance of caveolar clusters, pentads and heptads (close apposition of two or three T tubule elements with three or four elements with three or four elements of terminal cisternae of sarcoplasmic reticulum).

Apart mechanical stress, other mechanisms may contribute to muscle damage. In particular a metabolic impairment has been proposed as a result of ischemia or hypoxia during prolonged and intense resistance exercise. This insult leads to changes in ion concentration, accumulation of metabolic wastes, and adenosine triphosphate (ATP) deficiency which contribute to soreness and impaired function.

Importantly the early mechanical and metabolic mechanisms can promote biochemical changes within the affected area, leading to the generation of a secondary muscle damage including disruption of intracellular calcium homeostasis, local accumulation of inflammatory cytokines such as tumor necrosis factor-a, interleukin (IL)-1b, IL-6, and IL-1 receptor antagonist (IL-1ra) [17], *de facto* mimicking the sequential release of cytokines after trauma [18], and reactive oxygen species (ROS) that may further degrade muscle proteins and increase the local expression of cytokines [19, 20]. This condition may contribute to persistence of signs and symptoms of injury.

Although it is widely accepted that high intensity eccentric exercise is the fundamental exercise paradigm resulting in muscle damage and subsequent adaptation, structural and functional damage may also arise following long lasting endurance exercise paradigms as demonstrated by the appearance of ultrastructural alterations, as fibers necrosis, sarcolemmal disruption, Z discs streaming, contracture knots, and inflammatory infiltration in endurance athletes even before a race [21]. Anyhow even though the extent and location of damage may greatly vary according to the exercise paradigm and the previous conditioning of the muscoloskeletal system, the extent of damage observed with low intensity and long duration endurance exercise is often less pronounced than with higher intensities. This is the main reason of why most of works finalized to the identification of the physiological mechanisms that regulate the response to exercise-induced stress in skeletal muscle and the possible countermeasures, including the approach based on nutrient supplementation, have been focused on strength training exercise.

2. Nutritional intervention to minimize exercise-induced muscle injury

For decades, dietary supplementation has been proposed in various physiological or pathological conditions. Based on the recent progress in our understanding of the cell signaling and *in vivo* metabolism of nutrients and on accumulating experimental results, the concept that dietary supplementation might have effects in prevention or treatment of several disorders is experiencing a new revival. To date several investigations have been focused on accumulating experimental evidence aiming to extend the use of specific nutritional supplements in the prevention and/or treatment of exercise induced muscle injuries. Anyhow available outcomes on potentially efficacious supplements are mixed and often conflicting and confident conclusions cannot be drawn. Several variables may concur to contradictory results including the wide number of supplements to be considered, their combined use, their dose and timing of administration. Furthermore the choice of the proper indexes to be analyzed is certainly a major bias for several published studies on the topic as a misinterpretation of results may follow the analysis of indirect instead of direct signs of muscle injury. Thus, although many nutrients are potentially able to impact on the mechanisms underlying the appearance of muscle damage following exercise, the final efficacy and safety of their supplementation deserves future rigorous investigation.

The present chapter discusses the potential role of antioxidants, creatine, carnitine and branched chain amino acids on exercise induced muscle damage.

3. Antioxidant/vitamines

Nutritional antioxidants are non enzymatic compounds including the lipid-soluble vitamin E, β-carotene, co-enzyme Q10 (CoQ), and the water-soluble vitamin C, glutathione, and uric acid. These antioxidants either scavenge ROS into less reactive molecules or prevent their transformation into more highly reactive forms, having intracellular and extracellular sites of action [22].

During exercise and exercise-induced damage whole body oxygen consumption increases up to 20 fold and ROS are generated in excess [23]. The primary sources of ROS are endogenous sites within the skeletal muscle, whereas the secondary sites of production are exogenous [24]. Within the muscle the main font of ROS is reputedly through electron leakage in the mitochondria during mitochondrial phosphorylation and via xanthine oxidase metabolism in the capillary endothelium [25, 26] whereas the main secondary source of ROS is generated during the inflammation mainly by neutrophils.

Considering that increased ROS production could challenge the natural antioxidant defense system and that ROS play a major role in the initiation and progression of exercise-induced skeletal muscle injury [27, 28], it has been hypothesized that antioxidants supplementation may minimize its extent and this topic has been faced by a plethora of studies. However, to date, strong evidence to support significant reductions in structural or functional impairment due to antioxidants is missing. Inconsistencies of findings may relate to ununiformities in the experimental designs in terms of type, dose, time of administration and chosen indexes to evaluate and quantify muscle injury. In fact the majority of investigations have been focused on the effects of vitamin C and E and looked at changes in plasma concentrations in CK and LDH and oxidative stress markers. Much less studies have analyzed direct indexes of muscle damage as loss in muscle strength, soreness and structural/ultrastructural changes of the fibers [26, 29]. Indeed a not univocal strategy in the timing of supplementation (pre exercise, during exercise, post exercise) has been adopted demonstrating de facto a lack of a univocal and definite and generally accepted mechanism underlying the correlation between exercise, muscle damage, and antioxidant activity. As a matter of facts several studies have examined the effects of antioxidants on indices of ROS-induced muscle damage in exercise and suggested that antioxidant supplementation may exert some protection particularly in relation to bouts of resistance exercise in untrained or physically active individuals [30-35] as demonstrated by a reduced inflammation [35-39], force loss [30, 40, 41], and fatigue appearance [42, 43] and no evidence for any beneficial effect on performance [44]. On the contrary no significant effects of antioxidant supplements have been found by other authors on indices of inflammation [45-49], cell damage [45, 48, 50-53], oxidative stress [53], and muscle soreness [54-57]. The lack of effects appears to be particularly evident in highly trained individuals whose adaptation to increased exposure to oxidation is normally able to promote a secondary increase of the endogenous antioxidant defenses that reduce the risk of oxidative damage [58, 59] Therefore even following extreme exercise paradigms, unlike short periods of modest exercise [60], indications of oxidative damage may lack in well trained athletes [61]. Importantly in these conditions exposure to antioxidants may hinder the beneficial cell adaptations to exercise thereby promoting muscle damage instead of recovering from it [55, 62-64]. In fact there are concerns about possible adverse effects of megadose supplementation, as several of these nutrients have been shown to increase markers of exercise-induced oxidative stress thus serving as prooxidants instead of antioxidant nutrients. For example after intense exercise, supplementation with vitamin C, vitamin E, N-acetylcysteine and coenzyme Q10 was associated with oxidative stress, increased serum CK and, in some cases, reduced performance [63-67]. In another study prolonged (2 months) vitamin E supplementation increased lipid peroxidation and inflammation [68] whilst no effects on resting levels of oxidative stress were observed by others following vitamin C and E supplementation in ultraendurance athletes [69].

Vitamin C. To date there is no evidence to support the hypothesis that acute and prolonged supplementation with ascorbic acid before and/or after exercise may prevent/attenuate exercise induced muscle damage.

Although a long lasting supplementation with vitamin C before exercise bouts has met with conflicting results, some of them reporting a beneficial effect on lipid peroxidation and inflammation [70] probably due to an increase of the baseline response of antioxidant enzymes [71], nowhere a clear effect on muscle damage has been reported. Similar results have been obtained following acute supplementation prior to exercise. In particular an early study by Ashton and colleagues [72] demonstrated a protective effect of an acute dose of ascorbic acid against ROS production following exhaustive exercise. In this study no indices of muscle damage were measured. Later the effects of an identical dose of ascorbic acid 2 hours before 90 minutes of intermittent shuttle running were investigated by others [52]. Supplementation did not affect the increases in serum CK, serum aspartate aminotransferase, and delayed onset muscle soreness [52]. Importantly the same negative results were obtained when supplementation was performed after training. In particular vitamin C supplementation for 3 days after an intermittent shuttle running showed no effects on indexes of muscle damage, lipid peroxidation and inflammatory response [56]. In another study combination of vitamin C with n-acetylcysteine for 7 days after an eccentric bout of exercise exerted a prooxidant effect. Furthermore equivocal results emerged when supplementation was given before and after exercise bouts, as the smoothening effects on DOMS observed by some authors [34, 73] have been not confirmed by others [54, 55].

Overall, although conflicting results on the topic may result from ununiformities of supplementation strategies and inconsistencies in the experimental procedures adopted (for example the lack of crossover design or the missing measures of direct indexes of muscle damage), there is limited evidence of a protective effect of vitamin C on exercise induced muscle damage.

Vitamin E. Vitamin E, the most important lipid-soluble antioxidant vitamin, is known to stop the progression of the lipid peroxidation chain reaction and is an important scavenger of the superoxide, hydroxyl and lipid peroxyl radicals [74]. Vitamin E can be recycled from its radical form by vitamin C and less efficiently by other antioxidants (glutathione, CoQ, cysteine and a-lipoic acid). Importantly, this vitamin may also act as a prooxidant in the absence of these antioxidants [75]. Most of studies investigating the effects of vitamin E on exercise induced muscle damage have utilized a preexercise supplementation strategy starting from the assumption that vitamin E, contrarily to vitamin C, being lipid-soluble can be stored in tissues.

Anyhow direct indexes of muscle damage were not adequately measured in most cases and available results, albeit suggesting a minimal, unless absent [45], protection of vitamin E supplementation on oxidation, membrane damage [76, 77], and inflammation [76], do not provide enough evidence for a protective effect of vitamin E on exercise induced muscle damage.

In conclusion, there is little evidence to support the suggestion that supplementation with antioxidant nutrients can improve exercise performance, but there is a growing body of evidence to suggest that supplementation may reduce the extent of exercise induced oxidative damage. If this is indeed the case, it may be that the athlete undertaking a strenuous training programme may benefit in the long term by being able to sustain a higher training load (less fatigue). There is also evidence, however, that prolonged exposure to training increases the effectiveness of the endogenous antioxidant mechanisms, and it may be that supplementation is unnecessary or prooxidant and thus potentially unsafe.

4. Carnitine

Carnitine is the required carrier of fatty acids from the cytoplasm into mitochondria, where they undergo β-oxidation [78, 79]. In the cytoplasm carnitine combines with fatty acyl-coenzyme A (acyl-CoA) thus allowing that fatty acids may enter the mitochondrion. The first step of this process is catalysed by carnitine palmitoyl transferase 1 (CPT1) and the trans-membrane transport is facilitated by acylcarnitine transferase. Within the mitochondrion free carnitine is regenerated by the action of carnitine palmitoyl transferase 2 (CPT2) and the released fatty acyl-CoAs entry the β-oxidation pathway. Within the mitochondrion, carnitine also regulats the acetyl-CoA concentration and the concentration of free CoA. Considering that free CoA is involved in the pyruvate dehydrogenase reaction and in the process of β-oxidation it contributes to the coordinated integration of fat and carbohydrate metabolism. In fact when glucose oxidation increases, acetyl groups can be translocated from acyl-CoA within the mitochondrial matrix to the cytoplasm. The accumulation of cytosolic acetylcarnitine may result in a limitation of CPT-1 activity because of the decrease in availability of free carnitine. Consequently, there is fatty acid oxidation, since skeletal muscle predominantly expresses an isoform of CPT-1 with low affinity for L-carnitine [80].

In humans, 75% of carnitine is obtained from the diet. The primary dietary sources of carnitine are red meat and dairy products [81]. Dietary carnitine is absorbed from the intestinal lumen across the mucosal membrane by both passive and active transport mechanisms. Carnitine is also synthesized in the liver and in the kidneys (not in skeletal and cardiac muscle) [82] from the essential amino acids, lysine and methionine [83, 84] having ascorbic acid, ferrous iron, pyroxidine, and niacin as necessary cofactors [85]. More than 95% of the body's total carnitine store is within skeletal muscle tissue [86], and decreased plasma carnitine level has been related to low tissue concentrations [79, 87].

Considering the key roles of carnitine for normal skeletal muscle bioenergetics (long-chain fatty acid oxidation; removal of acyl groups from the mitochondria; detoxification), its availability may be the limiting factor for fatty acid oxidation and/or the removal of acyl-CoAs also during exercise [82]. Based on such considerations it has been proposed that carnitine consumption may improve exercise performance and/or recovery from exercise. Consistently the large majority of studies observed a beneficial effect of L-carnitine supplementation on maximum oxygen uptake or respiratory quotient in healthy athletes [88] whereas only a minority of studies failed to observe such effects [88]. In particular, several scientific reports highlight that carnitine supplement could be an ergogenic aid for endurance exercise [89, 90] as in presence of concomitant low carnitine concentration in skeletal muscle limiting carnitine acyltransferases to operate at a high rate, the oral ingestion of carnitine would result in an increase of the total carnitine concentration. This effect may be followed by increased rate of oxidation of intramuscular fatty acids and triacylglycerols during exercise thus reducing muscle glycogen breakdown and postponing fatigue appearance [88]. On the other hand a decrease of free carnitine concentration to very low levels is expected in skeletal muscles subjected to high-intensity training because the compound tends to react with acetyl- CoA. This decrease has been suggested as one of the mechanisms for the reduction of plasma fatty acid and intramuscular triacylglycerol oxidation during high-intensity exercise [91]. Accordingly most studies showed improved maximum oxygen consumption, reduced lactate accumulation, and increased high-intensity exercise performance in professional and nonprofessional athletes, especially when L-carnitine was supplemented for longer periods and at higher doses [92-95]. However, some investigations failed to show any effect of carnitine supplementation following on high-intensity training programs [96-101].

Recently a discrete bulk of research has provided the evidence to support the theoretical potential for the use of L-carnitine supplementation in exercise recovery. These studies demonstrated that supplemental carnitine is effective in attenuating tissue damage as directly assessed via magnetic resonance imaging, muscle soreness, and postexercise markers of metabolic stress following eccentric exercise training [102] or intense resistance exercise [103-105] thus leading to a quicker recovery (2 to 3 g/day of elemental carnitine being supplied by L-carnitine L-tartrate, LCLT). In particular Volek and colleagues [103] analyzed the effects of L-carnitine (2g/d for 3 wk before exercise and during 4d recovery) on markers of muscle damage in trained adult man following 5 sets of 15-20 repetitions of squats at 50% of 1-RM. Treated subjects experienced reduced muscle damage and decreased circulating CK compared to placebo. Similar results, recently obtained by the same authors, have clearly shown that LCLT is also effective in promoting recovery of tissue damage arising from the same protocol of high-repetition squat exercise in elderly individuals [106].

Overall the observed benefits of L-carnitine supplementation in preventing exercise-induced muscle injury have mostly been attributed to its potential as antioxidant. Increased generation of ROS is considered as a major cause of disruption/damage to the sarcolemma leading to leakage of cytosolic proteins into the circulation (CK, myoglobin, LDH). Furthermore ROS generated beyond physiological limits are found to reduce muscle force production by altering calcium ion sensitivity in muscle and thus contributing to muscle fatigue [107] [108, 109]. L-carnitine supplementation has been related to reduced postexercise CK [102, 103] and myoglobin [103, 105] concentrations suggesting that reduced oxidative stress may play a role in a quicker muscle recovery from strenuous exercise following supplementation. As a matter of fact early studies by Brass et al. (1993) [110] demonstrated that L-carnitine delays hypoxia-induced fatigue in electrically stimulated rat skeletal muscle in vitro through its key stimulatory role in muscle bioenergetics and antioxidant activity. Further evidence demonstrated that L-carnitine exhibits effective superoxide anion radical and hydrogen peroxide scavenging, total reducing power and metal chelating activities in vitro [111]. In vivo, in presence of high glycolytic rates as during strenuous resistance exercise, the stimulated formation of ATP and AMP from molecules of ADP results in the oxidation of AMP to hypoxanthine which is considered a marker of metabolic stress [112]. This oxidation reaction is mediated by xanthine oxidase. Accumulation of xanthine oxidase in spite of xanthine dehydrogenase is the consequence of the activation of calcium-dependent proteases, which cleave a portion of xanthine dehydrogenase and convert it into xanthine oxidase. This process is a direct consequence of raised intracellular calcium by inhibition of calcium ATPase pumps induced by insufficient supply of ATP. This response appears to be attenuated by L-carnitine supplementation which reduces intracellular hypoxanthine and xanthine oxidase following resistance exercise bouts [103, 106]. Indeed inhibition of xanthine oxidase with allopurinol during exercise has been shown to result in significantly less generation of ROS, reduced tissue damage after exhaustive exercise [112], and less accumulation of cytosolic enzymes CK and LDH [113, 114]. Furthermore a direct consequence of high-intensity training is hypoxia. Exercise under hypoxic conditions stimulates muscle glucose transport, increases the concentration of ammonia in blood, and lowers the concentration of free carnitine [115, 116]. It has been found that carnitine supplementation during exercise under hypoxic conditions may also prevent ammonia toxicity mainly through reduction of ROS production.

In summary, L-carnitine supplementation can beneficially affect postexercise markers of metabolic stress, muscle disruption, and muscle soreness in young and old healthy men and women. The attenuation of the side effects of high-intensity training mainly relate to its antioxidant potential and its capability to reduce the magnitude of exercise-induced hypoxia. Further research is needed to conclusively elucidate the mechanisms underlying its protective effects and whether these responses may also arise in exercised individuals affected by disorders of different origin as neuromuscular diseases.

5. Creatine

A large number of surveys indicate that creatine (n [aminoiminomethyl]-N-methylglycine) is one of the most widely used nutritional supplements [117-122]. Prevalence studies indicate that the use of creatine is particularly common in athletes and soldiers. Among the athletes population, powerlifters, boxers, weightlifters, and track/field athletes report the higher creatine consumption with prevalence ranging between 45 and 75% [122]. The major determinant of such a widespread consumption by resistance athletes mainly resides in the known ergogenic aid of creatine when supplementation is associated with repeated bouts of high intensity exercise. This combination leads to increased lean body mass (with no effect on fat mass), muscle strength and performance and accelerated post-exercise recovery [123].

Interestingly more pronounced effects of creatine supplementation have been found in strength trained older adults compared to the young adults [124] and in untrained compared to trained individuals whereas similar changes in muscle creatine content and exercise performance have been found between men and women [125, 126]. Besides no ergogenic effect of creatine has been found in a variety of endurance exercise paradigms [127-129].

Several mechanisms could explain the effects of creatine supplementation on muscle mass, strength and performance when supplementation is combined with strength training.

The hypertrophic response has been attributed to increased myosin heavy chain protein expression [130], changes in the expression of myogenic regulatory factors (MRF4 and myogenin) [131, 132], increased mitotic activity of satellite cells and swelling-induced protein synthesis [133-137] followed by net protein deposition. The most popular mechanism to explain the efficacy of creatine on muscle performance refers to a better match between ATP supply and fibers demands during physical exercise due to the enhancement of the resting high energy phosphate levels (total creatine, phosphocreatine, creatine and ATP) observed following supplementation. This change allows users to maintain a greater work intensity for longer durations of time (increased total training volume). In particular, the intracellular concentration of phosphocreatine is known to play a major role during the bioenergetic system mostly active during exercise at high intensities and short durations. Overall the dosing regimen that has been found to significantly increase the intracellular phosphocreatine is a loading phase of approximately 20 g/day for 5-7 days followed by a maintenance phase of 5 g/day for a period of several weeks [138, 139].

The known effects of creatine upon muscle cell function, structure and protein metabolism may represent the rationale for its potential use to prevent or treat muscle cell injuries. Nevertheless, although solid studies have examined the ergogenic potential of creatine, the current literature is very preliminary in relation to examining the effects of creatine supplementation in reducing the severity of exercise-induced muscle damage and/or promote recovery following strength training and endurance paradigms [140].

Considering that high-force eccentric exercise alters myofibre membrane structure and function [9, 141] leading to reductions in force, increased soreness, and impaired muscle function and that membrane stabilization due to decreased membrane fluidity is followed to increased intracellular concentration of phosphocreatine [142], the effects of creatine supplementation on markers of eccentric exercise damage have been assessed following resistance exercise sessions [143-146]. Initial studies conducted in rodents and humans agreed to demonstrate that creatine supplementation does not decrease muscle damage or enhance recovery after high intensity eccentric contractions. In particular Warren and colleagues [143] demonstrated that recovery of mouse anterior crural muscle strength after damage induced by 150 eccentric contractions was unaffected by creatine supplementation at 0.5 and 1% for two weeks. Following 3 minutes recovery, there was no effect of creatine supplementation on the isometric torque loss or on the torque loss at any eccentric or concentric angular velocity tested [143]. In 2001 Rowson and colleagues [146] evaluated the effects of short time creatine and dextrose supplementation (20 gr d-1 creatine and 28 gr d-1 for 5 days, a protocol previously shown to be effective in elevating muscle creatine and phosphocreatine levels [126]) before performing 50 maximal eccentric contractions of the elbow flexors on blood markers of muscle damage (CK and LDH), maximal isometric force, range of motion, arm circumference (an index of swelling), and muscle soreness. Despite the initial hypothesis, results showed nearly identical loss of maximal isometric force and range of motion, development of soreness, increase of the biceps circumference and change in blood CK and LDH in supplemented and placebo groups of subjects thus suggesting that creatine supplementation lacked to display significant improvement of membrane stabilization at the conditions analyzed. In a second study by the same authors male participants were supplemented with creatine for 5 days prior to, and 5 days following a hypoxic resistance exercise test (5 sets of 15-20 repetitions at 50% of 1 repetition maximum). Similarly to the first study creatine failed to have positive effects on the same criterion measures of muscle damage following the resistance exercise challenge [145]. More recently differing results have been obtained following creatine and carbohydrate supplementation to untrained male subjects by the scheme 5 days prior to, and 14 days following a resistance exercise training session consisting of 4 sets of 10 eccentric repetitions at 120% of maximum concentric 1-RM on the leg press, leg extension and leg flexion machine. Creatine supplementation produced significantly greater isokinetic and isometric knee extension strength during recovery from exercise-induced muscle damage. Furthermore, plasma CK activity was lower after 48, 72, 96 hrs, and 7 days recovery in the supplemented group [144]. As discussed by Cook such diverse observations could be in part attributed to the duration of supplementation period and/or post-exercise supplementation. In particular in the first study by Rawson the subjects enrolled were supplemented only for 5 days prior to the exercise protocol; with no continuation of supplementation following the exercise bout [146]. As it has been suggested that the effect of creatine on protein synthesis and muscle regeneration may be enhanced during the recovery period post-injury [130, 147], the time schedule of creatine supplementation respect to the exercise bout may be considered a potential limiter of the muscular protection against exercise-induced damage. This hypothesis seems to be confirmed by the observed increase of satellite cell number and myonuclei concentration following creatine supplementation in human skeletal muscle [147]. Indeed it can be hypothesized that this effect may sum to the known training-induced increase in muscle regeneration.

Notwithstanding supplementation was continued for 5 days after the exercise bout, in the second study by Rawson and colleagues no beneficial effects of creatine on criterion measures of muscle damage were observed [145]. Although it cannot be excluded that the resistance exercise paradigm used by Rawson, designed to be hypoxic in nature, may not have elicited enough muscle damage to unmask the anabolic effects of creatine supplementation, to date available conflicting data from a limited number of experimental works on the topic do not allow to safely draw conclusions on the beneficial effects of oral creatine supplementation on skeletal muscle damage and recovery following eccentric exercise challenge and new, more standardized, experimental works would help unravel this question in the next future.

Based on the fact that cell injury in running depends on cell volume integrity and that creatine potentially stabilizes the cell volume through an increase in cell water content, glycogen stores and/or myofibrillar content [135-137, 148], the effect of oral creatine supplementation has also been examined on markers of muscle damage, i.e. inflammatory and muscle soreness markers, following prolonged running exercise (30Km run) [149]. Marathon runners were supplement-ed for 5 days (20 g/day) prior to a 30km race. Blood samples were collected pre-race, and 24 hours following the end and CK, LDH, prostaglandin E2 (PGE2) and TNFalpha (TNF-α) were measured.

As expected, prolonged running provoked an increase in concentrations of all plasma markers tested, indicating the appearance of cell injury associated with an inflammatory response [6, 150]. Creatine supplementation was effective in significantly attenuate the observed increase in all muscle soreness markers analyzed, unlike CK, thus pointing this nutritional intervention as an effective strategy in maintaining muscle integrity during and after intense and prolonged endurance exercise. In fact the lack of effect upon plasma CK concentration might not reflect the overall positive effect of creatine on muscle damage as a strong variability of this parameter among athletes, its dependence from the training status and the weak correlation with changes in other markers of muscle damage [151-153] lessen its significance in comparison with other markers of cellular death and lysis as LDH [154]. Similar effects on plasma pro inflammatory markers (Interleukin (IL) 1 beta and IL-6, TNF-α, and Interferon alpha (INF alpha) and PGE2) [155] and on plasma markers of cellular integrity (CK, LDH aldolase (ALD), glutamic oxalo-acetic, acid transaminase (GOT), glutamic pyruvic acid transaminase (GPT), and C-reactive protein (CRP) [156] have been obtained in double blind trials following creatine supplemen-tation (20gr day-1) 5 days before a half-ironman and after ironman triathlon competition respectively.

These results confirm the hypothesis that creatine may have a protective effect against membrane cell disruption following prolonged and intense muscle contractions [156]. Indeed as skeletal muscle damage during an ironman competition mostly result from eccentric contractions, mainly related to the marathon segment of the race [157], it can be argued that creatine may be effective in preventing eccentric induced muscle injury. In fact exhaustive exercises involving eccentric contractions, as in triathlon competition, lead to more pro-nounced muscle damage than strenuous exercises involving concentric contractions [158]. Nevertheless other mechanisms but eccentric damage may contribute to muscle damage during triathlon competition including excessive metabolic workload, muscle fatigue, depletion of intramuscular glycogen, and oxidative stress which are generally implicated in prolonged exercise-induced muscle fiber disruption [157, 159, 160]. The observed reduction in plasma activities of GOT and GPT (markers of liver injury) observed in triathletes after an ironman competition may suggest that creatine supplementation can enhance the metabolic efficiency of skeletal muscle preventing the metabolic workload on the liver which has a critical role on the contractile activity-induced skeletal muscle injury. Indeed when eccentric contrac-tion is avoided as in electrically stimulated gastrocnemius muscle of the rat, creatine supple-mentation has been found to delay the fatigue appearance, preserve the force development, and prevent the rise of LDH and CK plasma activities and muscle vascular permeability evaluated with Evans blu staining [156]. Furthermore, although it cannot be excluded that in endurance settings the benefits of supplementation in preventing muscle damage may relate to the antioxidant potential that has been attributed to creatine in various oxidative stress-associated diseases, few studies have been published on the relationship between supplementation and oxidative stress and controversial and not conclusive results are currently available [161-163]. In particular creatine supplementation associated with resistance training or exhaustive exercise training has been associated either with reduced oxidative stress [162, 164], increased free radical generation and related consumption of antioxidant reserves [161] or no change of lipid peroxidation, resistance of low density lipoprotein to oxidative stress or plasma concentrations of non-enzymatic antioxidants [163]. Taken together these observations show that creatine supplementation before strenuous endurance exercise reduces the increase of markers of cell death/lysis and muscle soreness suggesting a positive effect of the supplementation strategy in maintaining muscle integrity after intense prolonged exercise. The mechanisms underlying such a protective effect are only partially known.

6. Essential amino acids

Considering that mechanical stimuli may induce skeletal muscle damage as a consequence of overload and/or eccentric actions causing cytoskeleton and subcellular disruption on muscle fibers, it appears that nutritional interventions finalized to maximize protein synthesis (MPS) or minimize protein catabolism (MPC) would be helpful in preventing and/or treating exercise induced muscle injuries.

As known MPS includes the complex process of mRNA translation which develops in three consecutive steps i.e. initiation, in which the initiator methionyl-tRNA and mRNA bind to 40S ribosomal subunit, elongation, by which tRNA-bound amino acids are incorporated into growing polypeptide chains according to the mRNA template, and termination, where the completed protein is released from the ribosome [165].

The first two steps of mRNA translation are highly regulated at two different levels: the binding of methionyl-tRNA to 40S ribosomal subunit to form 43S preinitiation complex, and recognition, unwinding, and binding of mRNA to the 43S, catalyzed by a multi-subunit complex of eukaryotic factors (eIFs), referred to as eIF4F. The mammalian target of rapamycin (mTOR) kinase which is now recognized as a key regulator of cell growth and a pivotal sensor of nutritional status, is a key regulator of MPS. In cells, mTOR forms two distinct complexes, mTORC1 and mTORC2, depending on the binding partners. When bound to raptor (regulatory associated protein of mTOR) mTOR forms mTORC1, which mediates the effects sensitive to rapamycin [166]. mTOR-mediated regulates protein synthesis is based on Activation of eIF4E binding protein-1 (4E-BP1) releases the inhibition on the eukaryotic factors complex eIF4F, which is responsible for the interaction with 40s ribosomal subunit and translation initiation [167]. In fact when 4E-BP1 is in its hypophosphorylated state it blocks the ability of eIF4E to bind to eIF4G and forms an inactive 4E-BP1-eIF4E complex. This interaction precludes mRNA to bind to the ribosome. mTORC1 is also responsible for the activation of downstream S6K1. S6K1 is a kinase which requires phosphorylation at two sites and its activation is necessary for muscle fibres to achieve normal size, since S6K1 knockout cells are smaller than control cells [168]. Following phosphorylation at Thr389 by mTORC1, S6K1 regulates the activity of eukaryotic elongation factor 2 kinase (eEF2k) [169].

Studies in animals models and humans showed that essential amino acids (EAA) [170, 171] unlike non EAA [170], are fundamental regulators of MPS and mitochondrial biogenesis [172]. It has been shown that hyperaminoacidemia stimulates amino acid transport and net MPS, unlike carbohydrate administration both in the young [173] and in the elderly [174]. The effects on protein synthesis arise independently of changes in anabolic hormone concentration [175, 176], although insulin is required for the effects of EAA on translation [177]. Among EAA, Branched chain amino acids (BCAA: leucine, isoleucine and valine) play a very important role as nutrient signals that regulates MPS through the stimulation of insulin-independent and rapamycin-sensitive pathways [178, 179]. In particular available data suggest that at least part of the postprandial translational activation is to be attributed to BCAAs through activation of mTOR and downstream signals (eIF4G, S6K1 and 4E-BP1). Although mTOR is the key integrator of the anabolic response to BCAA, mTOR itself may not be the direct target of EAA. It has been shown that inhibition by the upstream TSC1/2 complex represents the mechanism through which leucine and insulin upregulate mTOR and downstream targets.

The scenario arising from available studies indicates that the physiological anabolic response to BCAA may help counteracting the metabolic unbalance induced by exercise and in particular resistance training which has been linked to concurrent increase of MPS and MPC [180, 181] and negative changes in circulating free amino acids [182]. In these conditions the exercise-triggered hypercatabolism may be counteracted by amino acids supplementation which in turn has been related with net protein synthesis when combined with bouts of resistance exercise [173, 183, 184] and prevented BCAA exercise-induced oxidation [182].

Recent studies suggest that BCAA supplementation, by promoting MPS, may improve the repair of muscle damage induced by resistance exercise.

In particular Nosaka et al. [185] showed that an amino acid supplement containing around 60% BCAA was effective in reducing muscle damage and soreness when consumed immediately before (30 min) and during the four days of recovery following a damaging bout of lengthening contractions of the elbow flexors. Later Jackman and coworkers reported the effects of BCAA supplementation during recovery from intense eccentric exercise consisting in 12 x 10 repetitions of unilateral eccentric knee extension in male untrained subjects. A decrease in flexed muscle soreness was observed in supplemented compared with placebo group at 48 h and 72 h post exercise whereas the degree of force loss and the fluctuation of blood markers of muscle damage appeared unchanged between groups [186]. Similar results were obtained in female untrained young subjects by Shimomura et al. [187] examining the effects of BCAA supplementation on squat-exercise-induced DOMS. In this report the participants ingested either BCAA (isoleucine:leucine:valine = 1:2.3:1.2) or dextrin at 100 mg/kg body weight just before the squat exercise consisting of 7 sets of 20 squats/set with 3-min intervals between sets. The peak of DOMS was reached two or three days post exercise but the level of soreness was significantly lower in the BCAA trial than in the placebo. Interestingly three day post exercise the force decrease observed in the placebo appeared to be prevented by BCAA supplementation. Accordingly plasma myoglobin and elastase (index of neutrophil activation) appeared to be increased by exercise in the placebo but not in the BCAA group [187].

Interestingly the beneficial effects of BCAA mixtures supplementation has been reported also following moderate resistance training and endurance training both in rodents [188] and humans [189-191]. In these conditions the effect of supplementation seems to mainly reflected on a reduced rate of perceived exertion (RPE) [189] and reduced proteolysis as demonstrated by reduced phenyalanine release from the muscle [192], whereas no beneficial effects have been found in terms of changes in exercise performance [189]. In particular in the study by Greer and coworkers nine untrained male subjects where supplemented with a BCAA enriched beverage, an isocaloric, carbohydrate (CHO) beverage or a noncaloric placebo beverage. The subjects performed three 90-minute cycling bouts at 55% VO2 peak followed by 15-minute time trials and ingested a total of 200 kcal via the CHO or BCAA beverage before and at 60 minutes of exercise or the placebo beverage on the same time course. A greater distance was traveled during the CHO trial than the BCAA and placebo trial. On the contrary the RPE was reduced during the BCAA trial as compared with the placebo trial. This study clearly demonstrated that CHO supplementation improved performance compared with BCAA and PLAC beverage. Thus BCAA supplementation did not influence aerobic performance but attenuated RPE [189]. Accordingly BCAA supplementation (0.8% BCAA in a 3.5% carbohydrate solution; 2,500 mL/day for four days) effectively reduced the muscle soreness and fatigue sensation when supplementation was carried out during an intensive endurance training programme in male and female, and the perceived changes could be attributed to the attenuation of muscle damage as demonstrated by decreased LDH, CK and granulocyte elastase levels, and inflammation [190, 191].

Importantly a minority of works contradict the general findings from other research on the benefits of BCAA on resistance exercise muscle damage. In particular conflicting results have been reported by Stock et al. [193] showing that in a mixed sex group of trained participants there were no differences in damage indices of resistance exercise (6 sets of squats to fatigue using 75% of the 1 repetition maximum) between a carbohydrate versus a carbohydrate/ leucine supplement. The subjects enrolled consumed the carbohydrate beverage 30 minutes before and immediately after exercise with or without the addition of 22.5 mg kg-1 of leucine. Results showed that the addition of leucine did not significantly decrease CK and LDH activity or DOMS evaluated at different time points following exercise thus suggesting that adding leucine to carbohydrate beverages did not affect acute muscle recovery from exercise. Considering that in the study by Stock and coworkers the amino acid supplement consisted of leucine alone (and not of a mixture of BCAA), one can speculate that a methodological bias may account for the observed different outcome of this study compared to others.

In conclusion the overall effect of resistance exercise on circulating BCAA suggests that exercise induced muscle damage is followed by an increase of skeletal muscle BCAA uptake from the serum being used as energy source and/or participate in translation initiation signaling pathway involved in muscle remodeling. Functionally this appears to have some consequence in muscle pain. A similar effect on the rate of perceived exertion has been found following BCAA supplementation before and during endurance exercise, when muscle remodeling is reasonably much less than in resistance exercise. The mechanisms beyond the protective effects of BCAA supplementation on muscle damage deserve further investigations, to be mostly oriented on unraveling the effects of supplements on inflammation.

7. Conclusions

The skeletal muscle is placed under considerable stress during high repetitive eccentric, or lengthening, contractions.

Several studies have used a variety of nutritional supplementation strategies including macronutrients and micronutrients, with variations in dosage, timing and duration of supplementation, finalized to minimize exercise induced muscle injury. Although there is proper rationale and some evidence showing the efficacy of certain supplements such as creatine and essential amino acids, there is little evidence to support a role for others including the antioxidants. Indeed, antioxidant supplementation may interfere with the cellular signalling paths thereby unfavorably affecting muscle function, performance, and recovery from injury.

Author details

Giuseppe D'Antona*

Address all correspondence to: gdantona@unipv.it

Department of Molecular Medicine and Interdepartmental Research Centre in Motor Activities (CRIAMS), University of Pavia, Italy

References

[1] Hough T. Ergographic Studies in Muscular Fatigue and Soreness. Journal. 1900 Nov 20;5(3):81-92.

[2] McHugh MP. Recent advances in the understanding of the repeated bout effect: the protective effect against muscle damage from a single bout of eccentric exercise. Scandinavian journal of medicine & science in sports. 2003 Apr;13(2):88-97.

[3] Ciciliot S, Schiaffino S. Regeneration of mammalian skeletal muscle. Basic mechanisms and clinical implications. Current pharmaceutical design. 2010;16(8):906-14.

[4] Allen DG. Eccentric muscle damage: mechanisms of early reduction of force. Acta physiologica Scandinavica. 2001 Mar;171(3):311-9.

7

[5] Armstrong RB. Initial events in exercise-induced muscular injury. Medicine and science in sports and exercise. 1990 Aug;22(4):429-35.

[6] Clarkson PM, Hubal MJ. Exercise-induced muscle damage in humans. American journal of physical medicine & rehabilitation / Association of Academic Physiatrists. 2002 Nov;81(11 Suppl):S52-69.

[7] Ebbeling CB, Clarkson PM. Exercise-induced muscle damage and adaptation. Sports medicine (Auckland, NZ. 1989 Apr;7(4):207-34.

[8] Lieber RL, Friden J. Selective damage of fast glycolytic muscle fibres with eccentric contraction of the rabbit tibialis anterior. Acta physiologica Scandinavica. 1988 Aug; 133(4):587-8.

[9] Lieber RL, Thornell LE, Friden J. Muscle cytoskeletal disruption occurs within the first 15 min of cyclic eccentric contraction. J Appl Physiol. 1996 Jan;80(1):278-84.

[10] Armstrong RB, Ogilvie RW, Schwane JA. Eccentric exercise-induced injury to rat skeletal muscle. J Appl Physiol. 1983 Jan;54(1):80-93.

[11] Friden J, Seger J, Sjostrom M, Ekblom B. Adaptive response in human skeletal muscle subjected to prolonged eccentric training. International journal of sports medicine. 1983 Aug;4(3):177-83.

[12] Friden J, Sjostrom M, Ekblom B. Myofibrillar damage following intense eccentric exercise in man. International journal of sports medicine. 1983 Aug;4(3):170-6.

[13] Newham DJ, McPhail G, Mills KR, Edwards RH. Ultrastructural changes after concentric and eccentric contractions of human muscle. Journal of the neurological sciences. 1983 Sep;61(1):109-22.

[14] Ogilvie RW, Armstrong RB, Baird KE, Bottoms CL. Lesions in the rat soleus muscle following eccentrically biased exercise. The American journal of anatomy. 1988 Aug; 182(4):335-46.

[15] Armstrong RB, Warren GL, Warren JA. Mechanisms of exercise-induced muscle fibre injury. Sports medicine (Auckland, NZ. 1991 Sep;12(3):184-207.

[16] Takekura H, Fujinami N, Nishizawa T, Ogasawara H, Kasuga N. Eccentric exercise-induced morphological changes in the membrane systems involved in excitation-contraction coupling in rat skeletal muscle. The Journal of physiology. 2001 Jun 1;533(Pt 2):571-83.

[17] Pedersen BK. Special feature for the Olympics: effects of exercise on the immune system: exercise and cytokines. Immunology and cell biology. 2000 Oct;78(5):532-5.

[18] Ostrowski K, Hermann C, Bangash A, Schjerling P, Nielsen JN, Pedersen BK. A trauma-like elevation of plasma cytokines in humans in response to treadmill running. The Journal of physiology. 1998 Dec 15;513 (Pt 3):889-94.

[19] Filep JG, Beauchamp M, Baron C, Paquette Y. Peroxynitrite mediates IL-8 gene expression and production in lipopolysaccharide-stimulated human whole blood. J Immunol. 1998 Nov 15;161(10):5656-62.

[20] Li JJ, Oberley LW. Overexpression of manganese-containing superoxide dismutase confers resistance to the cytotoxicity of tumor necrosis factor alpha and/or hyperthermia. Cancer research. 1997 May 15;57(10):1991-8.

[21] Hikida RS, Staron RS, Hagerman FC, Sherman WM, Costill DL. Muscle fiber necrosis associated with human marathon runners. Journal of the neurological sciences. 1983 May;59(2):185-203.

[22] Packer L, Cadenas E. Oxidants and antioxidants revisited. New concepts of oxidative stress. Free radical research. 2007 Sep;41(9):951-2.

[23] McCord JM. The superoxide free radical: its biochemistry and pathophysiology. Surgery. 1983 Sep;94(3):412-4.

[24] Jackson MJ, Pye D, Palomero J. The production of reactive oxygen and nitrogen species by skeletal muscle. J Appl Physiol. 2007 Apr;102(4):1664-70.

[25] Jackson MJ, O'Farrell S. Free radicals and muscle damage. British medical bulletin. 1993 Jul;49(3):630-41.

[26] McGinley C, Shafat A, Donnelly AE. Does antioxidant vitamin supplementation protect against muscle damage? Sports medicine (Auckland, NZ. 2009;39(12):1011-32.

[27] Bloomer RJ, Goldfarb AH. Anaerobic exercise and oxidative stress: a review. Canadian journal of applied physiology = Revue canadienne de physiologie appliquee. 2004 Jun;29(3):245-63.

[28] McArdle A, Vasilaki A, Jackson M. Exercise and skeletal muscle ageing: cellular and molecular mechanisms. Ageing research reviews. 2002 Feb;1(1):79-93.

[29] Peternelj TT, Coombes JS. Antioxidant supplementation during exercise training: beneficial or detrimental? Sports medicine (Auckland, NZ. 2010 Dec 1;41(12):1043-69.

[30] Jakeman P, Maxwell S. Effect of antioxidant vitamin supplementation on muscle function after eccentric exercise. European journal of applied physiology and occupational physiology. 1993;67(5):426-30.

[31] Palazzetti S, Rousseau AS, Richard MJ, Favier A, Margaritis I. Antioxidant supplementation preserves antioxidant response in physical training and low antioxidant intake. The British journal of nutrition. 2004 Jan;91(1):91-100.

[32] Nakhostin-Roohi B, Babaei P, Rahmani-Nia F, Bohlooli S. Effect of vitamin C supplementation on lipid peroxidation, muscle damage and inflammation after 30-min exercise at 75% VO2max. The Journal of sports medicine and physical fitness. 2008 Jun; 48(2):217-24.

[33] Bloomer RJ, Goldfarb AH, McKenzie MJ, You T, Nguyen L. Effects of antioxidant therapy in women exposed to eccentric exercise. International journal of sport nutrition and exercise metabolism. 2004 Aug;14(4):377-88.

[34] Bryer SC, Goldfarb AH. Effect of high dose vitamin C supplementation on muscle soreness, damage, function, and oxidative stress to eccentric exercise. International journal of sport nutrition and exercise metabolism. 2006 Jun;16(3):270-80.

[35] Nieman DC, Peters EM, Henson DA, Nevines EI, Thompson MM. Influence of vitamin C supplementation on cytokine changes following an ultramarathon. J Interferon Cytokine Res. 2000 Nov;20(11):1029-35.

[36] Phillips T, Childs AC, Dreon DM, Phinney S, Leeuwenburgh C. A dietary supplement attenuates IL-6 and CRP after eccentric exercise in untrained males. Medicine and science in sports and exercise. 2003 Dec;35(12):2032-7.

[37] Funes L, Carrera-Quintanar L, Cerdan-Calero M, Ferrer MD, Drobnic F, Pons A, et al. Effect of lemon verbena supplementation on muscular damage markers, proinflammatory cytokines release and neutrophils' oxidative stress in chronic exercise. European journal of applied physiology. 2011 Apr;111(4):695-705.

[38] Peters EM, Anderson R, Nieman DC, Fickl H, Jogessar V. Vitamin C supplementation attenuates the increases in circulating cortisol, adrenaline and anti-inflammatory polypeptides following ultramarathon running. International journal of sports medicine. 2001 Oct;22(7):537-43.

[39] Senturk UK, Yalcin O, Gunduz F, Kuru O, Meiselman HJ, Baskurt OK. Effect of antioxidant vitamin treatment on the time course of hematological and hemorheological alterations after an exhausting exercise episode in human subjects. J Appl Physiol. 2005 Apr;98(4):1272-9.

[40] Nakazato K, Ochi E, Waga T. Dietary apple polyphenols have preventive effects against lengthening contraction-induced muscle injuries. Molecular nutrition & food research. 2010 Mar;54(3):364-72.

[41] Bowtell JL, Sumners DP, Dyer A, Fox P, Mileva KN. Montmorency cherry juice reduces muscle damage caused by intensive strength exercise. Medicine and science in sports and exercise. 2011 Aug;43(8):1544-51.

[42] Matsumoto H, Takenami E, Iwasaki-Kurashige K, Osada T, Katsumura T, Hamaoka T. Effects of blackcurrant anthocyanin intake on peripheral muscle circulation during typing work in humans. European journal of applied physiology. 2005 May;94(1-2):36-45.

[43] Reid MB, Stokic DS, Koch SM, Khawli FA, Leis AA. N-acetylcysteine inhibits muscle fatigue in humans. The Journal of clinical investigation. 1994 Dec;94(6):2468-74.

[44] Kanter M. Free radicals and exercise: effects of nutritional antioxidant supplementation. Exercise and sport sciences reviews. 1995;23:375-97.

[45] Beaton LJ, Allan DA, Tarnopolsky MA, Tiidus PM, Phillips SM. Contraction-induced muscle damage is unaffected by vitamin E supplementation. Medicine and science in sports and exercise. 2002 May;34(5):798-805.

[46] Thompson D, Bailey DM, Hill J, Hurst T, Powell JR, Williams C. Prolonged vitamin C supplementation and recovery from eccentric exercise. European journal of applied physiology. 2004 Jun;92(1-2):133-8.

[47] Silva LA, Pinho CA, Silveira PC, Tuon T, De Souza CT, Dal-Pizzol F, et al. Vitamin E supplementation decreases muscular and oxidative damage but not inflammatory response induced by eccentric contraction. J Physiol Sci. 2010 Jan;60(1):51-7.

[48] Mastaloudis A, Morrow JD, Hopkins DW, Devaraj S, Traber MG. Antioxidant supplementation prevents exercise-induced lipid peroxidation, but not inflammation, in ultramarathon runners. Free radical biology & medicine. 2004 May 15;36(10):1329-41.

[49] Nieman DC, Henson DA, Gross SJ, Jenkins DP, Davis JM, Murphy EA, et al. Quercetin reduces illness but not immune perturbations after intensive exercise. Medicine and science in sports and exercise. 2007 Sep;39(9):1561-9.

[50] Kaikkonen J, Kosonen L, Nyyssonen K, Porkkala-Sarataho E, Salonen R, Korpela H, et al. Effect of combined coenzyme Q10 and d-alpha-tocopheryl acetate supplementation on exercise-induced lipid peroxidation and muscular damage: a placebo-controlled double-blind study in marathon runners. Free radical research. 1998 Jul;29(1): 85-92.

[51] Dawson B, Henry GJ, Goodman C, Gillam I, Beilby JR, Ching S, et al. Effect of Vitamin C and E supplementation on biochemical and ultrastructural indices of muscle damage after a 21 km run. International journal of sports medicine. 2002 Jan;23(1): 10-5.

[52] Thompson D, Williams C, Kingsley M, Nicholas CW, Lakomy HK, McArdle F, et al. Muscle soreness and damage parameters after prolonged intermittent shuttle-running following acute vitamin C supplementation. International journal of sports medicine. 2001 Jan;22(1):68-75.

[53] Jowko E, Sacharuk J, Balasinska B, Wilczak J, Charmas M, Ostaszewski P, et al. Effect of a single dose of green tea polyphenols on the blood markers of exercise-induced oxidative stress in soccer players. International journal of sport nutrition and exercise metabolism. 2012 Dec;22(6):486-96.

[54] Connolly DA, Lauzon C, Agnew J, Dunn M, Reed B. The effects of vitamin C supplementation on symptoms of delayed onset muscle soreness. The Journal of sports medicine and physical fitness. 2006 Sep;46(3):462-7.

[55] Close GL, Ashton T, Cable T, Doran D, Holloway C, McArdle F, et al. Ascorbic acid supplementation does not attenuate post-exercise muscle soreness following muscle-

damaging exercise but may delay the recovery process. The British journal of nutrition. 2006 May;95(5):976-81.

[56] Thompson D, Williams C, Garcia-Roves P, McGregor SJ, McArdle F, Jackson MJ. Post-exercise vitamin C supplementation and recovery from demanding exercise. European journal of applied physiology. 2003 May;89(3-4):393-400.

[57] Ganio MS, Armstrong LE, Johnson EC, Klau JF, Ballard KD, Michniak-Kohn B, et al. Effect of quercetin supplementation on maximal oxygen uptake in men and women. Journal of sports sciences. 2010 Jan;28(2):201-8.

[58] Gomez-Cabrera MC, Domenech E, Vina J. Moderate exercise is an antioxidant: upregulation of antioxidant genes by training. Free radical biology & medicine. 2008 Jan 15;44(2):126-31.

[59] McArdle F, Spiers S, Aldemir H, Vasilaki A, Beaver A, Iwanejko L, et al. Preconditioning of skeletal muscle against contraction-induced damage: the role of adaptations to oxidants in mice. The Journal of physiology. 2004 Nov 15;561(Pt 1):233-44.

[60] Tiidus PM, Pushkarenko J, Houston ME. Lack of antioxidant adaptation to short-term aerobic training in human muscle. The American journal of physiology. 1996 Oct;271(4 Pt 2):R832-6.

[61] Margaritis I, Tessier F, Richard MJ, Marconnet P. No evidence of oxidative stress after a triathlon race in highly trained competitors. International journal of sports medicine. 1997 Apr;18(3):186-90.

[62] Teixeira VH, Valente HF, Casal SI, Marques AF, Moreira PA. Antioxidants do not prevent postexercise peroxidation and may delay muscle recovery. Medicine and science in sports and exercise. 2009 Sep;41(9):1752-60.

[63] Childs A, Jacobs C, Kaminski T, Halliwell B, Leeuwenburgh C. Supplementation with vitamin C and N-acetyl-cysteine increases oxidative stress in humans after an acute muscle injury induced by eccentric exercise. Free radical biology & medicine. 2001 Sep 15;31(6):745-53.

[64] Avery NG, Kaiser JL, Sharman MJ, Scheett TP, Barnes DM, Gomez AL, et al. Effects of vitamin E supplementation on recovery from repeated bouts of resistance exercise. Journal of strength and conditioning research / National Strength & Conditioning Association. 2003 Nov;17(4):801-9.

[65] Malm C, Svensson M, Sjoberg B, Ekblom B, Sjodin B. Supplementation with ubiquinone-10 causes cellular damage during intense exercise. Acta physiologica Scandinavica. 1996 Aug;157(4):511-2.

[66] Malm C, Svensson M, Ekblom B, Sjodin B. Effects of ubiquinone-10 supplementation and high intensity training on physical performance in humans. Acta physiologica Scandinavica. 1997 Nov;161(3):379-84.

[67] Lamprecht M, Hofmann P, Greilberger JF, Schwaberger G. Increased lipid peroxidation in trained men after 2 weeks of antioxidant supplementation. International journal of sport nutrition and exercise metabolism. 2009 Aug;19(4):385-99.

[68] Nieman DC, Henson DA, McAnulty SR, McAnulty LS, Morrow JD, Ahmed A, et al. Vitamin E and immunity after the Kona Triathlon World Championship. Medicine and science in sports and exercise. 2004 Aug;36(8):1328-35.

[69] Knez WL, Jenkins DG, Coombes JS. Oxidative stress in half and full Ironman triathletes. Medicine and science in sports and exercise. 2007 Feb;39(2):283-8.

[70] Thompson D, Williams C, McGregor SJ, Nicholas CW, McArdle F, Jackson MJ, et al. Prolonged vitamin C supplementation and recovery from demanding exercise. International journal of sport nutrition and exercise metabolism. 2001 Dec;11(4):466-81.

[71] Khassaf M, McArdle A, Esanu C, Vasilaki A, McArdle F, Griffiths RD, et al. Effect of vitamin C supplements on antioxidant defence and stress proteins in human lymphocytes and skeletal muscle. The Journal of physiology. 2003 Jun 1;549(Pt 2):645-52.

[72] Ashton T, Rowlands CC, Jones E, Young IS, Jackson SK, Davies B, et al. Electron spin resonance spectroscopic detection of oxygen-centred radicals in human serum following exhaustive exercise. European journal of applied physiology and occupational physiology. 1998 May;77(6):498-502.

[73] Kaminski M, Boal R. An effect of ascorbic acid on delayed-onset muscle soreness. Pain. 1992 Sep;50(3):317-21.

[74] Packer L. Oxidants, antioxidant nutrients and the athlete. Journal of sports sciences. 1997 Jun;15(3):353-63.

[75] Bowry VW, Mohr D, Cleary J, Stocker R. Prevention of tocopherol-mediated peroxidation in ubiquinol-10-free human low density lipoprotein. The Journal of biological chemistry. 1995 Mar 17;270(11):5756-63.

[76] Cannon JG, Orencole SF, Fielding RA, Meydani M, Meydani SN, Fiatarone MA, et al. Acute phase response in exercise: interaction of age and vitamin E on neutrophils and muscle enzyme release. The American journal of physiology. 1990 Dec;259(6 Pt 2):R1214-9.

[77] McBride JM, Kraemer WJ, Triplett-McBride T, Sebastianelli W. Effect of resistance exercise on free radical production. Medicine and science in sports and exercise. 1998 Jan;30(1):67-72.

[78] Rebouche CJ. Synthesis of carnitine precursors and related compounds. Methods in enzymology. 1986;123:290-7.

[79] Rebouche CJ, Paulson DJ. Carnitine metabolism and function in humans. Annual review of nutrition. 1986;6:41-66.

[80] Weis BC, Cowan AT, Brown N, Foster DW, McGarry JD. Use of a selective inhibitor of liver carnitine palmitoyltransferase I (CPT I) allows quantification of its contribu-

tion to total CPT I activity in rat heart. Evidence that the dominant cardiac CPT I iso-form is identical to the skeletal muscle enzyme. The Journal of biological chemistry. 1994 Oct 21;269(42):26443-8.

[81] Vaz FM, Wanders RJ. Carnitine biosynthesis in mammals. The Biochemical journal. 2002 Feb 1;361(Pt 3):417-29.

[82] Brass EP. Supplemental carnitine and exercise. The American journal of clinical nu-trition. 2000 Aug;72(2 Suppl):618S-23S.

[83] Bremer J. Carnitine--metabolism and functions. Physiological reviews. 1983 Oct; 63(4):1420-80.

[84] Rebouche CJ, Bosch EP, Chenard CA, Schabold KJ, Nelson SE. Utilization of dietary precursors for carnitine synthesis in human adults. The Journal of nutrition. 1989 Dec;119(12):1907-13.

[85] Kendler BS. Carnitine: an overview of its role in preventive medicine. Preventive medicine. 1986 Jul;15(4):373-90.

[86] Brass EP. Pharmacokinetic considerations for the therapeutic use of carnitine in he-modialysis patients. Clinical therapeutics. 1995 Mar-Apr;17(2):176-85; discussion 5.

[87] Proulx F, Lacroix J, Qureshi IA, Nadeau D, Gauthier M, Lambert M. Acquired carni-tine abnormalities in critically ill children. European journal of pediatrics. 1997 Nov; 156(11):864-9.

[88] Karlic H, Lohninger A. Supplementation of L-carnitine in athletes: does it make sense? Nutrition (Burbank, Los Angeles County, Calif. 2004 Jul-Aug;20(7-8):709-15.

[89] Arenas J, Huertas R, Campos Y, Diaz AE, Villalon JM, Vilas E. Effects of L-carnitine on the pyruvate dehydrogenase complex and carnitine palmitoyl transferase activi-ties in muscle of endurance athletes. FEBS letters. 1994 Mar 14;341(1):91-3.

[90] Huertas R, Campos Y, Diaz E, Esteban J, Vechietti L, Montanari G, et al. Respiratory chain enzymes in muscle of endurance athletes: effect of L-carnitine. Biochemical and biophysical research communications. 1992 Oct 15;188(1):102-7.

[91] Brass EP, Hiatt WR. The role of carnitine and carnitine supplementation during exer-cise in man and in individuals with special needs. Journal of the American College of Nutrition. 1998 Jun;17(3):207-15.

[92] Dragan IG, Vasiliu A, Georgescu E, Eremia N. Studies concerning chronic and acute effects of L-carnitina in elite athletes. Physiologie. 1989 Apr-Jun;26(2):111-29.

[93] Dragan GI, Wagner W, Ploesteanu E. Studies concerning the ergogenic value of pro-tein supply and 1-carnitine in elite junior cyclists. Physiologie. 1988 Jul-Sep;25(3): 129-32.

[94] Vecchiet L, Di Lisa F, Pieralisi G, Ripari P, Menabo R, Giamberardino MA, et al. Influence of L-carnitine administration on maximal physical exercise. European journal of applied physiology and occupational physiology. 1990;61(5-6):486-90.

[95] Arenas J, Ricoy JR, Encinas AR, Pola P, D'Iddio S, Zeviani M, et al. Carnitine in muscle, serum, and urine of nonprofessional athletes: effects of physical exercise, training, and L-carnitine administration. Muscle & nerve. 1991 Jul;14(7):598-604.

[96] Barnett C, Costill DL, Vukovich MD, Cole KJ, Goodpaster BH, Trappe SW, et al. Effect of L-carnitine supplementation on muscle and blood carnitine content and lactate accumulation during high-intensity sprint cycling. International journal of sport nutrition. 1994 Sep;4(3):280-8.

[97] Vukovich MD, Costill DL, Fink WJ. Carnitine supplementation: effect on muscle carnitine and glycogen content during exercise. Medicine and science in sports and exercise. 1994 Sep;26(9):1122-9.

[98] Colombani P, Wenk C, Kunz I, Krahenbuhl S, Kuhnt M, Arnold M, et al. Effects of L-carnitine supplementation on physical performance and energy metabolism of endurance-trained athletes: a double-blind crossover field study. European journal of applied physiology and occupational physiology. 1996;73(5):434-9.

[99] Nuesch R, Rossetto M, Martina B. Plasma and urine carnitine concentrations in well-trained athletes at rest and after exercise. Influence of L-carnitine intake. Drugs under experimental and clinical research. 1999;25(4):167-71.

[100] Trappe SW, Costill DL, Goodpaster B, Vukovich MD, Fink WJ. The effects of L-carnitine supplementation on performance during interval swimming. International journal of sports medicine. 1994 May;15(4):181-5.

[101] Oyono-Enguelle S, Freund H, Ott C, Gartner M, Heitz A, Marbach J, et al. Prolonged submaximal exercise and L-carnitine in humans. European journal of applied physiology and occupational physiology. 1988;58(1-2):53-61.

[102] Giamberardino MA, Dragani L, Valente R, Di Lisa F, Saggini R, Vecchiet L. Effects of prolonged L-carnitine administration on delayed muscle pain and CK release after eccentric effort. International journal of sports medicine. 1996 Jul;17(5):320-4.

[103] Volek JS, Kraemer WJ, Rubin MR, Gomez AL, Ratamess NA, Gaynor P. L-Carnitine L-tartrate supplementation favorably affects markers of recovery from exercise stress. American journal of physiology. 2002 Feb;282(2):E474-82.

[104] Kraemer WJ, Volek JS, French DN, Rubin MR, Sharman MJ, Gomez AL, et al. The effects of L-carnitine L-tartrate supplementation on hormonal responses to resistance exercise and recovery. Journal of strength and conditioning research / National Strength & Conditioning Association. 2003 Aug;17(3):455-62.

[105] Spiering BA, Kraemer WJ, Vingren JL, Hatfield DL, Fragala MS, Ho JY, et al. Responses of criterion variables to different supplemental doses of L-carnitine L-tar-

trate. Journal of strength and conditioning research / National Strength & Conditioning Association. 2007 Feb;21(1):259-64.

[106] Ho JY, Kraemer WJ, Volek JS, Fragala MS, Thomas GA, Dunn-Lewis C, et al. l-Carnitine l-tartrate supplementation favorably affects biochemical markers of recovery from physical exertion in middle-aged men and women. Metabolism: clinical and experimental. 2010 Aug;59(8):1190-9.

[107] Reid MB, Haack KE, Franchek KM, Valberg PA, Kobzik L, West MS. Reactive oxygen in skeletal muscle. I. Intracellular oxidant kinetics and fatigue in vitro. J Appl Physiol. 1992 Nov;73(5):1797-804.

[108] Westerblad H, Allen DG. Cellular mechanisms of skeletal muscle fatigue. Advances in experimental medicine and biology. 2003;538:563-70; discussion 71.

[109] Bruton JD, Place N, Yamada T, Silva JP, Andrade FH, Dahlstedt AJ, et al. Reactive oxygen species and fatigue-induced prolonged low-frequency force depression in skeletal muscle fibres of rats, mice and SOD2 overexpressing mice. The Journal of physiology. 2008 Jan 1;586(1):175-84.

[110] Brass EP, Scarrow AM, Ruff LJ, Masterson KA, Van Lunteren E. Carnitine delays rat skeletal muscle fatigue in vitro. J Appl Physiol. 1993 Oct;75(4):1595-600.

[111] Gulcin I. Antioxidant and antiradical activities of L-carnitine. Life sciences. 2006 Jan 18;78(8):803-11.

[112] Vina J, Gimeno A, Sastre J, Desco C, Asensi M, Pallardo FV, et al. Mechanism of free radical production in exhaustive exercise in humans and rats; role of xanthine oxidase and protection by allopurinol. IUBMB life. 2000 Jun;49(6):539-44.

[113] Duarte JA, Appell HJ, Carvalho F, Bastos ML, Soares JM. Endothelium-derived oxidative stress may contribute to exercise-induced muscle damage. International journal of sports medicine. 1993 Nov;14(8):440-3.

[114] Heunks LM, Vina J, van Herwaarden CL, Folgering HT, Gimeno A, Dekhuijzen PN. Xanthine oxidase is involved in exercise-induced oxidative stress in chronic obstructive pulmonary disease. The American journal of physiology. 1999 Dec;277(6 Pt 2):R1697-704.

[115] Casas H, Murtra B, Casas M, Ibanez J, Ventura JL, Ricart A, et al. Increased blood ammonia in hypoxia during exercise in humans. Journal of physiology and biochemistry. 2001 Dec;57(4):303-12.

[116] Parolin ML, Spriet LL, Hultman E, Hollidge-Horvat MG, Jones NL, Heigenhauser GJ. Regulation of glycogen phosphorylase and PDH during exercise in human skeletal muscle during hypoxia. American journal of physiology. 2000 Mar;278(3):E522-34.

[117] Greenwood M, Farris J, Kreider R, Greenwood L, Byars A. Creatine supplementation patterns and perceived effects in select division I collegiate athletes. Clin J Sport Med. 2000 Jul;10(3):191-4.

[118] LaBotz M, Smith BW. Creatine supplement use in an NCAA Division I athletic program. Clin J Sport Med. 1999 Jul;9(3):167-9.

[119] McGuine TA, Sullivan JC, Bernhardt DA. Creatine supplementation in Wisconsin high school athletes. Wmj. 2002;101(2):25-30.

[120] McGuine TA, Sullivan JC, Bernhardt DT. Creatine supplementation in high school football players. Clin J Sport Med. 2001 Oct;11(4):247-53.

[121] Juhn MS, O'Kane JW, Vinci DM. Oral creatine supplementation in male collegiate athletes: a survey of dosing habits and side effects. Journal of the American Dietetic Association. 1999 May;99(5):593-5.

[122] Ronsen O, Sundgot-Borgen J, Maehlum S. Supplement use and nutritional habits in Norwegian elite athletes. Scandinavian journal of medicine & science in sports. 1999 Feb;9(1):28-35.

[123] Volek JS, Duncan ND, Mazzetti SA, Staron RS, Putukian M, Gomez AL, et al. Performance and muscle fiber adaptations to creatine supplementation and heavy resistance training. Medicine and science in sports and exercise. 1999 Aug;31(8):1147-56.

[124] Tarnopolsky MA. Potential benefits of creatine monohydrate supplementation in the elderly. Current opinion in clinical nutrition and metabolic care. 2000 Nov;3(6): 497-502.

[125] Tarnopolsky MA, MacLennan DP. Creatine monohydrate supplementation enhances high-intensity exercise performance in males and females. International journal of sport nutrition and exercise metabolism. 2000 Dec;10(4):452-63.

[126] Harris RC, Soderlund K, Hultman E. Elevation of creatine in resting and exercised muscle of normal subjects by creatine supplementation. Clin Sci (Lond). 1992 Sep; 83(3):367-74.

[127] van Loon LJ, Oosterlaar AM, Hartgens F, Hesselink MK, Snow RJ, Wagenmakers AJ. Effects of creatine loading and prolonged creatine supplementation on body composition, fuel selection, sprint and endurance performance in humans. Clin Sci (Lond). 2003 Feb;104(2):153-62.

[128] Van Schuylenbergh R, Van Leemputte M, Hespel P. Effects of oral creatine-pyruvate supplementation in cycling performance. International journal of sports medicine. 2003 Feb;24(2):144-50.

[129] Izquierdo M, Ibanez J, Gonzalez-Badillo JJ, Gorostiaga EM. Effects of creatine supplementation on muscle power, endurance, and sprint performance. Medicine and science in sports and exercise. 2002 Feb;34(2):332-43.

[130] Willoughby DS, Rosene J. Effects of oral creatine and resistance training on myosin heavy chain expression. Medicine and science in sports and exercise. 2001 Oct;33(10): 1674-81.

[131] Willoughby DS, Rosene JM. Effects of oral creatine and resistance training on myogenic regulatory factor expression. Medicine and science in sports and exercise. 2003 Jun;35(6):923-9.

[132] Hespel P, Op't Eijnde B, Van Leemputte M, Urso B, Greenhaff PL, Labarque V, et al. Oral creatine supplementation facilitates the rehabilitation of disuse atrophy and alters the expression of muscle myogenic factors in humans. The Journal of physiology. 2001 Oct 15;536(Pt 2):625-33.

[133] Bemben MG, Bemben DA, Loftiss DD, Knehans AW. Creatine supplementation during resistance training in college football athletes. Medicine and science in sports and exercise. 2001 Oct;33(10):1667-73.

[134] Haussinger D, Roth E, Lang F, Gerok W. Cellular hydration state: an important determinant of protein catabolism in health and disease. Lancet. 1993 May 22;341(8856): 1330-2.

[135] Ingwall JS. Creatine and the control of muscle-specific protein synthesis in cardiac and skeletal muscle. Circulation research. 1976 May;38(5 Suppl 1):I115-23.

[136] Demant TW, Rhodes EC. Effects of creatine supplementation on exercise performance. Sports medicine (Auckland, NZ. 1999 Jul;28(1):49-60.

[137] Lawler JM, Barnes WS, Wu G, Song W, Demaree S. Direct antioxidant properties of creatine. Biochemical and biophysical research communications. 2002 Jan 11;290(1): 47-52.

[138] Green AL, Hultman E, Macdonald IA, Sewell DA, Greenhaff PL. Carbohydrate ingestion augments skeletal muscle creatine accumulation during creatine supplementation in humans. The American journal of physiology. 1996 Nov;271(5 Pt 1):E821-6.

[139] Schoch RD, Willoughby D, Greenwood M. The regulation and expression of the creatine transporter: a brief review of creatine supplementation in humans and animals. Journal of the International Society of Sports Nutrition. 2006;3:60-6.

[140] Bloomer RJ. The role of nutritional supplements in the prevention and treatment of resistance exercise-induced skeletal muscle injury. Sports medicine (Auckland, NZ. 2007;37(6):519-32.

[141] Yasuda T, Sakamoto K, Nosaka K, Wada M, Katsuta S. Loss of sarcoplasmic reticulum membrane integrity after eccentric contractions. Acta physiologica Scandinavica. 1997 Dec;161(4):581-2.

[142] Konorev EA, Medvedeva NV, Dzhaliashvili IV, Stepanov VA, Saks VA. [Membrano-tropic effect of phosphocreatine and its structural analogs]. Biokhimiia (Moscow, Russia). 1991 Sep;56(9):1701-9.

[143] Warren GL, Fennessy JM, Millard-Stafford ML. Strength loss after eccentric contractions is unaffected by creatine supplementation. J Appl Physiol. 2000 Aug;89(2): 557-62.

[144] Cooke MB, Rybalka E, Williams AD, Cribb PJ, Hayes A. Creatine supplementation enhances muscle force recovery after eccentrically-induced muscle damage in healthy individuals. Journal of the International Society of Sports Nutrition. 2009;6:13.

[145] Rawson ES, Conti MP, Miles MP. Creatine supplementation does not reduce muscle damage or enhance recovery from resistance exercise. Journal of strength and conditioning research / National Strength & Conditioning Association. 2007 Nov;21(4): 1208-13.

[146] Rawson ES, Gunn B, Clarkson PM. The effects of creatine supplementation on exercise-induced muscle damage. Journal of strength and conditioning research / National Strength & Conditioning Association. 2001 May;15(2):178-84.

[147] Olsen S, Aagaard P, Kadi F, Tufekovic G, Verney J, Olesen JL, et al. Creatine supplementation augments the increase in satellite cell and myonuclei number in human skeletal muscle induced by strength training. The Journal of physiology. 2006 Jun 1;573(Pt 2):525-34.

[148] van Loon LJ, Murphy R, Oosterlaar AM, Cameron-Smith D, Hargreaves M, Wagenmakers AJ, et al. Creatine supplementation increases glycogen storage but not GLUT-4 expression in human skeletal muscle. Clin Sci (Lond). 2004 Jan;106(1):99-106.

[149] Santos RV, Bassit RA, Caperuto EC, Costa Rosa LF. The effect of creatine supplementation upon inflammatory and muscle soreness markers after a 30km race. Life sciences. 2004 Sep 3;75(16):1917-24.

[150] Noakes TD. Effect of exercise on serum enzyme activities in humans. Sports medicine (Auckland, NZ. 1987 Jul-Aug;4(4):245-67.

[151] Lev EI, Tur-Kaspa I, Ashkenazy I, Reiner A, Faraggi D, Shemer J, et al. Distribution of serum creatine kinase activity in young healthy persons. Clinica chimica acta; international journal of clinical chemistry. 1999 Jan;279(1-2):107-15.

[152] Janssen GM, Kuipers H, Willems GM, Does RJ, Janssen MP, Geurten P. Plasma activity of muscle enzymes: quantification of skeletal muscle damage and relationship with metabolic variables. International journal of sports medicine. 1989 Oct;10 Suppl 3:S160-8.

[153] Sorichter S, Mair J, Koller A, Gebert W, Rama D, Calzolari C, et al. Skeletal troponin I as a marker of exercise-induced muscle damage. J Appl Physiol. 1997 Oct;83(4): 1076-82.

[154] Moran JH, Schnellmann RG. A rapid beta-NADH-linked fluorescence assay for lactate dehydrogenase in cellular death. Journal of pharmacological and toxicological methods. 1996 Sep;36(1):41-4.

[155] Bassit RA, Curi R, Costa Rosa LF. Creatine supplementation reduces plasma levels of pro-inflammatory cytokines and PGE2 after a half-ironman competition. Amino acids. 2008 Aug;35(2):425-31.

[156] Bassit RA, Pinheiro CH, Vitzel KF, Sproesser AJ, Silveira LR, Curi R. Effect of short-term creatine supplementation on markers of skeletal muscle damage after strenuous contractile activity. European journal of applied physiology. 2010 Mar;108(5):945-55.

[157] Hausswirth C, Lehenaff D. Physiological demands of running during long distance runs and triathlons. Sports medicine (Auckland, NZ. 2001;31(9):679-89.

[158] Neubauer O, Konig D, Wagner KH. Recovery after an Ironman triathlon: sustained inflammatory responses and muscular stress. European journal of applied physiology. 2008 Oct;104(3):417-26.

[159] Newham DJ, Mills KR, Quigley BM, Edwards RH. Pain and fatigue after concentric and eccentric muscle contractions. Clin Sci (Lond). 1983 Jan;64(1):55-62.

[160] Wood SA, Morgan DL, Proske U. Effects of repeated eccentric contractions on structure and mechanical properties of toad sartorius muscle. The American journal of physiology. 1993 Sep;265(3 Pt 1):C792-800.

[161] Percario S, Domingues SP, Teixeira LF, Vieira JL, de Vasconcelos F, Ciarrocchi DM, et al. Effects of creatine supplementation on oxidative stress profile of athletes. Journal of the International Society of Sports Nutrition. 2012;9(1):56.

[162] Rahimi R. Creatine supplementation decreases oxidative DNA damage and lipid peroxidation induced by a single bout of resistance exercise. Journal of strength and conditioning research / National Strength & Conditioning Association. 2011 Dec; 25(12):3448-55.

[163] Kingsley M, Cunningham D, Mason L, Kilduff LP, McEneny J. Role of creatine supplementation on exercise-induced cardiovascular function and oxidative stress. Oxidative medicine and cellular longevity. 2009 Sep-Oct;2(4):247-54.

[164] Coco M, Perciavalle V. Creatine ingestion effects on oxidative stress in a steady-state test at 75% VO(2max). The Journal of sports medicine and physical fitness. 2012 Apr; 52(2):165-9.

[165] Vary TC, Lynch CJ. Nutrient signaling components controlling protein synthesis in striated muscle. The Journal of nutrition. 2007 Aug;137(8):1835-43.

[166] Wullschleger S, Loewith R, Hall MN. TOR signaling in growth and metabolism. Cell. 2006 Feb 10;124(3):471-84.

[167] Flati V, Pasini E, D'Antona G, Speca S, Toniato E, Martinotti S. Intracellular mechanisms of metabolism regulation: the role of signaling via the mammalian target of rapamycin pathway and other routes. The American journal of cardiology. 2008 Jun 2;101(11A):16E-21E.

[168] Ohanna M, Sobering AK, Lapointe T, Lorenzo L, Praud C, Petroulakis E, et al. Atrophy of S6K1(-/-) skeletal muscle cells reveals distinct mTOR effectors for cell cycle and size control. Nature cell biology. 2005 Mar;7(3):286-94.

[169] D'Antona G, Nisoli E. mTOR signaling as a target of amino acid treatment of the age-related sarcopenia. Interdisciplinary topics in gerontology. 2010;37:115-41.

[170] Smith K, Reynolds N, Downie S, Patel A, Rennie MJ. Effects of flooding amino acids on incorporation of labeled amino acids into human muscle protein. The American journal of physiology. 1998 Jul;275(1 Pt 1):E73-8.

[171] Smith K, Barua JM, Watt PW, Scrimgeour CM, Rennie MJ. Flooding with L-[1-13C]leucine stimulates human muscle protein incorporation of continuously infused L-[1-13C]valine. The American journal of physiology. 1992 Mar;262(3 Pt 1):E372-6.

[172] D'Antona G, Ragni M, Cardile A, Tedesco L, Dossena M, Bruttini F, et al. Branched-chain amino acid supplementation promotes survival and supports cardiac and skeletal muscle mitochondrial biogenesis in middle-aged mice. Cell metabolism. 2010 Oct 6;12(4):362-72.

[173] Biolo G, Tipton KD, Klein S, Wolfe RR. An abundant supply of amino acids enhances the metabolic effect of exercise on muscle protein. The American journal of physiology. 1997 Jul;273(1 Pt 1):E122-9.

[174] Volpi E, Ferrando AA, Yeckel CW, Tipton KD, Wolfe RR. Exogenous amino acids stimulate net muscle protein synthesis in the elderly. The Journal of clinical investigation. 1998 May 1;101(9):2000-7.

[175] Svanberg E, Moller-Loswick AC, Matthews DE, Korner U, Andersson M, Lundholm K. Effects of amino acids on synthesis and degradation of skeletal muscle proteins in humans. The American journal of physiology. 1996 Oct;271(4 Pt 1):E718-24.

[176] Svanberg E, Zachrisson H, Ohlsson C, Iresjo BM, Lundholm KG. Role of insulin and IGF-I in activation of muscle protein synthesis after oral feeding. The American journal of physiology. 1996 Apr;270(4 Pt 1):E614-20.

[177] Preedy VR, Garlick PJ. The response of muscle protein synthesis to nutrient intake in postabsorptive rats: the role of insulin and amino acids. Bioscience reports. 1986 Feb; 6(2):177-83.

[178] Lynch CJ, Halle B, Fujii H, Vary TC, Wallin R, Damuni Z, et al. Potential role of leu-
       cine metabolism in the leucine-signaling pathway involving mTOR. American jour-
       nal of physiology. 2003 Oct;285(4):E854-63.

[179] Lynch CJ, Patson BJ, Anthony J, Vaval A, Jefferson LS, Vary TC. Leucine is a direct-
       acting nutrient signal that regulates protein synthesis in adipose tissue. American
       journal of physiology. 2002 Sep;283(3):E503-13.

[180] Biolo G, Maggi SP, Williams BD, Tipton KD, Wolfe RR. Increased rates of muscle
       protein turnover and amino acid transport after resistance exercise in humans. The
       American journal of physiology. 1995 Mar;268(3 Pt 1):E514-20.

[181] Phillips SM, Tipton KD, Aarsland A, Wolf SE, Wolfe RR. Mixed muscle protein syn-
       thesis and breakdown after resistance exercise in humans. The American journal of
       physiology. 1997 Jul;273(1 Pt 1):E99-107.

[182] Shimomura Y, Harris RA. Metabolism and physiological function of branched-chain
       amino acids: discussion of session 1. The Journal of nutrition. 2006 Jan;136(1 Suppl):
       232S-3S.

[183] Tipton KD, Ferrando AA, Phillips SM, Doyle D, Jr., Wolfe RR. Postexercise net pro-
       tein synthesis in human muscle from orally administered amino acids. The American
       journal of physiology. 1999 Apr;276(4 Pt 1):E628-34.

[184] Brooks GA. Amino acid and protein metabolism during exercise and recovery. Medi-
       cine and science in sports and exercise. 1987 Oct;19(5 Suppl):S150-6.

[185] Nosaka K, Sacco P, Mawatari K. Effects of amino acid supplementation on muscle
       soreness and damage. International journal of sport nutrition and exercise metabo-
       lism. 2006 Dec;16(6):620-35.

[186] Jackman SR, Witard OC, Jeukendrup AE, Tipton KD. Branched-chain amino acid in-
       gestion can ameliorate soreness from eccentric exercise. Medicine and science in
       sports and exercise. 2010 May;42(5):962-70.

[187] Shimomura Y, Inaguma A, Watanabe S, Yamamoto Y, Muramatsu Y, Bajotto G, et al.
       Branched-chain amino acid supplementation before squat exercise and delayed-onset
       muscle soreness. International journal of sport nutrition and exercise metabolism.
       2010 Jun;20(3):236-44.

[188] Pellegrino MA, Brocca L, Dioguardi FS, Bottinelli R, D'Antona G. Effects of voluntary
       wheel running and amino acid supplementation on skeletal muscle of mice. Europe-
       an journal of applied physiology. 2005 Mar;93(5-6):655-64.

[189] Greer BK, White JP, Arguello EM, Haymes EM. Branched-chain amino acid supple-
       mentation lowers perceived exertion but does not affect performance in untrained
       males. Journal of strength and conditioning research / National Strength & Condi-
       tioning Association. 2011 Feb;25(2):539-44.

[190] Matsumoto K, Koba T, Hamada K, Sakurai M, Higuchi T, Miyata H. Branched-chain amino acid supplementation attenuates muscle soreness, muscle damage and inflammation during an intensive training program. The Journal of sports medicine and physical fitness. 2009 Dec;49(4):424-31.

[191] Koba T, Hamada K, Sakurai M, Matsumoto K, Hayase H, Imaizumi K, et al. Branched-chain amino acids supplementation attenuates the accumulation of blood lactate dehydrogenase during distance running. The Journal of sports medicine and physical fitness. 2007 Sep;47(3):316-22.

[192] Matsumoto K, Mizuno M, Mizuno T, Dilling-Hansen B, Lahoz A, Bertelsen V, et al. Branched-chain amino acids and arginine supplementation attenuates skeletal muscle proteolysis induced by moderate exercise in young individuals. International journal of sports medicine. 2007 Jun;28(6):531-8.

[193] Stock MS, Young JC, Golding LA, Kruskall LJ, Tandy RD, Conway-Klaassen JM, et al. The effects of adding leucine to pre and postexercise carbohydrate beverages on acute muscle recovery from resistance training. Journal of strength and conditioning research / National Strength & Conditioning Association. 2010 Aug;24(8):2211-9.

Chapter 2

Etiology, Biology and Treatment of Muscular Lesions

Gian Nicola Bisciotti and Cristiano Eirale

Additional information is available at the end of the chapter

1. Introduction

The detrimental event on a muscular level, founds one of the most recurring traumatic insults in sporting environment. The entity of the lesion can go from simple sprain, often associated with the breakage of small vessels, with appearance of pain and swelling, to complete muscular tear. The consequences for the athlete, which appear linked with the entity of the lesion, are always unpleasant and involve suspension, more or less long, of sporting activity, not to mention suitable therapy.

In this chapter we will try to clear up the different physiological aspects which normally characterize the traumatic event and to describe, even if only summarize, the mechanism of muscular repair.

2. The definition of muscular lesion

Few authors have explicitly defined the term "muscular lesion", even though some have attempted to link the concept of lesion to that of the loss of proper muscular function (Brooks et al., 1995). However, identifying muscular lesion with the simple loss of function isn't altogether correct, indeed muscular function may be nullified by events, such as tiredness or atrophy, which have nothing to do with the detrimental mechanism. For these reasons, even though the concept of functionality loss represents one of the main characteristics of the lesion of the muscle, we believe that the correct definition of muscular lesion cannot overlook the concept of "damage" towards the muscular structure. Therefore, a correct definition in this sense could be the following: " muscular lesion is identifiable by the loss of functionality of the muscle caused by damage, more or less severe, on a level of muscular structure or on a level of anatomical sites assigned to transmit strength", intending with the last explanation the damage on a level of tendon-muscular passage. This definition clears the concept that in the field of muscular lesion the loss of function cannot be separated from the concept of structural damage.

3. The connection of the contractile apparatus to the extra-cellular matrix

The link of the muscle fibers to the tendon or to the fascia, must have the capacity to resist considerable strength which can go above 1000 kg during maximum type strain (Tidball and Daniel, 1986; Tidball, 1991;). To possess such a great strength, each fiber contains specific molecule chains: integrin and the complex distrofin-glycoprotein (Mayers,2003; Michele and Campbell, 2003). These two complex proteins connect the contractor myofilamentous apparatus to the extracellular matrix(ECM) through the sarcolemma. (Brown, 1996; Giancotti and Rouslathi,1999; Chiquet, 2003; Chargé and Rudnicki, 2004; Ervasti, 2004; Sunada and Campbell,1995; Kääriäinen et al., 2000;). It is necessary to remember briefly that ECM is made up of an intricate network of macromolecules formed by fibrous protein included in an gel of polysaccharides, L'ECM, apart from being particularly present on a skeletal muscle level, it also results in abundance in the connective tissue. The integrins are a family of "adhesion molecules" positioned in the cellular membrane, which cover a fundamental role in many biological processes tied related to the tissue survival, at growth and regeneration. In addition, the integrins actively participate in the cellular communication, for example in the case of signal between cell and cell, of interaction between cell and ECM or in the process of translation of the signal inside and outside the cell itself (Giancotti, 1999, Mayer, 2003; Rouslathi, 1996). In a healthy muscular fiber the majority of integrins are positioned on a level with the junction of tendon muscle (MTJs) (Bao et al., 1993; Kääriäinen et al., 2000a; 2000b; Mayer, 2003) and are organized in a structure specifically named "integrin associated-complex" (figure1). In this complex the sarcomerica terminal ties, through different sub-sarcolemmal molecules, to the sub-unit B1 of the transmembral integrin muscle specific x7B1 (Otey et al., 1990; Song et al., 1994; Yao et al., 1996; Kääriäinen et al., 2000a; Mayer, 2003), which in turn connects the intracellular contractor apparatus with the surrounding ECM by means of the link with the proteins ECM (Burkin and Kaufman, 1999) (Figure1). On the contrary what we can observe for the integrin, whose accumulation is met in proximity of the distal of the muscular fiber the molecules of the complex distrofin-glycoprotein(figure1) are relatively distributed along the entire sarcolemma, even though they result more abundant on a level of the MTJs and the neuro-muscular junction (Sunada and Campbell, 1995; Brown,1996; Hoffman,1996; Cohn and Campbell, 2000; Kääriäinen and et al., 2000a; Michele and Campbell, 2003). The terminal actin ties with the distrofin which in turn ties with three proteic complexes: the distroglicans, the sarcoglicans and the sintrofins (Cohn and Campbell, 200; Ground, 1991; Michele and Campbell, 2003, of these the x-distroglicans tie with the ECM proteins (Michele and Campbell, 2003). The integrins therefore form true " adhesion focal complexes", which form articulated biological systems which show themselves extremely sensitive in comparison with mechanical strengths which stimulate the muscular complex and could, for this reason, perform a key role in the inducing mechanism of hypertrofic phenomena (FLuk et al., 1991). The formation of new systems of focal adhesion, could in fact induce a modification of the transcription and translation processes of mRNA, inducing the muscular cell to raise the proteic synthesis and induce the variation the characteristics of the expressed isoforms from the heavy chain of the myosin (Lee et al.., 1991).

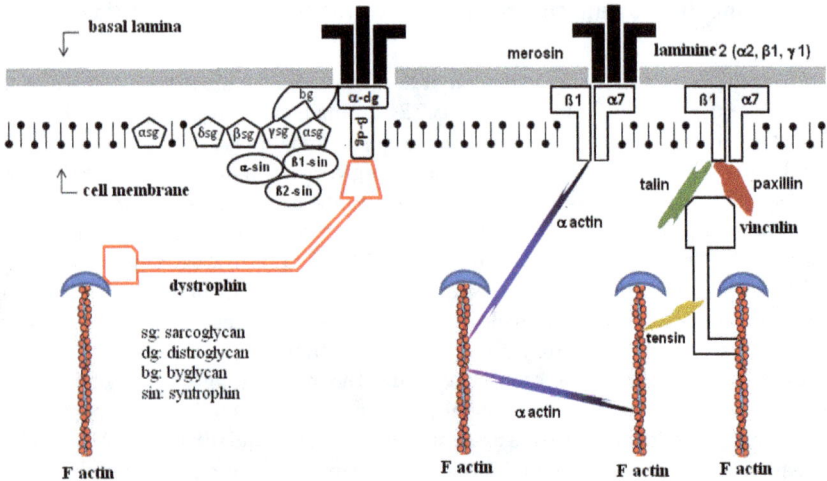

Figure 1. Schematic representation of the adhesion of muscle fiber to extracellular muscular-matrix (ECM). Each fiber contains specific chains of molecules defined integrin and dystrofin, which connect the myofilamentous contractor apparatus to the ECM through the sarcolemma. The main part of the integrin is located in the neuro-muscular junction. The sarcomeric actin ties itself through several molecules, located on a sarcomeral level, to β1 sub-unit of the trasn-membranal muscle specific integrin 7 β1, which is then tied to the ECM protein. The molecules of the dystrofin associated complex, are relatively distributed in a homogenous way along the whole sarcolemma, even though they are particularly abundant in the muscle-.tendon junction and the neuro-muscular junction. The actin ties itself to the dystrofin which is in turn associated with three complex proteins: distroglicans, sarcoglicans and sintrofins.

In the end we have to remember the role of dystrofin as a marker of muscular lesion. Some research conducted on animal models show a conspicuous decrease in coloration of the dystrofin in the muscle immediately after an eccentric contraction (Koh and Eswcobedo, 2004; Lovering and Deyne, 2004). In these studies the loss of dystrofin was associated with the decrease of another membrane protein, the beta-spectrin whose role would seem similar to that of the dystrofin in the stabilization of the membrane. On the other hand the role of dystrofin in maintaining membrane integrity as well as its stability is confirmed by the fact that its missing genetics is at the base of the onset of the Duchenne muscular dystrophy (Hoffman et al., 1987; Zubrycka-Gaarn et al., 1998).

All the same, it is not entirely correct to consider the loss of membrane integrity as a negative event able to compromise muscular homeostasis through the destruction of the barrier which allows the maintenance of an ideal balance between intra and extra cells molecules. In effect a reduced and transitory destruction of the membrane may allow a normal pathway for the

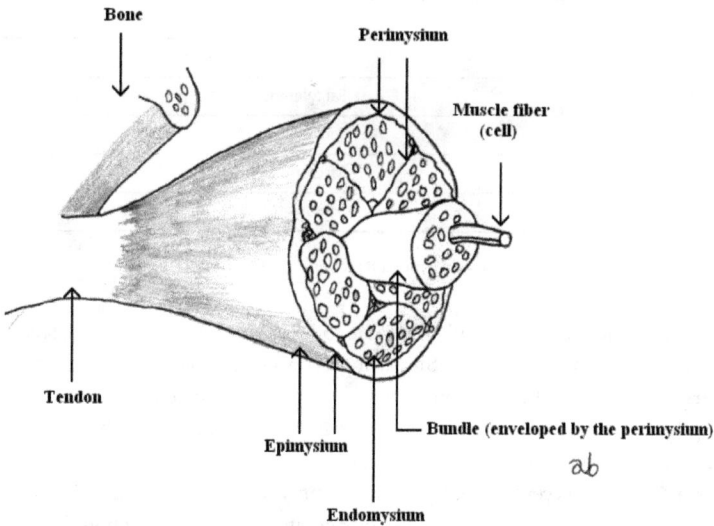

Figure 2. Schematic representation of the skeletal muscle

release and for the assumption of some molecules, above all in tissue exposed to repetitive mechanical stress (McNeil and Khakee, 1992). The muscular tissue in effect shows undeniable capacity in repairing quickly minor entity damage dependent on the membrane structure, limiting in such a way the possible negative consequences. A molecule whose pathway depends on a transitory disturbance of the membrane integrity is the Basic Fibroblast growth factor (bFGF), growth factor strongly concerned in tissue repair processes and in adaptation processes of the muscular tissue regarding strenuous physical exercise. In conclusion a transitory and modest loss of the membrane integrity, can be interpreted also as a physiological answer to the muscular tissue in comparison to intense exercise, answer which is seen in function of the release and transfer of essential growth factors for the repair and functional and biological adaptation of the muscle. If the destruction process of the membrane integrity hesitates towards repair and adaptation, or towards cell death it will depend, obviously, on the entity of the detrimental event in itself and from all the other factors which will contribute to the lesion and repair process.

4. Structural damage and contraction types: An overall vision

The structural damage of muscular fiber may be caused by a singular muscular contraction or by a series of contractions (Armstrong et al., 1991b). In any case the mechanism mainly linked to the possible damage of muscular fiber would be the eccentric contraction (Garret, 1990; Armstrong, 1991b;). The reason of main traumatic incidence on a muscular level, seen during

General term	Specific muscle term
Muscular cell	Muscular fiber or fiber cell
Cellular membrane	Sarcolemma
Cytoplasm	Sarcoplasma
Mitochondria	Sarcosoma
Endoplasmic reticulum	Sarcoplasmic reticulum

Table 1. Equivalent terminology of the principal muscular terms

an eccentric contraction is above all ascribable to the main production of registered strength, as opposed to how much happens in the during a concentric or isometric contraction (Stauber, 1989; Garret, 1990). In fact during an eccentric contraction, carried out at the speed of 90 s^{-1}, the strength expressed from the muscle appears to be three times more than that produced, at the same speed, during a concentric contraction (Middleton et al., 1994). This higher strength production during an eccentric contraction, is mainly due to the elastic capacity of the tail of the myosin; in fact from the moment that, during an eccentric contraction the production of strength occurs during the detachment of the acto-myosinic bridges, the fact that the tail of the myosin is capable of resisting the detachment thanks to its elastic characteristics, allows a substantial increase in the capacity of strength production during the course of the eccentric phenomena (Middleton et al., 1994). In addition, during an eccentric contraction, the strength appears higher generated by the passive elements of the connective tissue of the muscle undergoing extension (Elftman, 1966). Above all, with reference to this last data we have to underline that also the purely mechanical phenomena of the extension, may play an important role in the onset of traumatic event, seeing as this latter one may prove, either in an active muscle during the lengthening phase, or in a muscular area which, during the extension phase, is totally passive (Garrett et al., 1987). However, the rate of extension in which the muscle risks its structural integrity is quite broad, being between 75 and 225% of its length at rest (Garret, 1990). This data underlines the fact that the muscular injury, due to elongation, does not appear at an relatively constant extension but may depend on many other factors, for example the level of electric activation of the muscle undergoing elongation, or the structural weakness of the latter following previous structural damage. In any case, it is important to notice the fact that some authors sustain the hypothesis that the length at which the muscle comes under extension represents a key factor in the entity of the possible damage, in that a superior initial muscle length corresponds with a superior extension and, consequently, a possible superior structural damage (Talbot and Morgan, 1998). The fact that at a superior length of extension the muscle may produce superior structural damage could depend on the heterogeneously of the length of the various sarcomeres of minor dimension which compose the muscular fiber. In fact, in superior length of extension the sarcomeres of minor dimension undergo a phenomena of "overstretching" whose magnitude would be directly linked to the muscle length which triggers the process of elongation(Morgan,1990).

Regarding the level of muscular activation during the course of extension it is important to know that an active muscle is capable of absorbing much more energy- in terms of tensile energy- in comparison to a passive muscle. So the potential energetic absorption of a muscle is increased drastically when the latter contracts actively (Garret, 1990). This introduces the concept of how a muscle, contracting actively, may put into action a kind of self-blocking strategy following damage due to excessive extension. The capacity of a muscle to resist a lengthening force absorbing energy is represented graphically, in mechanical terms of the underlying area of the stress-strain curve, as shown in figure 3.

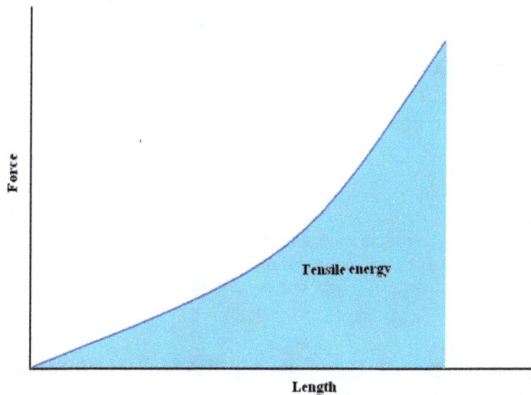

Figure 3. A biological material such as the skeletal muscle, lengthened over a certain length produces a certain quote of tensile energy which, in the graph that shows the rapport strength-length, is represented by the underlying area of the curve.

We may consider that inside the biological muscular structure, there are two structural components able to absorb tensile energy: the passive component and the contractile component. The possibilities of energetic absorption on behalf of the passive component don't depend on the muscular activation, but are essentially attributed to the connective tissue which is found inside the muscular belly but also in the "dumping factor" composed of fiber itself and to the connective associated tissue. The muscle shows however an increase of its capacity to absorb tensile energy thanks to its contractile characteristics, which obviously depend on the level of contraction at the time of extension, as we can see represented in the graph in figure 4.

So there could exist conditions able to diminish the contractile capacity of the muscle and thus reduce its capacity to absorb energy during an extension phase. The muscular fatigue and the structural weakness following a previous lesion, could be two determining factors. It is also important to note that an optimal capacity of absorption of extension strength represents an important protection factor, not only for the muscle itself but also as far as articulation and capsule-ligamentous apparatus is concerned (Radin et al., 1979) In addition, it is interesting to observe that at low levels of elongative tension, the energy absorbed by a muscle is almost totally dependent on the contractile component and, since the normal eccentric muscular

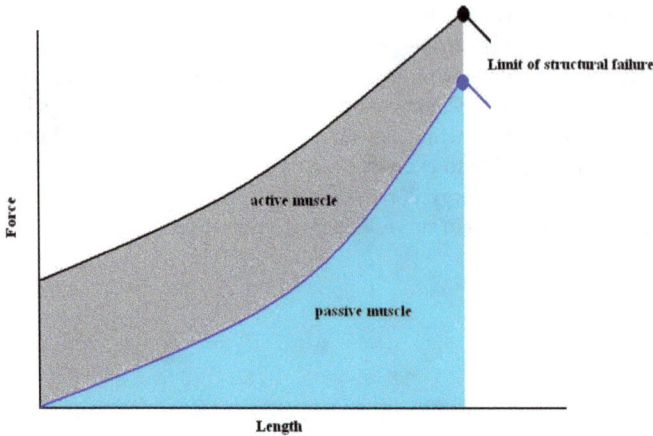

Figure 4. Graphic representation of the force-length relationship in an elongated muscle up to its breakpoint either in passive condition, or in contraction. As is easily recognizable from the graph, the peak of strength of breakage is supe- rior, in the contracted muscle in comparison to the same muscle in relaxed conditions, by a quota equal to only 15%. However, the tensile energy absorbed by the contracted muscle appears superior to that of the same muscle in re- laxed conditions. In addition, it is interesting to note that the absorbed energy is superior at low levels of extension (from Garret, 1990, modified).

activity entails quite reduced tensile levels, almost all energy due to tensile stress is absorbed in this case by the contractile component. (Radin et al.,1979)

During the eccentric contraction the muscle undergoes an "overstretching" phenomena which, as such, may determine the onset of lesions on a level of tendon insertion, of the muscle – tendon junction, or on a level of a muscular area rendered more fragile by a deficit of vascu- larization (Middleton et al., 1994). It is interesting to note how the pluriarticular muscles are the ones mostly exposed to traumatic insult, precisely due to the fact of having to control, through the eccentric contraction, the articular range of one or more articulations (Brewer, 1960). Also the different type of muscular fibers presents a different incidence of harmful event. Fast contraction fibers (FT) are in fact more highly exposed to structural damage in comparison to those of slow contraction(ST), probably due to their superior contractile capacity which translates itself into an increased production of strength and contraction speed, in comparison to fibers type ST (Garret et al., 1984; Friden and Lieber,1992).Furthermore the muscles which present a high percentage of FT, are generally more superficial (Lexell et al., 1983) and are normally interested by two or more articulations, both factors made ready for structural damage (Brewer, 1960; Garret, 1990). To this we can add several studies (Potvin, 1997), which show how in the course of the eccentric phase of movement, the electromyographic activity shows a preferential recruitment of FT fibers.

As well as these hypotheses, it is interesting to note several studies, available in bibliography, which ascribe superior susceptibility to structural damage on behalf of the glycolytic fibers to their particular metabolism (Patel et al., 1998). According to this theory the low oxidative potential, typical of glycolytic fibers, would predispose the latter to structural damage in the course of repeated eccentric contractions because of the depletion of the highly energetic phosphates. This situation would cause the formation of actomyosinic bridges in "rigor state" particularly exposed, because of their excessive rigidity, to the potentially induced structural damage from the eccentric contraction. However, this hypothesis even though engaging and not void of rationality, wasn't supported by experimental evidence in the course of ulterior studies conducted by the same author, during which it wasn't possible to show, on an animal model, that a superior oxidative potential of the glycolytic fibers, induced by a specific training plan, could represent a protective factor for the possible damage induced by eccentric contraction. Beyond the undoubted differences of metabolic type between the gylcolytic and oxidative fibers, other theories which attempt to discuss a superior predisposition to the traumatic insult of the FT single out the different contents of the latter regarding the level of some cytoskeletal proteins(Koh,2002). These particular cytoskeletal proteins, which are fewer in glycolytic fibers in comparison to those of oxidative fibers, would provide a kind of structural support for sarcomeres and the cellular membrane, contributing in such a way to maintain the integrity of such anatomical structures towards mechanical stress represented by eccentric contraction. Koh himself moreover identified in other particular proteic molecules, named "heat shock proteins" which would head to a family of "stress proteins", once again contained in superior quantity in oxidative fibers rather than glycolytic ones, substances able to carry out a protective role towards the muscular structure still during the "induced injury contraction" represented by eccentric contraction.

Another risk factor is represented by the heterogeneity of the sarcomeral length. The sarcomers of minor length represent in fact, the "weak point of the chain" during the eccentric over-stretching phenomena (Morgan,1990). To this end it's important to remember that after a muscular lesion we can note, in an animal model, an increase of the heterogeneity of the sarcomeral length (Patel et al.,), this could, at least in part, explain why, a previously damaged muscle, presents a higher risk of traumatic recurrence. In addition, it is interesting to note how the traumatic event is mainly located on a muscle-tendon junction level, witnessing the fact that in this area, just as in the rest of the final portion of muscle fiber, appears the most mechanical stress (Garrett et al., 1987; Garrett,1990; Lieber etal., 1991). Even though to this end we have to remember that some studies (Huxley and Peachey, 1961) show how muscle fiber, in proximity of the muscle-tendon junction, shows a minor lengthening during an eccentric phase, in comparison to the one in its central area. This data could lead us to the hypothesis that the following damage in an eccentric contraction, on a muscle-tendon level, is not so attributable to the size of elongation as such, but to the application of forces of tangential type on a less vascularized area, and thus structurally more fragile. We need to underline the particular metabolic aspect connected to the eccentric type of contraction. During this type of contraction, since the muscular perfusion is drastically diminished with consequential functional deficit of the aerobic mechanism, the physiological activity is mainly anaerobic type; this determines, either an increase in local temperature, or acidosis, in addition to a marked cellular anoxia. These metabolic events translate themselves into an increased muscular fragility and into a possible cellular necrosis, both on a muscular level as on connective tissue (Middleton et al., 1994).

5. The calcium overload phase

From close examination of international literature it appears clear that, if on the one hand muscular exercise represents a potential source of traumatic events, on the other hand a correct conditioning of the same muscle and its functionality, may reduce considerably the risk of lesion (Ebbeling and Clarkson 1989; Stauber, 1989; Scwane and Armstrong, 1983; Armstrong, 1984). The majority of the studies agrees on the fact that muscular damage is produced, practically in most cases, through an eccentric contraction, during which the muscle elongates at the same time in which it is activated from a contractile point of view (Armstrong et al., 1983b; McCully and Faulkner, 1985; Lieber and Friden, 1988), in addition the muscular damage would seem linked both to the intensity and the duration of exercise (Tiidus and Inauzzo, 1983; McCully and Falukner, 1986).The traumatic event is generally accompanied by a series of clinical and functional problems which are identifiable in : loss of contractile strength, pain, swelling and /or edema, diminution of the contractual capacity, alteration in the proprioceptive muscular pattern and alteration in the strategy of neuro-muscular activation (Davies and White, 1981; Newman et al., 1983; Riden et al., 1983; Armstrong, 1984; Ogilvie et al., 1985; Ebbeling and Clarkson 1989; Darren et al., 1990). The indirect muscular trauma must be visibly distinguished from DOMS (Delayed Onset Muscle Soreness), in fact, if the two biological descriptions present many common points, the DOMS must be anyway understood as a physiological process which poses itself to all effect as a natural forerunner of a process of muscular adaptation aimed at the better functioning of the muscle towards an external load, represented by the training process (Armstrong,1984; Armstrong 1990). The initial detrimental event, drives rapidly to a loss, located inside the injured muscle fiber of the homeostasis of CA^{++} which is named "Ca^{++} overload phase". The muscular cells possess several specific mechanisms deputed to the regulation of the levels of cytosolic Ca^{++} (Carafoli, 1985; Klug and Tibbis, 1988); at the moment in which these buffering and translocation mechanisms are inhibited by the excessive intracellular level of Ca^{++}, caused by the breakage of the sarcoplasmatic reticulum following the injury, we may assist with the activation of numerous pathways of degradation inside the muscular fiber of the injured area. In such a way it activates, on the injured area, a mechanism of autogenetic degradation which includes the activation of the phosfolipase A_2 (PLA_2) with consequent production of arachidonic acid, prostaglandin, leukotrien, Ca^{++} dependent proteases and lysomial proteases. In addition, the increase of intracellular Ca^{++} levels, apart from provoking a sarcomeral contraction reflex (i.e. not interposed from the SNC), may inhibit, or even suppress, the normal mitochondrial breathing. This series of autogenetic factors inside the damaged fiber comes about before the invasion, inside the injured fiber of the macrophages and continues, anyway, also after the appearance of the latter on the damaged area.

6. The hypotheses of onset of muscular damage

Even if the etiology of the event or specific events able to induce damage on skeletal muscle fiber they aren't fully understood, the hypotheses can be, in any case, divided into two typologies, the first of physical type and the second of metabolic type, even though in many cases these etiological descriptions overlap not allowing, in fact, an unmistakable distinction.

7. The hypotheses of physical type

The possible mechanisms of physical type capable of inducing initial structural damage to the muscular fiber, may be divided into two categories. The first includes the hypothesis of mechanical nature, whereas the second includes those induced by change of temperature. The fact that the muscular damage recognizes in an eccentric contraction its *"primum movens"*, is a widely spread concept amongst many authors (Armstrong, 1984; Ebbeling and Clarkson, 1989; Stauber, 1989, Kano et al., 2008; Schache et al., 2008, Chang et al., 2009), so for this reason the mechanical theory of the fibrillary damage, underlines the substantial difference, in terms of strength production, between the eccentric and concentric and isometric contraction, whereas the theory which identifies the damage as consequence of a "temperature-dependent" mechanism is based on the hypothesis that, during an eccentric contraction, the local temperature of the muscle is higher, factor which would predispose the muscular fiber to structural and /or metabolic changes, potentially harmful.

8. The hypotheses of physical type: The theory of mechanical factors

The mechanical theory is essentially based on the central role which covers the eccentric contraction in a harmful process. The skeletal muscle may be defined as a flexible biological material, or a material able to sustain elongation which can also go over 5% of its at rest length (Popov, 1990). However, the skeletal muscle is, at the same time, a compound biological material of complex type and, for this exact reason, the study of its components of structural weakness, which can determine the mechanical yielding, appears extremely difficult. As previously implied, the structural damage depending of muscular fiber may be the consequence, both of a single muscular contraction and of a cumulative series of contractions (Armstrong et al., 1991). During a contraction the muscular fiber may mechanically give way, at the moment in which the tensile stress, to which its structural components are undergone, overtake the maximum production of strength of the same components and goes beyond the said" maximum theoretical stress value" (MTSV). If the tensile stress to which the fiber is subjected, overtakes the MTSV, the structural components give way; in other words an irreversible lesion is produced in the muscular fiber (Figure 5). In a way such as we can see in the course of a monodirectional elongation, such as that described in a stress-strain curve, the muscular structure may give way irreversibly also at the moment in which it undergoes through a stress cutting (i.e. an oblique strength stress), in accordance with what is stated from the "maximum stress-shear theory" said also "maximum distortion-energy theory" (Popov, 1990), in which the acting forces on muscular fiber are considered in a three-dimensional way.

However, the studies of the mechanisms which may cause structural damage to the muscular fiber, have aimed and still aim, also to the cumulative effect of the mechanical tensions to which

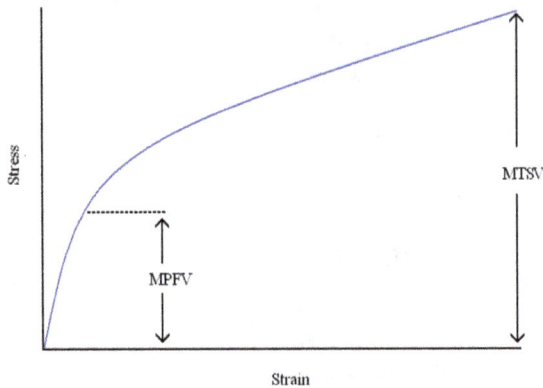

Figure 5. A stress-strain curve, typical of a flexible biological material undergoing tension. The material shows, before the stress which it undergoes surpasses the value of maximum production of strength (VMPF), an elastic type behavior. Once the MPFV is overtaken, the material undergoes a permanent change in form, in other words it undergoes a "plastic deformation". Once the value of maximum force is reached (MTSV) the material gives way irreversibly. From a traumatological point of view we can therefore indentify three different zones in the stress-strain curve of a muscular fiber undergoing tension in the course of an eccentric contraction. The first is included between the beginning of elongation and the value of MPFV, inside which, despite the lengthening stress, the muscular fiber shows elastic behaviour thus not risking structural damage. The second is included between the value of MPFV and the value of MTSV, inside which the fiber surpasses its elastic limits, in which the fiber doesn't show loss of its structural integrity and undergoes a plastic deformation. In this zone the fiber doesn't show loss of its structural integrity. And the last an area which goes beyond the value of MTSV, in which the same fiber gives way. In this last case, *we can observe a muscle tear which severity* - first, second or third degree -is directly linked to the magnitude of the tensile stress to which the fiber undergoes.

the fiber is exposed, focalizing in such a way on the important aspect of the resistance of biological material to the fatigue phenomena. In this particular investigation we study the answer of the biological material at the moment in which the latter is exposed to a high amount of tension and relaxation, up until its breakpoint. For the materials which present a high degree of flexibility, the relationship between the stress to which it is exposed and the number of tension-relaxation cycles which guide to their breakage, is of exponential type (figure 6). To an increase in stress to which the material is exposed, corresponds a drop in the number of cycles which lead to the structural weakening of the same material (Ashby and Jones, 1988). In accordance with what is stated from the theories of the resistance to the fatigue of the biological materials, the energy absorbed by a muscle in the course of a strong elongation, may be eliminated both under form of heat and plastic deformation, intending the latter term a permanent change in the form and in the dimensions of the structural components of the muscular fiber. A plastic deformation, in a biological structure such as the one represented by muscular fiber, may begin with an initial weakening of one or more of its ultrastructural components, which can lead to perpetual tension-relaxation cycles and to a breakage of the structures exposed to tensile stress. In addition, we must underline that the increase in the rate of development of stress tends to reduce the number of cycles which lead to structural weakening, underlining in this way that the speed of lengthening of muscular fiber may play an important role in the onset of the damage (Armstrong et al., 1991).

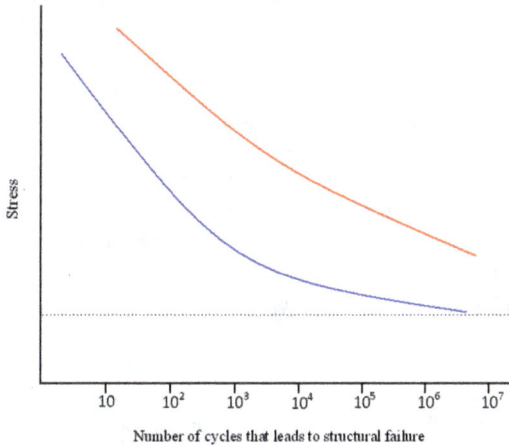

Number of cycles that leads to structural failure

Figure 6. A fatigue curve typical of a flexible biological material. At the moment in which the stress applied during a tension relaxation cycle- also defined from a mechanical point of view as a tension-compression cycle- increases, there is a drop in the number of cycles which lead to the structural weakening. In the graph the dotted horizontal line represents the limit of resistance of the material, (i.e. the stress value under which the considered biological material can support an infinite number of tension-relaxation cycles without incurring structural damage). The red line represents the behavior of a higher resistant material to fatigue in comparison to that of the behavior represented by the blue line (from Armstrong et al.,1991, modified).

The analysis of muscular lesions faced through the given perspective of related literature of the science of materials, appears difficult. The first difficulty which we face is represented by the fact that no data regarding the relationship between the entity of tensile or shear forces and the degree of the lesion doesn't exist. Few studies have in fact investigated, from this point of view, the forces directly expressed inside the muscular structure and even if this type of investigation had been done, the derived values always refer to the registration of forces effected on a tendon structure level. It is important to remember that, in this specific case, the values of such calculated forces represent the sum of values of stress of each single structural component, multiplied by their respective section area (cross-sectional area,CSA). In this way it appears clear that like, from this "global" value, it is difficult, if not impossible, to carry out an analysis of the factors and values of structural weakening for each single component of the considered biological system. A second problem is represented by the fact that individual values of MPSV and of MTSV of the single elements that make up the muscular fiber are, in effect, unknown. A last aspect, problematic in this field, is made up of scarce knowledge of the total capacities of work, in relation to risk lesion, that the skeletal muscle can support during a cycle of eccentric contractions. Above all in this specific field, certain data concerning the loss of percentage of energy absorbed by the muscle and which is dispersed in the form of plastic deformation,. Despite the undoubted conceptual difficulties, from a careful examination of literature we may glean some important data regarding the capacity of tensile resistance of the muscular fiber towards the eccentric contraction. The first interesting data is represented by the fact that during an eccentric contraction the strength production may surpass a percentage between 50 and 100% the isometric strength maximum value (P0) of the considered muscle (Woledge et al., 1985), in addition, as previously said, during an eccentric contraction, carried out at a speed of 90 degrees, the strength expressed of the muscular area appears to be three times higher than that produced, at the same speed, during a concentric contraction (Middleton et al., 1994). We must remember that this higher production of force during an eccentric contraction, is mainly due to the elastic capacity of the tail of the myosin, which thanks to its elastic characteristics, allows a substantial increase in the capacity of the force production during the elongating phase of the contraction (Middleton et al., 1994). Another interesting aspect is given by the fact that, during an eccentric contraction, to be able to satisfy the principle of an isovolumetric contraction, the CSA of each fiber drops in function of the degree of lengthening to which the fiber is exposed. From a careful analysis of this data, we may presume that the medium value of tensile stress that a muscular fiber actively lengthened during an eccentric contraction of 130% of its length at rest (L0), may be higher from 100 to 160% in comparison to one which appears during an maximum isometric contraction carried out at L0. For this reason regarding the turnover of formation and detachment of the acto-myosinic bridges, it is possible to presume from specific literature some interesting information. The number of acto-myosinic bridges would seem in fact decreasing at the increase of the speed of lengthening of the muscle (McMahon, 1984).This phenomena could involve an increase of the produced force on a level of every single acto-myosinic bridge, predisposing in such a way the contractile proteins of the muscle to the traumatic damage (McMahon,1984). In addition, certain experimental evidence carried out like this would confirm the so far mentioned theories. On preparations of isolated frog sartorious muscle, after only three eccentric contractions, the rate of development of force drops significantly and we may observe a movement of the length-tension curve of the muscle towards superior muscle lengths. However, these changes appear only following a contraction of certain magnitude, and anyway not before force values exceeding 180% (McCully and Faulkner, 1985; 1986). Even though, in current practice, the majority of muscular lesions would seem to occur in the course of particularly fast eccentric contractions, the degree, in terms of severity, of the structural damage of the fiber is mainly linked to the peak of force expressed during an eccentric contraction and not at its intrinsic speed (McCully and Faulkner, 1986). In addition, it is interesting to note that eccentric contractions of magnitude equal to 85% of P0, are able to cause structural damage to the architecture of the muscular fiber, this does not happen during isometric or concentric contractions of the same leve. This particular mechanical behavior, may be explained by the fact that the same peak of force, during an eccentric contraction, is produced at a superior muscular length in comparison to that of one in the course of an isometric or concentric contraction, a factor which would drop the capacity of tensile resistance of the fiber. In fact, the peak of force during an eccentric contraction is reached at a superior length in comparison to that during an isometric or concentric contraction, or on average at 110% versus the 100% of L0 (McCully and Faulkner, 1986; Newham et al., 1988). Since 1939 (Katz,1939) we could state that the harmful process concerning the skeletal muscle was of "length-dependent" type, meaning by this that the majority of damage to muscular structure happened at the moment in which the eccentric contraction appeared as important muscular lengths and higher than L0; the same data found by Katz was later confirmed by other authors (McCUlly and Faulkner 1985; 1986) So we can affirm that eccentric contractions carried out at higher lengths of L0, cause an excessive tensile stress potentially harmful not only for active elements of the muscular ultrastructure but also for the passive ones, like for example the connective support tissue. In effect this sort of innate structural weakness which the streaked muscle fiber shows during an eccentric contraction, is probably attributable to the fact that, during the amounting of the force peak force in an eccentric contraction The number of active actomyosinic bridges is probably less in comparison to that which we may observe during the peak force fulfillment in an isometric and /or concentric contraction. It is important to underline that in the tension-length curve of the isolated muscular fiber it is proved, by exceeding lengths of L0, a decrease in active tension, which is compensated by a contextual increase of the expressed tension by the passive elements, which in this case contribute to the production of the level of total force, giving at the same time an idea of how much they are stimulated from a tensile point of view during the lengthening of the muscle. For this reason, during the lengthening phase a muscular complex- intended both in active and passive components – is exposed to the harmful event, not only when is electrically active but also in an electrically silent phase. Many authors have underlined the fact that, for a given level of production of force, the generated stress on a level of passive elements of the muscle, is higher during an eccentric contraction in comparison to an isometric or concentric contraction (McCully and Faulkner, 1986; Faulkner et al., 1989). However, it is also true that during a lengthening carried out at the same speed of a lengthening at which an eccentric contraction is carried out- considered in this case like a sort of active lengthening of the muscle- a harmful event does not occur on a structural level (McCully and Faulkner,1986; Faulkner et al., 1989), this means that despite the fact that structural damage is theoretically possible also in the course of lengthening of an electrically silent muscle, it is also true the fact that the tensile load to which the passive elements of the muscle are exposed is not the same during an active or passive lengthening. In effect, there is not much practical or experimental evidence which witness the fact that the passive elements may be damaged during an eccentric contraction. In fact, in these cases the majority of the passive tension, up to higher sarcomeral lengths of 140-150% of L0, is absorbed by the sarcolemma (Casella,1951; Rapoport,1972; Higuchi and Umazume,1986). Due to the inhomogeneities of the sarcomeral length, in the course of an eccentric contraction, the sarcomeres of minor dimension may sustain an excessive lengthening, even if the change in the muscular belly in full is relatively scarce. (Julian and Morgan, 1979; Colomo et al., 1988). In this particular situation, the sarcomeres of minor dimension, due to this undergo a real mechanism of overstretching, they may be harmed or cause a lesion in the nearby sarcomeres. The importance of the sarcomeral integrity, is well illustrated in the diseases associated with of Duchenne muscular dystrophy where we assists in the development in a series of defects on a sarcomeral level. (Bhattacharya et al., 1989) essentially ascribable to a deficiency of dystrofin (Hoffman et al., 1987; Zubrycka-Gaarn, 1988). To this end, some authors (Karpati and Carpenter, 1989) have underlined, for a long time, the fundamental importance of dystrofin for the mechanical stability of plasmalemma, above all what concerns the maintenance of a correct alignment between basal lamina and the same plasmalemma. Some experiments carried out on frog semitendinosus muscle, show how an important loss of energy at the same time as an increase of the sarcomeral length appears, postulating in such a way that the so dispersed energetic quota may be dispersed under heat form, or in plastic deformation of the sarcolemma, of the sarcoplasmatic reticulum, of the basal lamina or of the cytoskeleton (Tidball and Daniel,1986). Globally from the same data, we may deduct that about 77% of the total energetic dissipation, which happens in the course of a stretching-shortening cycle, is dissipated on a basal membrane level. This same data was confirmed by other experimental studies (Stauber, 1989), which showed histochemistry and immune histochemistry evidence of damage on a basal lamina and endomysium level in a muscle undergoing a eccentric contraction. Also, the theory of the inhomogeneity of the sarcomeral length- and consequently of the phenomena of overstretching to which they were exposed, during an eccentric contraction, the sarcomeres of minor structural length- was later confirmed also by following studies (Morgan, 1990). Morgan also proposed a sequence of well defined events in this sense:

a. The eccentric contraction carries some sarcomeres whose length is minor in comparison to the average sarcomeral length- to be over-tensioned.

b. The over-tensioned sarcomeres are not able to relax conveniently during a contraction-time/relaxation-time cycle.

c. Above all, in the course of a cycle of particularly fast eccentric contractions the over-tensioned sarcomeres, and for this reason incapable of reaching sufficient relaxation during a succession of contractions, transfer the tensile stress onto the nearby myofibrils.

d. Following the transfer of an excessive tensile stress, the sarcolemma and the sarcoplasmatic reticulum of the nearby fibers to the over-tensioned sarcomeres it structurally gives in.

This theory is, at least partially, supported by data supplied by McCully and Faulkner (1986) who showed how there was no evidence of structural damage when the lengthening speed was reduced under a certain limit. In any case, the data supplied from the experimental studies of McCully and Faulkner, give evidence that the structural components of the muscular fiber may meet up with a fatigue phenomena connected to the repetition of an eccentric contraction. Of particular interest is the strong link, shown by the same authors, between the increase in number of the eccentric contractions, the decrease of the peak of maximum eccentric force of the muscle and the increase of the areas of structural weakness inside the same muscle. This data suggests how the degree of lesion may be proportional to the complex amount of eccentric work carried out by muscular fibers. From the data of the work of McCully and Faulkner, we could draw two important conclusions, which have considerable relapses on a practical/rehabilitative plane and that is:

i. The muscle would have a maximum limit of eccentric contractions beyond which a progressive phenomena of structural weakness would start which could lead to structural damage.

ii.   From the time that a progressive increase of the number of eccentric contractions, it
            would lead to a contextual progressive decrease of the peak of maximum eccentric
            force, due to the fatigue phenomena, expressed by the muscle, there would exist a
            limit of the value of eccentric force, below which the muscle would be exposed to the
            risks of structural damage. According to McCully and Faulkner, such a limit would
            be between 60 and 80% of the maximum value of eccentric force. In other words when
            the decrease of the production of eccentric force drops below 20-40% the muscle runs
            the risk of injury.

From a practical but above all rehabilitative /preventive point of view, this data underlines the
importance of:

i.   Increasing the muscle capacity in the field of specific stamina regarding the eccentric
            contraction, in such a way to increase the quantity of eccentric work supported by
            the same muscle, moving the curve of structural weakness of the relation "stress-
            number of cycles leading to structural weakness", up and to the right,

ii.   Increasing the maximum value of eccentric force, limiting the decrease of the latter
            in conjunction with the increase of the number of cycles. To this end it is important
            to remember how the value of stamina- in this case of stamina in eccentric regime-
            depends on the values of maximum force- and so in this specific case of maximum
            eccentric force.

9. The hypotheses of physical nature: The role of the increase in temperature in muscular damage

Numerous studies (Nielsen 1969; Nadel et al.,1972; Pahud et al., 1980) witness the fact of how
the intramuscular temperature is higher during the negative work (i. e. eccentric contraction)
in comparison to that seen in the course of positive work (i.e. concentric contraction) when
the data is compared to a metabolic equivalent or to a ratio of heat production (for further in-
depth analysis please see the specific box). In equivalent experimental conditions the eccentric
contraction, in comparison to the concentric one, produces an increase in heat superior of about
1.2 degrees Celsius (Nadel et al., 1972), sufficient increase to determine a decrease of the
viscosity of the sarcolemma equal to about 7% (Nagamoto et al., 1984). Such decrease in
viscosity, although modest, would be able to activate the phospholipase A_2, triggering in such
a way an increase in the ratio of degradation of the cellular membrane (Chang et al., 1987).
Other studies, carried out on muscle in vitro, would highlight as an increase of the temperature
from 25 to 35 ° Celsius obtained by placing the muscle under a series of eccentric contractions,
increases the risk of structural damage by a good 50% (Zerba et al., 1990) However, we must
adopt care in interpreting the role of the increase of the muscle temperature in the field of its
structural damage. Such care is obligatory above all considering the fact that, in the mentioned
studies, the difference between the peak of temperature obtained during negative and positive
work is essentially modest; secondly the absolute metabolic ratio would not seem, in this
specific field, the most discriminating parameter. In addition to this, we must consider that

the Fenn effect would theoretically foresee a ratio of minor heat during an eccentric contraction, in comparison to the theoretically predictable one in the course of an isometric and concentric contraction. In effect, the theoretic forecast carried out based on the Fenn effect, which would foresee a minor heat production during an eccentric contraction, would be confirmed also in some experimental data (Abbot and Aubert, 1951). All these observations could lead us to consider the highest production of heat observed in the course of negative work, not so much as an increase in the ratio of heat production on behalf of the muscle itself in similar conditions, but as the consequence of the drop of the ratio or heat removal by the muscle, which is registered during an eccentric contraction (for further information please refer to the specific box.)

9.1. Eccentric contraction and heat dispersion

The production of metabolic heat and its disposal, may be modeled through a central "heat producer" nucleus, made up of skeletal muscles, bowels, internal organs and the central nervous system, a "means of transport", made up of the circulatory system and of a "cooling surface", made of skin. During an eccentric contraction we can see a transient and intermittent mechanism of vasoconstriction which strongly limits the capacity of transporting heat, produced by the muscular contraction, on the part of the circulatory system. For this reason the highest production of heat during negative work, in comparison to the production of heat during positive work, it is essentially attributable to the reduced ratio of degradation of heat which occurs during negative work, caused by the aforementioned vasoconstriction mechanism.

10. The metabolic hypotheses: The role of insufficient mitochondrial respiration

In the course of physical exercise the mitochondrial respiration appears high together with the synthesis and hydrolysis of the ATP. This situation is well balanced from a physiological point of view in the course of moderate exercise in which, the muscular fibers in activity, manage to maintain the concentration of ATP near to the base values (Krisanda et al.,1988). However, in the course of intense and prolonged exercise, a certain reduction in the concentration of energetic phosphates constantly occurs (Krisanda et al.,1988) and the possibility that this event occurs inside some specific compartments of the fiber represents a concrete and reasoned hypothesis which could explain the initial events of the mechanism of muscular lesion. For example, in the case in which a drop in ATP levels occurs near the Ca^{++} - ATPase on a level of the sarcoplasmatic reticulum or of the sarcolemma, the removal of Ca^{++} from the cytoplasm could result compromised, causing in such a way an increase in cytosolic Ca^{++}. To this end there exists important experimental evidence which show that, to maintain an optimal state of cellular function, it is of vital importance to maintain an optimal functionality of the Ca^{++} pump (Duncan, 1987). Also in this field, some studies have shown how a drop in the cellular energetic provision may lead to a release of Ca^{++} from the sarcoplasmatic reticulum (Duchen et al., 1990). Some physiological evidence would show that the deficit of mytochondrial respiration inside the muscular fiber, cannot be considered the same way as an initial event in the onset of muscular damage; these affirmations are based on the fact that, a given level of production of force and /or mechanical power by the muscle, generated through an eccentric contraction, would result less costly than it is for the same level of production of force and /or generated power through a concentric or isometric contraction (Infante et al., 1964; Curtin and Davies, 1970; Bonde- Peterson et al., 1972) Despite this, it is the eccentric contraction the type of contractile muscular behavior which show higher harmful potential towards the integrity of the muscular structure (Asmussen, 1956; Armstrong et al., 1983; Newham et al., 1983; Armstrong, 1984; Ebbeling and Clarkson, 1989; Stauber, 1989). This lack of linking between metabolic cost and harmful event in the course of an eccentric contraction, would indicate, according to some authors, that the etiology of the muscular lesion would not lead to an insufficient production of ATP. Some authors have shown how there are no changes in levels of ATP, CP or in the pH after an injury, even though 24 hours after intense exercise we may register a significant increase in inorganic phosphate levels (Aldridge et al., 1986) At the same time, it is reasonable to expect that during a series of concentric contractions the muscular pH is lower than what it would be during an eccentric contraction. This could represent another indirect test of the fact that the lowering of the pH cannot, in itself, make up the initial factor of muscular damage. In this sense there exist experiments which show how, on isolated muscle, we may induct muscular damage also in the presence of neutral pH (between 7.3 and 7.6) with an average of 3mmol of lactate per liter (Duncan, 1987) Despite this it is of extreme importance to underline that these studies, and the consequential hypotheses, even though logical and rational, do not make up the indisputable test of the fact that the depletion of ATP or the lowering of the pH, are not implied in the process which carries to the muscular damage, but how rather they show that the muscular damage can come about also in absence of these assumptions of metabolic order (Armstrong et al., 1991). Particular attention must be placed on the fact that these specific situation of " metabolic unevenness", may be focal inside the fiber, reason for which in a well defined area of muscular fiber we may observe essential depletions of energetic phosphates and /or accumulation of lactate, which, on the contrary, are not observed in the rest of the muscular belly. So, even though definite demonstrations are missing of the fact that muscular damage recognizes its etiological cause in an insufficient mytochondrial respiration ratio, in bibliography there are not missing studies which speculate how the muscular damage, above all against the pure glycolytic fibers, at least on an animal model, is amenable to the contextual eccentric mechanism to a metabolic situation predisposing the damage itself (Liebere and Friden, 1988). In effect, a higher rational hypothesis in this sense is that which sees the intermittent anoxia, of which the muscle suffers during an intense series of eccentric contractions, as the cause of the drop in muscle pH to which follows a potential structural fragility situation both of the contractile tissue and of the connective tissue inside the muscle itself (Armstrong et al., 1991). So generally, a marginal fatigue may make up, at least from a theoretical point of view, a predisposing situation to muscular damage, even if a precise estimate of the role of fatigue in the harmful mechanism at the expense of the skeletal muscle, is objectively difficult.

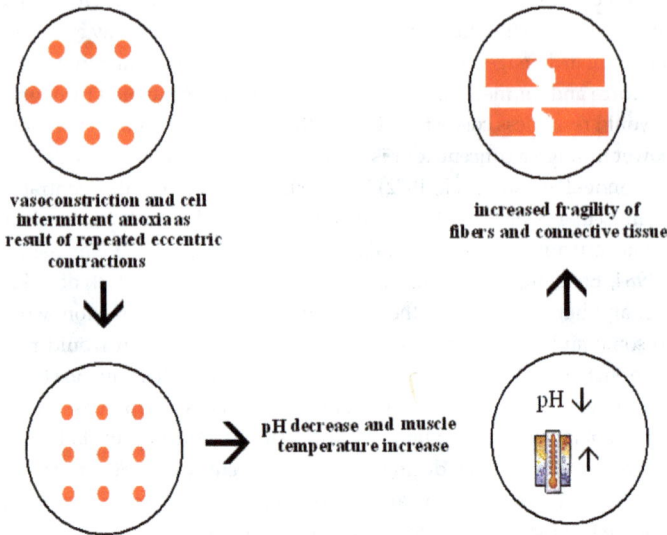

vasoconstriction and cell
intermittent anoxia as
result of repeated eccentric
contractions

increased fragility of
fibers and connective tissue

pH decrease and muscle
temperature increase

pH ↓

Figure 7. In a muscle exposed to a series of intense eccentric contractions, a capillary vasoconstriction may happen which can, in itself, be the cause of an intermittent and transitory anoxia inside the muscle belly itself. The drop if the efficiency of the mechanism of mitochondrial respiration, would cause a drop in the production of ATP provided by the aerobic mechanism, which would induce an even higher involvement in the energetic production of the anaerobic lactate mechanism. This, together with the loss of efficiency of the heat regulator mechanisms due to the phenomena of vasoconstriction, would cause a drop in the pH and an increase of the muscular temperature, factors which would lead to an increase in the fragility both of the myofibrils and the of the sustaining connective tissue predisposing, in such a way, the muscle to harmful event (Armstrong et al., 1991).

11. The production of free radicals

Another consequence of the increase in metabolism during exercise is represented by the high production of free radicals (Packer, 1986; Jenkins, 1988; Matsunaga et al., 2003; Kon et al., 2008). Even though in many situations the increased production of free radicals is controlled by a wide variety of enzymes and of anti-oxidant molecules (Xu et al., 1997; Kon et al.,2008), in other circumstances this protective mechanism may result inefficient (Demopoulos, 1973b; Jenkins, 1988; Horakova et al., 2005). An uncontrollable production of free radicals may cause damage on a cellular level through an oxidation mechanism of phospholipids (Demopoulos, 1973; Blake et al., 1987) of DNA, (Cochrane et al., 1988), of carbohydrates (Blake et al., 1987) and of proteins (Tappel, 1973; Wolffe et al., 1986). The lipoperoxidation of the lipidic membrane may alter the normal permeability of the barrier of the sarcolemma (Quintanihla et al., 9182), allowing in such a way an abnormal molecular diffusion, in particular of Ca^{++} and of intra-muscular enzymes (Braughler, 1988); the inactivity of this enzyme can in fact perturb the homeostasis of the Ca^{++} inside the muscular fiber and cause, consequentially, the activity of a series of cellular degradation processes. However, research which supports in an evident way the role of free radicals in the etiology of muscular lesion, is quite limited, above all if linked to an eccentric contraction as principal mechanical cause. One of the most convincing studies in this field is represented by that of Zerba in 1990 (Zerba et al., 1990), in which the authors showed how, in a murine model, an intraperitoneal injection of superoxide-dismutase limits, after the imposition of a series of eccentric contractions in situ, the drop in the value of P0 of the considered muscle. The treatment based on superoxide-dismutase was able to reduce the drop in the value of P0 for a period of three days following the eccentric exercise. Other experiments, carried out on animal models have further corroborated the hypothesis formulated by Zerba (Strosova et al., 2005; Kon et al., 2007), so for this it appears reasonable to extend this theoretical model also in a human field (Castilho et al., 1996; Close et al., 2005; Clanton, 2007; Kerkweg et al., 2007; Voss et al., 2008). There is not missing, however, in literature studies which deny the thesis that the administration of anti-oxidant agents may reduce muscular damage connected with high intensity exercise (Warren et al., 1990; Childs et al., 2001; Sacheck and Blumberg, 2001; Kerkweg et al., 2007). It is also important to remember some interesting experiences (Brooks et al., 2008) which underline the fact that the production of free radicals, on behalf of the skeletal muscle, and consequently their control and their regulation, are in function of precise physiological stimuli and how these parameters play a very important role in the field of physiological adaptation of the muscle during the contraction mechanism. These adaptations would include an optimization of the contraction mechanism, and in addition they would represent the beginning of adaptation processes and changes of gene expression regarding stress induced by the muscular contraction. Evidently these beneficial effects of the free radicals in the field of muscular contraction, contrast with contrary scientific evidence, which see the beginning and /or the cause of free radicals of a pathway of degenerative type which would appear fundamental, not only in the field of possible structural damage regarding the skeletal muscle, but also, more in general, in its aging process. This only apparent contradiction, underlines the necessity of deeper understanding in the role covered by the free radicals in the field of both physical exercise and the sarcopenia. Anyway, despite the relative lack of convincing and undisputable scientific evidence concerning the role of free radicals in the field of initial mechanisms, and /or predisposition of muscular lesion, it is without doubt legitimate to ask ourselves this question: is it reasonable to be able to support an increase in production of free radicals during an eccentric exercise? To answer this interesting and legitimate query, it is useful to remember that some studies (Brand and Lehninger, 1975) show how during an ischemic phenomena, in a model of ischemic /reperfusion damage, we can see in the cardiac muscle a destruction of the normal tight association between the elements of the chain of transport of the electrons. This would provide a particularly evident production of free radicals during the reperfusion phase, phase in which we may find high concentrations of O_2 of the tissue(Hess et al., 1982; Arkhipenko et al., 1983; Faust et al., 1988; Fisher, 1988). It is possible to speculate that the high and specific muscular tensions which happen during of eccentric contraction, may alter the normal cytoskeletal structure, of which whose functions are to stabilize the position of the mitochondria (BIgland-Richie and Woods, 1976). The destruction of the cytoskeleton l could, in its turn, cause a disruption of the spatial configuration of the elements which compose the electron transport chain (Demopoulos, 1973a). This structural disruption of the electron transport chain could lead to an excessive production of free radicals and so to a dramatic increase of the lipoperoxidation phenomena. So, in general, every disruption of the electron transport chain, may lead to an increase in the production of free radicals and potentially represent an initial mechanism in the field of the phenomena which we can name as "Exercise-induced muscle fiber injury".

12. The loss of Ca^{++} homeostasis

If the initial events of harmful mechanism are of mechanical and metabolic nature, the immediately successive phases leading to the same harmful event, are characterized by an elevation of the levels of intracellular Ca^{++} in the injured area (Statham et al., 1976; Publicover et al., 1978; Kameyana and Etlinger, 1979; Baracos et al., 1984; Carpenter, 1989; Boobis et al., 1990). It is interesting to note how also in patients affected by muscular dystrophy and other muscular pathologies, we may find an increase in the intracellular levels of Ca^{++} (Jackson et al., 1985 ; Turner et al., 1988). The importance of maintaining the concentration of free cytosolic Ca^{++}, is indirectly underlined by the number of the Ca^{++} transport mechanisms from the cytosolic compartment which the cell possesses (Gillis, 1985; Klug and Tibbits, 1988). There exists, in fact, at least seven membrane transport systems of Ca^{++}. In the actual state of knowledge in the specific field, it would seem that there exists, until today, direct evidence of the fact that the elevation of the intracellular levels of Ca^{++} is involved in the mechanism of "exercise-induced muscle fiber injury" (Hall-Craggs, 1980; Steer and Mastaglia 1986; Childs et al., 2001), even if studies exist which show how in the condition of DOMS, they are present inside the muscle of high contextual levels of Ca++ to a same increased level of mitochondrial Ca^{++} (Duan et al., 1990a). The hypothesis that would justify an increase of intracellular levels, are essentially based on to the destruction of the sarcolemma found during the harmful event. The sarcolemma in fact represents a suitable barrier for the maintenance of concentration and of the electric gradient between the intra and extra cellular spaces; its destruction so permits the Ca^{++} to invade the intracellular space. The concentration of free extracellular Ca^{++} oscillates between 2 and 3 mmol.1^{-1} whereas that of cytosolic Ca^{++}, in the muscle fiber at rest, is about 0.1 umol1^{-1}. So it evidently appears how, at the expense of Ca^{++}, there exists and important gradient between the intra and extra cellular space and that how each loss of normal permeability of the barrier, represented by the sarcolemma, may cause an important influx of Ca^{++} in the intracellular space. In experiments carried out on muscular fibers treated with saponin and incubated in Ca^{++} solution in concentration between 0.5 and umol- 1^{-1}, we may observe a destruction of the myofibrils and a hyper-contraction of the sarcomeres. (Duncan, 1987). From the moment in which such concentrates enter in the same physiological range seen during an "*in vivo*" muscular contraction, this experimental data could induce us to believe that also during normal contractile activity the level of free cytosolic Ca^{++} could be high enough to start the degradation of the muscular ultrastructure. However, this event does not happen above all because the increase of the level of cytosolic Ca^{++} in the course of an *in vivo* muscular contraction is of transient type; In other words at the moment in which the Ca^{++} is released from the sarcoplasmatic reticulum in the course of the contraction itself, its level is readily limited by the regulating proteins, in such a way that its level seems high only for a short amount of time, and too scarce to allow the activation of proteolytic enzymes (Robertson et al., 1981) ; in addition the proteolytic enzymes inside the fiber are in compartments and for this reason are not influenced by the increase of the level of Ca^{++} which happens during the stimulus- contraction cycle. So, the damage to the muscular membrane or to the sarcoplasmatic reticulum, may be caused by an increase of the concentrate Ca^{++} only in those compartments, inside the muscular fiber, where Ca^{++} is allowed to arrive in contact with the areas of degrading enzymes. (Duncan, 1987). So essentially, it would not be the absolute level of Ca^{++} which can represent an important starting factor of the process of muscular damage, rather than the temporary length of the magnitude of active movement of Ca^{++} through the muscular fiber (Duncan, 1987). In some experiments which simulated an injury, similar to that which can happen following an eccentric contraction obtained by using micro injections on the sarco-lemma, we observed the area of necrosis corresponding to the place of insertion, was literally "surrounded" by a sort of barrier, made up of hyper-contracted filaments, in which we could find an increase in the concentration of Ca^{++} (Armstrong et al.,1983b; Ogilvie et al., 1988). A similar mechanism may probably be observed also following an "exercise-induced muscle fiber injury" (Armstrong et al., 1983b; Kuipers et al., 1983; Ogilvie et al., 1988). Many muscular disease show an increase of the levels of intracellular Ca^{++}, caused by the disturbance of the normal barrier permeability of the sarcolemma regarding the Ca^{++} itself. For example in muscles affected by the of Duchenne muscular dystrophy, the proteic degradation is directly linked to the increase in intracellular levels of Ca^{++} (Turner et al., 1988). Another example in which we can observe a high concentration of Ca^{++} is represented by the malignant hyperther-mia, in which a specific agent causes a prolonged increase of the concentration of intracellular Ca^{++} which, in its turn, provokes a massive and uncontrollable muscular contraction, whose consequence is an increase in body temperature which can reach 46° C (Cheah and Cheah, 1985). A second mechanism responsible for the elevation of free cytosolic levels of Ca^{++} is represented by the malfunction of the sarcoplasmatic reticulum. Apart from the fact that this happens, following an eccentric contraction which has caused muscular damage, represented by a flux of Ca^{++} from the extracellular space (Duan et al, 1990b) it would still seem certain that the malfunction on behalf of the sarcoplasmatic reticulum in re-absorbing Ca^{++}, may contribute to the increase of its cytosolic concentration. In effect the sarcoplasmatic reticulum reduces its re-absorbing capacities of Ca++ reduced in the course of exercise, both in the case that the intensity of the latter is moderate or maximal (Byrd et al., 1999). However, there is no certain data which can enlighten us in regards to the different possible effects of eccentric, concentric or isometric exercise on the functionality of the sarcoplasmatic reticulum. In any case, it is plausible to put forward the hypothesis that the inhomogeneity of the sarcomeral length can negatively influence on the adjacent segments of the sarcoplasmatic reticulum itself (Arm-strong et al., 1991). Some experiments on isolated muscle would go into effect in this sense. When an isolated muscle is incubated with caffeine- a substance which stimulates the Ca^{++} inducing its release on behalf of the sarcoplasmatic reticulum - it is possible to observe a deterioration of the myofibril structure (Duncan,1987); in other respects also the incubation of isolated muscle in ruthenium red - substance which inhibits the Ca^{++}-ATPase - is able to induce significant damage of the myofibril (Duncan et al., 1980). This experimental data witnesses the fact that a loss in the homeostasis of Ca^{++}, as in the case of muscular injury, could be, at least in part, due to a malfunction and/or and drop in the efficiency or normal re-absorbing machanisms of Ca^{++} on behalf of the sarcoplasmatic reticulum. Some authors, to this end, emphasize the fact that the mechanisms which cause the destruction of the membrane, are mainly responsible for the increase in levels of intracellular Ca^{++} inside the injured fibers (Armstrong et al. 1991), even if we have to admit the existence of other numerous factors able to perturb the homeostasis of the latter. For example some studies (Snowdowne and Lee, 1980; Lopez et al., 1985) would evidence the existence, inside the skeletal muscle, of "stretch-sensitive calcium channels" ; so - from the moment the muscle during an eccentric contraction is mechanically elongated at the same time in which it is electrically active- the hypothesis appears more than plausible that these specific channels are involved in mechanisms which induce, during the eccentric contraction itself, the increase in intracellular Ca^{++} levels. Another mechanism which could be implied in the increase of intracellular Ca^{++} would be the pathway of Na^+: Ca^{++}, through which the mechanism of uptake and the release of Ca^{++} on cellular level is completed, (Allen et.al., 1989), even if in truth there isn't any unequivocal evidence of its involvement in the field of Ca^{++} overload mechanism observable in the injured skeletal muscle.

It has also been shown how the inhibition of the acetylcholinesterase on a level of neuro-muscular junctions, causes and influx of Ca^{++} inside the muscular area, contextual to contraction of the fibers and local necrosis of the latter (Leonard and Salpeter, 1979). Also other similar experiments, which have induced an increase in the release of Ca^{++} on behalf of the sarcoplasmatic reticulum have permitted to observe an increase in the contraction of the fibers, together with a rapid process of destruction of the myofibril structure- which happen in less than 30 minutes- in addition to a drop of the intramuscular enzymes (Duncan, 1987). This data underlines the importance which the role of an increase in intracellular Ca^{++} levels could have in the field of construction of the theoretical model of "exercise-induced muscle fiber injury". One of the consequences of the elevation of the level of intracellular Ca^{++} is represented by the phenomena called "blebbing" which consists in the formation of cytoplasmic vesicular enlargements on the cellular surface. We retain that these alterations are to be put in relation with a possible disturbance of the relationship which runs between the cytoskeletal proteins (in particular actin and tubulin) and the cell of the membrane (Orrenius et al., 1989). The "blebbing " phenomena is furthermore observable also outside the model represented by the skeletal muscle, like for example in the cells of the myocardium in the field of the model of "ischemia-reperfusion" (Ganote and Humphrey, 1985; Ariel et al., 2008). In the light of what we have already said, in the field of the theoretical model of "exercise-induced muscle fiber injury" we may think that, during exercise itself, an initial damage occurs, of probable mechanical nature, at the expense of the designated components for the maintenance of a correct permeability of the barrier regarding extracellular Ca^{++}. This alteration would allow a massive diffusion, through the damaged membrane site, of Ca^{++}, giving origin, in such a way, to the said phenomena of "Ca^{++} overload", whose consequence is represented by the annihilation of the tampon systems of the muscular fiber (like for example the Ca^{++} binding proteins, the functionality of the sarcoplasmatic reticulum and the mitochondria). Once the level of cytosolic Ca^{++} has reached a critic level, which remains for a sufficiently long level of time- and above all if the latter stays high inside the specific compartments of the fiber - different degradation mechanisms start inside the injured muscle fiber which are represented by:

- The mechanism of the myofibrillar reflex contraction

- The phenomena of mitochondrial Ca^{++} overload

- The mechanism of activation of the dependent Ca++ protease

- The lysosomal protease

- The pathway of the A^2 phospholipase

13. The mechanism of the reflex myofibrillar contraction

The loss of the homeostasis of the Ca^{++} involves an uncontrollable contractionreflex (or not through the SNC) by the sarcomeres inside the injured area (Ogilvie et al., 1988). We need however to specify that the myofibrillar contraction reflex phenomena, does not have to be necessarily understood as a degradation phenomena in the strict meaning, like for example the enzymatic pathway could be. Even if some authors have put forward the hypothesis that this zone of concentration may make up a sort of barrier apt to block the degradation processes preventing the latter to extend to the sarcomeres adjacent to the injured zone (Carpenter and Karpati, 1989), we need to consider that this uncontrolled state of contraction of the sarcomeres may have serious consequences in the field of aggravation of structural damage. The first negative effect is represented by the local depletion of ATP following the endurance of the contraction itself, which would give origin to a vicious circle, and so, capable of auto sustainment, identifiable in "depletion of ATP- increase in levels of Ca^{++}" and vice versa (Goodman, 1987). The second negative outcome of the mechanism of myofibrillar contraction reflex is made up of the fact that such a phenomena produces mechanical forces, inside the fibers able to damage further both the membrane and the same contractile components, contributing in such a way to further deterioration of the clinical situation (Armstrong et al., 1991).

14. The phenomena of mitochondrial Ca^{++} overload

The mitochondria inside the muscular fiber have, among their tasks, also that which to react to "buffer", or to tampon mechanism, regarding the increase of the concentration of cytosolic Ca^{++}. However the hypothesis is generally creditable that the uptake of Ca^{++} on a mitochondrial level is quite modest, and in any case insufficient to be able to consider as fundamental, or at least important, the role taken on the mitochondria itself in the field of the mechanism of relaxation of the muscular fiber. Even though we need to remember that the mitochondria, in particular pathologic situations, are capable of accumulating a large quantity of ions (Gillis, 1985). Between all the types of fibers, the oxidative ones show marked capacity of mitochondrial buffering regarding the Ca^{++} which can exceed the registered ones by 2-3 times on a glycolitic fiber level (Sembrowich and Quintinskie, 1985). An excess in uptake of Ca^{++} on behalf of the mitochondria is accompanied by a contemporary uptake in phosphates causing, in such a way, a precipitation of calcium phosphate which can deposit itself in the intra-mitochondrial spaces (Gillis,1985). So, on the one hand, an increase in the level of mitochondrial Ca^{++}, which stays in a nano-molar range, appears useful in stimulating the mitochondrial respiration, whereas on the other hand an accumulation of Ca^{++}, in a micro-molar range, causes a depression of the respiratory functions on a level with the mitochondria itself (Wrogemann and Pena, 1976; Hansford, 1985; McMillin and Madden, 1989).

15. The mechanism of the dependent Ca^{++} protease

The Ca^{++} dependent protease is of two types: type 1 and type 2: this division is based on the level of Ca^{++} necessary for their activation. The type 1 isoform is activated in presence of micro-molar levels of Ca^{++}, whereas the type 2 form needs quantities in milli- molars for its activation (Murachi et al., 1981). Unlike not for the lysosomal protease, this enzyme has it optimal pH in the field of neutrality. Its activation is associated with the degradation of particular structures inside the myocell and in particular in the degradation of the Z band (Bush et al., 1972; Ishiura et al., 1980), of the myofilaments (Daytona et al., 1976; 1979; Cullen and Fulthorpe, 1982) and of the A band (Friden et al., 1981; Newham et al., 1983; Ogilvie et al., 1988). All these alterations are observable in an injured muscle following eccentric exercise. Also the proteins of the cytoskeleton would represent a preferential underlayer for the action of the Ca^{++} dependent protease (Pontremoli and Melloni, 1986) To this end, there has been a hypothesis that the proteolysis of the vinculin (a protein of the cytoskeleton which anchors the cellular membrane to the cytoskeleton) on behalf of the Ca^{++} dependent protease, causes a fragility of the sarco-lemma of the myocardium cells in the course of the ischemic process (Steenbergen et al., 1987a).

16. The lysosomal protease

Since the myofibrillar protein may be degraded by the proteolytic enzymes contained in the lysosomes of the muscular fibre (Schwartz and Bird,1977), it is reasonable to suppose that the lysosomial protease plays an important role in the field of the successive autogenic phase to the muscular damage. This supposition is corroborated by the evidence of a strong increase in the lysosomal protease, following exhaustive exercise in an animal model (Vinko et al., 1978). There is also evidence of the fact that the lysosomal enzymes are activated by the increase of the level of intracellular Ca^{++} (Rodemann et al., 1982).

17. The pathway of the phospholipase A_2

The phospholipase A_2 (PLA_2) uses the phospholipidic membrane as an underlayer for the production of arachidonic acid, prostaglandin – in particular the prostaglandin E_2 (PGE_2)-

leukotrienes and thromboxanes. This enzyme is located in the sarcolemma, in the mitochondrial membrane, in the cytosolic compartment and in the lysosomes (Van der Vusse et al., 1989). In particular we suppose that the PLA_2 present in the mitochondrial membrane may be implied in the mechanisms that induce the loss of the homeostasis of Ca^{++} (Cheah and Cheah, 1985). Likewise an increase of the concentrate of intracellular Ca^{++} would involve an activation of PLA2(Vane and Botting, 1987) The arachidonic acid and the lysophospholipids produced by the activation of PLA_2, would cause a destabilization of the membrane structure assuming, in such a way, an important role in the field of autogenic processes following the harmful event (Jackson and Edwards, 1986; Chang et al., 1987). In addition the PLA_2 would contribute to the loss of intramuscular enzymes observable in a muscular injury (Jackson et al., 1987). It is interesting to know that the PLA2 is one of the most important active principals of snake and bee poison. In fact the injection of poison of the coral snake (*Micrurus fulvius*) in the muscle of a mouse, provokes similar damage to that of an eccentric contraction (Arroyo et al., 1987) even if we need to underline the fact that the muscular necrosis induced by the snake's poison is much faster and larger than that seen in eccentric exercise. It is enough to think that an injection of only two micrograms of poison of the Australian tiger snake (*Notechis scutatus*) on rat muscle, leads to the total destruction of fiber in only 24 hours (Harris, 1989). It is also interesting to know that PLA possesses a protective role regarding oxidative stress (Van Kuijk et al., 1987)

18. The pathobiology of muscular lesion

The distinctive element which differentiates a muscular lesion and a lesion at bone level, is represented by the fact that the skeletal muscle heals through a phenomena of "repair", whereas the bone damage heals thanks to a process of "regeneration"- The main part of biological body tissue, at the moment in which it is damaged, heals through a process which hesitates in the formation of a scar area, which represents a biologically different tissue in comparison to the pre-existing one. On the contrary, when a bone segment becomes injured the regenerated tissue results identical in comparison to the pre-existent tissue. The process of repair of an injured skeletal muscle inescapably follows a constant pattern, independently of the cause which provoked the injury itself, whatever the injury may be contusion, elongation or tear (Hurme et al., 1991; Kalimo et al., 1997). In this type of process we may essentially identify three phases:

1. The destruction phase, which is characterized by the breakage and by the consequent necrosis of the muscular fibers, by the formation of a hematoma between the stumps of the injured fibers and by the inflammatory cellular reaction.

2. The repair phase, which consists in the phagocytosis of the necrotic tissue, in the repair of fibers and the contextually production of healing connective tissue, contextual to the capillary growth in the injured area.

3. The remodeling phase, a period during which the maturation of the repaired fibers, the contraction, or the reduction and the re-organization of the scar tissue and lastly, the recovery of the functional capacities of the muscle come about.

The last two phases, of repair and re-modeling, are usually associated or overlapping (Kalimo et al., 1997).

19. The three post-lesion weeks

The processes of muscular repair are completed in a period of about three weeks during which follow precise and expiring biological stages which we can schematically illustrate in six fundamental phases as follows:

Second post-lesion day: the necrotic parts of muscular fibers have been removed by the macrophages whereas, contextually, the formation, on behalf of the fibers-blasts, of the healing connective tissue inside the central zone (CZ) has started.

Third day: the satellite cells have already started their activation which takes place inside the cylinders of the basal lamina in the zone of repair (RZ).

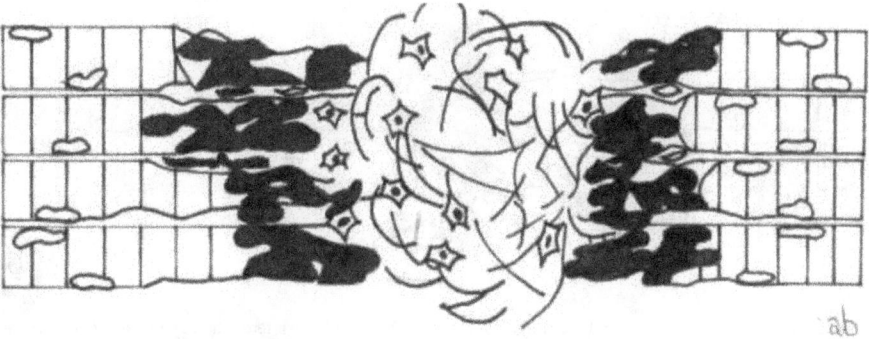

Fifth day: the myoblasts collect inside the myotubes of the RZ and the connective tissue of the CZ starts to become more dense.

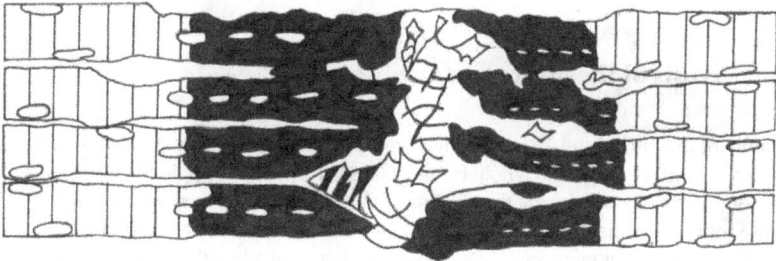

Seventh day: the repair processes of the muscular cells extend outside the old cylinders of the basal lamina up to the CZ area and start to penetrate through the scar area.

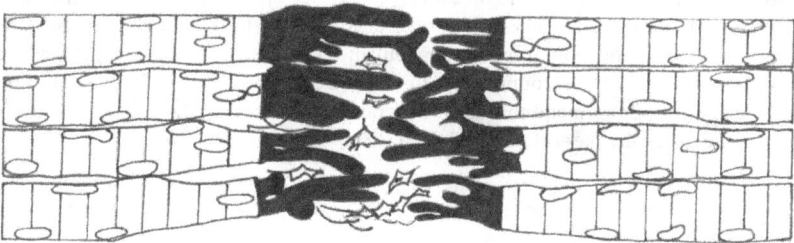

Fourteenth day: the healing area in the CZ area is further condensed and reduced in dimension and the repaired myo-fibres fill the remaining gap of the CZ area itself.

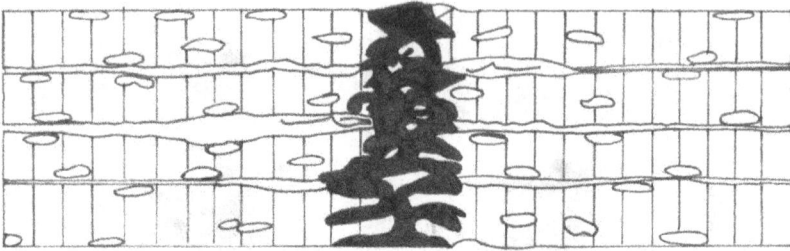

Twenty-first day: the twining of the myo-fibres is virtually complete with the interposition of a small quantity of scar tissue. The quantity of scar tissue is linked to the quality of the repair processes themselves. The remodeling phase of the injured area may lengthen for a period of up to 60 days, depending on the anatomic and functional entity of damage. It is interesting to note that some authors have shown that, in the case which when the muscular lesion extends to more than 50% of the anatomic surface, the complete tissue repair comes about in a period not inferior to five weeks (Pomeranz and Heidt, 1993).

20. The necrosis of the muscular fibre

At the moment in which the skeletal muscle is injured, we can generally observe a mechanical force which extends through the whole transversal section of each single fiber and causes the breakage of the sarcolemma inside the stumps of already injured fibers; leaving the latter amply open. From the moment that the myofibrillars (and consequently the muscular fibers)are, from a structural point of view, cells of notable length and of a lengthened and tapered form, there exists a real risk that the process of necrosis, begun in the location of the injury, extends along the whole length of the fiber itself. However, there exists a special anatomic structure named "contraction band" made up of a particularly dense cytoskeletal material, which behaves as a true "fire door" (Hurme et al., 1991). Some hours following the traumatic event, the propagation of the necrotic process is blocked by a local phenomena represented by a sort of seal carried out by the contraction band on a level of modified areas of the cellular membrane. In such a way, a sort of protective barrier is created inside which starts the repair processes regarding the laceration of the cellular membrane (Hurme et al., 1991). Recent studies have also shown that the lysosomal vesicles found inside the site of destruction of the cellular membrane, cover the role of a temporary membrane and carry out a central task in the healing process of the cellular membrane (Miyake et al., 2001; McNeil, 2002).

21. The inflammatory phase

Contextually into the muscular fiber injury, in the traumatic event, also the blood vessels of the injured muscle tissue are lacerated. In such a way the inflammatory cells, transported by the blood flow, have direct access to the injured site. The inflammatory reaction is "amplified" by the fact that the satellite cells and the necrotic parts of the injured muscular fibers, release several substances defined "wound hormones", which behave as chemo-attractant increasing in such a way the overflowing of the inflammatory cells (Tidball, 1995; Chazaud et al., 2003; Hirata et al., 2003;). Inside the injured muscle, we may observe macrophages and fibro-blasts whose activation gives origin to the additional chemo-tactic signals (as growth factor, chem-iochins and citochines) directed at the circulating inflammatory cells. In addition to this quota of growth factors, produced *ex-novo*, the main part of the muscle tissue contains growth factors stocked in active form inside its ECM, ready to be used in cases of urgent necessity; like for example in the repair of a lesion. (Ragk and Kerbel, 1997). In the case of tissue injury the capacity of biological tissue repair depends on the release of the activation of the growth factors ECM-dependent (or to the growth factors tied to the ECM) and of their capacity to start repair processes (Ragk and Kerbel, 1997). In particular, direct evidence exists that the Tumor Necrosis factor-α (TNF-α) covers and important physiological role in the repair process of the injured skeletal muscle, which is shown by the fact that, if its activity is inhibited during the healing process, there is a slight deficit of the repair capacity of the skeletal muscle itself (Warren et al., 2002). In addition, a large number of growth factors and citochine, as member of the family of Fibroblastic Growth Factors (FGF) of Insulin-Like Growth Factors (IGF), and of the family of Transforming Growth Factors-β (TGF-β), the Hepatocyte Growth factors (HGF), the Interleukin 1β (IL-1β) and the Interleukin-6 (IL-6), are amply known for their expression during muscular injury. After all it is also certain that many other factors, like the Plateled –Derived Growth-Factors are present in the course of various stages which are registered in a muscular injury (Mishra et al., 1995; Burkin and Kaufman, 1999). We should also note the fact that their expression may be induced, in the field of the skeletal muscle by physiological stimuli similar to those which cause micro-traumatic lesions, such as the phenomena of overstretching, or those relative to non-appropriate external mechanical loads (Burkin and Kaufman, 1999; Perrone et al., 1995). Considering the fact that these growth factors make up powerful mytogenic activators for numerous types of cells, it is now an acquired fact that the latter may also be involved in the activation of regenerative processes of the injured skeletal muscle (Burkin and Kaufman, 1999; Best et al., 2001; Chargè and Rudnicki, 2004). A certain number of these growth factors, like FGFs, IGF1, IGF2, TGF-β, HGF. TNF-α and the IL-6,are potential activators of the proliferation of the myogenic precursor cell (MPC,Myogenic Precursor Cells or satellite cells) (Chargè and Rudnicki, 2004). Some of these are also powerful stimulators for the differentiation of the MPC and after, in the course of regenerative processes, regarding the fusion of myotubes in multi-nuclear mature myo-fibers (Burkin and Kaufman, 1999; Best et al., 2001; Chargé and Rudnicki, 2004). In the acute phase, following a harmful muscular event, the polymorphonuclear leukocytes are the most abundant cells present on the injured area (Hurme et al., 1991; Thorsson et al., 1998; Brickson et al., 2001; Schneider et al., 2002; Bricksona et al., 2003) but, before the first day, the latter are substituted by the monocytes. In relation to the basic principles of an inflammatory process, these monocytes are eventually transformed into macrophages, which are employed in proteolysis and phagocytosis of the necrotic material, thanks to the release of lysosomal enzymes (Hurme et al., 1991; Best and Hunter, 2001; Farges et al., 2002 ; Timballi, 1995) The phagocytosis on behalf of the macrophages depending on the necrotic material, makes up a highly specific process. In this phase the intact cylinders of the basal lamina, surround the necrotic part of the survived cells which have been left intact by the macrophages attacks and which, consequently, will be used as a scaffold inside which the satellite cells, able to survive, will start the formation of new myofibres (Grounds, 1991; Hurme and Kalimo, 1991; 1992). A fascinating demonstration of the incredible exactness and of its high biological co-ordination of this process, is given by the fact that the macrophages, at the same time that they phagocyte the necrotic residue that surrounds the satellite cells, simultaneously send specific survival factors to the satellite cells themselves (Chazaud et al., 2003). It is also important to remember how the trauma involves a contextual breakage of the sarcoplasmatic reticulum and a consequent leakage of the calcium ions contained in it. The drastic increase of calcium ions inside the muscular fiber determines, in the 24-48 post-lesion hours, a reflex contraction of the myofibrils inside and around the injured area. This phenomena involves an auto worsening phase of the injury prolonged in function of the period of muscular reflex contraction due to the phase defined by the name of "calcium overload" (Armstrong et al., 1991a) which we have amply spoken about previously.

22. The role of lactate in the process of muscular healing

A few hours from the injury, the consumption of oxygen at rest, inside the injured muscular area, rises drastically, generating as a consequence an imbalance between the storing and the request of O_2, which in its turn determines a rapid descent in the tension of O_2 inside the injured area. Contextually to this, we assist in an increase in the concentration of lactate inside the lesion. All this series of events is well shown in the process of repair tissue in the ear of the rabbit observed at 15 days from the traumatic event(Hunt and Hussain, 1993) At the moment in which the tension of the O_2 falls, the process of accumulation of lactate starts (Wasserman et al., 1990); to this end it is important to remember that the muscle produces a superior quantity of lactate than that which it consumes, in all conditions, including at rest (Graham et al., 1986). In this physiological context, the lactate assumes a sort of "guide role", inducing the fibroblasts to produce collagen and influencing the macrophages, and eventually also the lymphocytes, to excrete angiogenic substances. The repair components which we could describe as "lactate-guided" would seem to assume an even further importance, above all at the moment in which the inflammatory component diminishes notably, or starting, approximately, from the seventh post-lesion day (Hunt and Hussain, 1993). The accumulation of lactate in the injured area is substantially ascribable to three factors. The first of these is made up of the fact that the vascular damage, following the tissue damage, inhibits the diffusion of O_2 inside the injured tissue, from this follows a quota of lactate which is produced by anaerobic glycolysis (Im and Hoopes, 1970a: 1970b). The second of these, the vascular damage limits the external diffusion of lactate (Hunt et al., 1967) and the last reason, fact which makes up the most important aspect, is the activation of the leucytes which causes the release of a large quantity of lactate, both of hypoxic nature and not (Calwell et al., 1984). The macrophages which appear on the site of lesion a few hours before the harmful event- playing the role of "guided cells" in the field of the first repair processes they are not only able to supply the injured area with lactate, but are also influenced by the quota of lactate present. In fact, confirming this hypothesis, it is possible to note how the concentration of lactate inside the injured area, diminishes only slightly at the moment in which the concentration of O_2 rises (Hunt et al., 1978). To this end, it is worth it to mention how some authors report values of lactate concentration, inside the injured muscle, between 8 and 18 mmol.1^{-1} (Hunt and Hussain, 1993). On the other hand, the hypothesis, that lactate was implied in the synthesis of collagen, it had already been put forward by some authors more than forty years ago (Green and Goldberg, 1963; Levine and Bates, 1976). In these experiments, it was described how lactate was implied in the synthesis of collagen, the authors noted how in their experiments the fibroblats put into culture, produced a higher quantity of collagen, in comparison with the control group when the concentration of lactate surpassed 20mmol.1^{-1}. In these, just as in other successive experiments of such kind, it was observed in a hypoxic regime, the production of collagen is delayed up until the moment in which the hypoxic cells are not supplied with oxygen. In other words, the production of collagen only starts when there is the contextual presence of oxygen and lactate. This data suggests how the effect of lactate is independent in comparison to that of oxygen (Comstock and Udenfriend, 1970). However, in spite of the first stimulating results, this line of research has been practically abandoned since 1976. After nearly 20 years, other authors speculated that the lactate could work as a regulator in the process of collagen synthesis inside the injured tissue (Hunt and Hussain, 1993). According to these authors, the maximum ratio of collagen production, would occur in the presence of a high concentration of lactate, included between 8 and 18 mmol.1^{-1}, concurrent with an high value of PO_2, equal to about 100 mm Hg. This data, at a first look, would seem paradoxical, since we can usually consider logical a strong presence of lactate where there are scarce conditions of O_2. However, we need to remember that the leucocytes are responsible for the production, in aerobic conditions, for an important quantity of lactate inside the injured tissue area, and that the production of lactate on behalf of the leucocytes inside the injury remains high also in the presence of a high value of PO_2 (Levine and Bates, 1976). This type of biological model, characterized by a high concentration of contextual lactate to a high value of PO_2, would establish a favorable condition, not only to the collagen synthesis but also to the angiogenesis (Hunt and Hussain, 1993) and in addition it is also probable that the lactate serves as stimulus for the secretion of TGF-β in the injured area (Falanga et al., 1991).

23. The repair and re-modeling phase of the muscular fibers

Once the phase of destruction has dropped in intensity, the real repair process of the injured muscle begins, which shows itself through two concurrent processes, which show between themselves, at the same time, complementary and antagonistic: the repair of the destroyed myofibers and of their respective innervations and the formation of healing tissue. A balanced progression of these two processes, makes up an essential pre-requisite for an optimal reactivation of the contractile functions of the skeletal muscle (Kalimo et al., 1997; Hurme and Kalimo, 1991;). In spite of the fact that the muscular fibers are, in general, considered as fibers of irreversibly post-mitotic type, the notable repair potential of the skeletal muscle is guaranteed by an innate mechanism able to reactivate the injured contractile apparatus. Consequently, a reserve pool of undifferentiated cells, defined satellite cells are, during the fetal development, dislocated under the basal lamina of each singular muscular fibre (Hurme and Kalimo, 1992; Rantenen et al., 1995; Kalimo et al., 1997;). In answer to the harmful event, these particular cells, initially proliferate, then differentiate into myoblasts and at the end of the process, they connect to the remaining fibers forming multinuclear myotubes. The multinuclear myotubes of recent formation fuse, in a second moment, with the part of the injured fiber which survived the initial trauma (Hurme and Kalimo, 1992). In the end, the part of regenerated myofiber acquires its mature form, with normal streaking and with the myonuclei peripherally dislocated (Hurme and Kalimo, 1992). Curiously, in answer to t very balad traumas, like for example in a singular eccentric elongation which provokes trauma of light entity, the satellite cells immediately respond starting to proliferate, but due to the limitation of trauma and of the rapid "innate" answer of repair on behalf of the fibres of the injured muscle, they auto-block their activation before myoblasts are formed (Aarimaa et al., 2004). In the mature skeletal muscle there exists at least two principle populations of satellite cells (Rantenen et al., 1995; Jancowski et al., 2002; Kalimo et al., 1997; Qu-Peterson et al., 2002;; Rouger et al., 2004; Zammit et al., 2004). The "classic" satellite cells which reside under the basal lamina of the muscular fiber and which can be divided into"committed satellite cells" which are ready to differentiate themselves into myoblasts immediately after the harmful event and the "stem sateliite cells" which have to first undergo cellular division to be able to differentiate (Kalimo et al., 1997; Rantenen et al., 1995; Zammit et al.,2004). Through this cellular division (which may be seen form a biological point of view as a true and proper proliferation process), the population of stem satellite cells, again builds up the reserve of satellite cells for a future possible regenerative request (Rantenen et al., 1995; Zammit et al., 2004). In this population of satellite cells, we may note the existence of and under-population of cells capable of differentiation, beyond the myogenic lines, not only in mesenchymal lines but also in neural or endothelial ones (Jankowski et al., 2002; Qu-Peterson et al., 2002). Up until to today the satellite cells were retained the only resource of the myonucleus in the course of muscular repair (Chargé and Rudnicki, 2004), recent discovery has shown the presence of a different population of multi-powerful stem cells, which can contribute to the reparation of the injured skeletal muscle; the "non-muscle-resident stem cells" (Chargé and Rudnicki, 2004). In fact, even some isolated progenitor cells of the bone marrow (BM), the neuronal compartment, and different mesenchymal tissue, are able to differentiate in myogenic lines. The cells derived from BM, not only contribute to the regeneration of the muscles fibers in the injured skeletal muscle, but they are also able to re-integrate the pool of the satellite cells in the injured skeletal muscle (Labarge and Blau, 2002). In each case, it is important to note that the frequency at which these events happen seems to be very low, also in the case of serious lesion, if compared to the number of regenerated myoblasts derived from the "muscle-resident" satellite cells (Grounds et al., 2002; Labarge and Blau, 2002). So, it is quite disputable the fact that the "non muscle-resident" stem cells may give a significant contribution to the repair of injured skeletal muscle (Ground et al., 2002) In addition to the classic satellite cells, resident in the lower part of the basal lamina, there also exists a distinct population of extra-lamina collocated stem cells, inside the connective tissue of the skeletal muscle (Dreyfus et al., 2004). In answer to a harmful event on the skeletal muscle, these cells take part in the formation of myoblasts and in the differentiation of myotubes (Chargé and Rudnicki, 2004). After the cylinders of the old basal lamina have been filled with new myofibers, the myofiber itself extends, through the opening of the basal lamina, towards the healing connective tissue, which has been formed between the stumps of the survived myofibers (Hurme et al., 1991; Kalimo et al., 1997). On both parts of the scar of connective tissue, the myofibers and the stumps of the survived fibers, in the attempt to pass through the scar which separates them, form multiple branches (Hurme et al., 1991). After trying to extend, for a short distance, the branches start to adhere to the connective tissue with their final points, forming mini MTJs with the scar tissue. In time, the scar area progressively diminishes in dimension, conducting the stumps to join with each other (Vaittinen et al., 2002). Even so it is still not well known the stumps of the sheared fibers on the opposite parts of the scar tissue, fuse totally between themselves at the end of the regeneration process or if, on the contrary, there remains some form of septum of connective nature (Vaittinene et al., 2002; Aarima at al., 2004). It has also been amply shown how the repair capacity of the skeletal muscle, in answer to trauma, is significantly reduced in the course of life. (Järvinen et al., 1983). This drop in regenerative capacity is not apparently attributable to a drop in the number or of the activity of the satellite cells (Järvinen et al., 1983) but rather to a complex drop in repair capacity of the muscles in an elderly person, such as it seems that each phase of repair process slows down and deteriorates with age (Järvinen et al., 1983).

24. The formation of connective scar tissue

Immediately after a muscular trauma, the gap formed in correspondence with the fibers, is filled with a hematoma, within the first day the pro-inflammatory cells, including the phagocytes, invade the hematoma itself and start to form blood coagulation (Hurme et al., 1991b; Tidball, 1995; Cannon and Pierre, 1998). The fibrin and the fibronectin tie together to form both an initial granulation tissue and an initial ECM, which will serve as a scaffold and as an anchorage site for the successive invasion on behalf of the fibroblasts (Hurme and Kalimo, 1991). We need to remember, to this end, how some fibroblasts present in the granulation tissue, may also derive from the myogenic cells (Li and Huard, 2002). It is very important to underline the fact that this neo-formed tissue bestows upon the tissue of the injured area the initial resistance to be able to support the contraction forces applied to the latter (Lehto et al.,1985; 1986; Hurme et al., 1991c). Following this, the fibroblasts start the synthesis of the proteins and of the proteo-glycans of the ECM, to restore the integrity of the framework of the connective tissue (Lehto et al., 1985; 1986; Hurme et al., 1991c; Goetsch et al., 2003). Amongst the first synthesized proteins of the ECM, there is tenacin- C (TN-C) and fibronectin (Lehto et al., 1986; Hurme and Kalimo, 1991; 1992; Goetsch et al., 2003) which initially change direction in multimeric fibrils to then form super-fibronectin, a protein which has much better adhesive properties (Morla et al., 1994; Wierzbika- Patynowski and Schwarzbauer, 2003). Both the fibronectin and the TN-C, due to their elastic properties, are able to support a remarkable number of elongation cycles, in respect to their rest length. These elongations, which are due to mechanical loads applied on a tissue level, play an important role both in the production of force and for the apparition of the first precocious elastic behavior on behalf of the neo-granulation tissue of the injured skeletal muscle (Järvinen et al., 2000; 2003a; 2003b). The expression of the fibronectin is later followed by the type III collagen (Lehto et al., 1985; 1986; Goetsch et al., 2003; Hurem et al., 1991; Best et al., 2001; Ground et al., 2002), the production of type I collagen, on the contrary, only starts a couple of days later, to then remain elevated for several weeks (Lehto et al., 1985a; 1985b; Hurme et al., 1991; Best et al., 2001; Yan et al., 2003). The initial ample granulation tissue (i.e. the scar which forms between the stumps of the injured fibers) concentrates a high degree of mechanical efficiency in a particularly reduced area of connective tissue, an area which is mainly composed of type I collagen (Järvinen, 1975; Lehto et al., 1985a; 1985b; Hurme et al., 1991; Järvinen and Lehto, 1993). Despite the diffused preconception that the formation of fibrosis makes up an inevitable process in the natural history of muscular damage (Huard et al., 2002), the increase in the connective intramuscular tissue, in effect, does not increase in a substantial manner in an injured muscle, unless the muscle itself is not completely immobilized for an excessive length of time (Järvinen 1975; Lehto et al., 1985a; Järvinen and Lehto, 1993). The connective tissue scar, which is formed in the injury area represents the weak point of the injured muscle in the immediate post-traumatic phases (Hurme et al., 1991; Kääriäinen et al., 1998); however, its capacity of tensile force, increases considerably with the production of type I collagen (Lehto et al., 1985a ; 1985b; Kääriäinen et al., 1998). The mechanical stability of collagen, in its turn, is due to the formation of intermolecular cross-links, which form during the maturity of the scar tissue (Lehto et al., 1985b). Approximately ten days after the trauma, the maturity of the scar has reached a phase in which it no longer represents the structurally weak ring of the chain inside the injured muscle, so that, if the latter is stretched until break point, the damage generally occurs inside the adjacent tissue rather than where new mini MTJs have been formed between the repaired myofibers and the scar tissue (Järvinen, 1975; Järvinen, 1976; Kääriäinen et al., 1998). In any case, it will still need a long period of time before the strength of the muscle has completely recovered. (Järvinen, 1975; 1976; Kääriäinen et al., 1998). Even though a large part of harmful events on the skeletal muscle heals without the formation of a debilitating fibrotic scar from a functional point of view, the proliferation of fibroblasts can be excessive and hesitate in the formation of thick scar tissue inside the injured muscle. In these cases, which are generally associated with superior levels of muscular trauma, and above all to those which are recurring, the scar can create a mechanical barrier which delays, or sometimes strongly limits, the repair of the myofibers through the gap formed by the damage (Järvinen, 1975; 1976). Some of these experimental studies have recently given interesting clarification regarding the scar formation in the injured skeletal muscle; we have been able to ascertain in fact, how direct application is of a particular form of small leucine-rich proteoglycan (SLRP), of decorin and of an antifibrotic agent like suramin or the γ-interferon, are able to inhibit the scar formation in the injured skeletal muscle (Fukushima et al., 2001; Chan et al., 2003; Foster et al., 2003). The decorin, the suramin and the γ-interferon are all specific inhibitors of the TGF-β (Yamaguchi et al., 1990; Grounds, 1991; Hildebrand et al., 1994; Chan and Foster, 2003) a growth factor which is held responsible for the scar formation during the repair processes of the muscle. In addition to the inhibiting action towards the TGF-β, the decorin and the SLRP, even though they can't tie themselves to the different collagens, are however able to regulate the fibrillogenesis and the assembly of the type I collagen fibrils (Frank et al., 1999; Nakumura et al., 2000; Corsi et al., 2002).

25. The re-vascularization of the injured muscle

A fundamental process in the field of reparation of the injured muscle, is represented by the re- vascularization of the injured area (Snow, 1973; Järvinen, 1976; Józsa et al., 1980;). The restoration of vascularization in the injured area, represents the first sign of reparation and it is a pre-requisite for the successive morphological and functional recuperation of the injured muscle. The new capillary network has origin of the survived trunks of the blood vessels which go towards the centre of the trauma area (Järvinen, 1976) and they go to supply the same area with an adequate amount of oxygen allowing, in such a way, the successive functional restoration of the aerobic metabolism, which represents, in its turn, a fundamental stage in the field of repair process of the myofibers. The young myotubes are supplied with few mito-chondria and only show a moderate functional capacity in the field of the energetic aerobic restoration mechanism but they contextually present a clear increase in the energetic anaerobic restoration mechanism (Järvinen and Sorvari, 1978). In any case, during the final phases of tissue repair, the aerobic metabolism makes up the principle energetic resource for the multi-nuclear myofibers (Järvinen and Sorvari, 1978). This particular repair procedure, also supplies a plausible explanation of why the regeneration of the myofibres doesn't progress further than the precocious formation phase of slim myotubes, up until when the growth of a sufficient capillary network can't assure the necessary oxygen contribution to a satisfying functional restoration of the aerobic mechanism.

26. The regeneration of intramuscular nerves

Similarly to what happens in the course of the process of re-vascularization, the healing of the skeletal muscle may be blocked by a failure in the regeneration of intramuscular nerves (Hurme et al., 1991; Rantenen et al., 1995; Vaittinen et al., 1999; Vaittinen et al., 2001). The regeneration of the myofiber continues from the phase of myotubes formation also in absence of innervations; but if innervations were not completed correctly, a process of atrophy would inevitably occur (Rantanen et al., 1995). In the case of neurogenic denervation, or the breakage of the axon, the re-innervation process requires the growth of a new axon, distally with respect to the breakage area. However, since the moment the axons usually undergo go thorug a breakage inside or around the muscle, the nerve-muscle contact is, generally, rapidly raidly restabilized.

27. The adherence of the myofiber to the ECM

At the moment in which a myofiber loses its continuity also the continuity of the unit "tendon-muscle-tendon" is interrupted at the point of breakage itself and the contractile force cannot be transmitted through the gap which has been created between the stumps of the fibers. In such a situation, in fact, during muscular contraction the stumps are simply pushed further

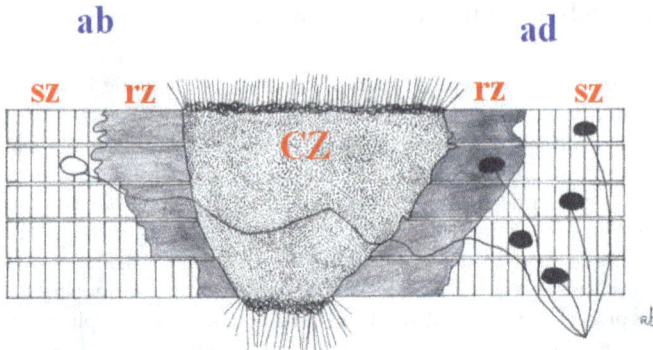

Figure 8. Schematic representation of a breakage trauma of the skeletal muscle. The injured muscle fiber contract and the gap between the stumps, or the central zone CZ; initially begins to fill with the hematoma. The muscular fibers are necrotic inside their basal lamina, of a distance which is usually between 1 and 2 millimeters. Inside this segment generally, with time, complete repair occurs (repair zone RZ; we prefer, in this case, the term "repair zone" to the term "regeneration zone" used by anglo-saxon autors. The reason of this choice derives from the different biological concept between the term "repair" and "regeneration", already illustrated at the beginning of the chapter), whereas in the part of the muscle which is not injured by trauma, we may observe only changes of reactive type (survival zone SZ). Each muscular fiber is innerved, in a single and precise site,by a neuromuscular junction (NMJs, full point in the diagram). Since the muscular fibbers generally break from one or the other side with respect to the line of NMJs of the same fiber, the accessory stumps of fibre 1 and of the fibres that go from 3 to 5, of the "ad" side (right), remain innerved, whereas their accessory stumps on side"ab" (left), remain denerved. At the same time the accessory stump of fibre 2 has remained denerved, because its NMJ is found in the RZ zone. The re-innervation of the accessory stump will come about through the penetration of a new axon sprout through the scar zone in formation (CZ) and so thanks to the formation of a new NMJ (represented by the white point in the diagram). Fibre 2 will go back to its normal re-innervation when the repair process in zone RZ is completed.

aside. The final part of the myofibers in repair which attempt to pass through the scar tissue, maintains a visible growth cone for a relatively long period during the repair process (Hurme et al., 1991; Hurme and Kalimo, 1992), this represents a period of time during which the final part of the myofibers cannot adhere firmly to the scar tissue. However, the myofibers in the course of repair strengthen their adherence to the ECM in both parts of their lateral profile, both in their intact part and in the part of re-growth (Kääriänen et al., 2000; Sorokin et al., 2000; Allikian et al., 2004) (Figure 9), This strengthening of the lateral adherence reduces both the movement of the stumps and the push on the still fragile scar, reducing in such a way the risk of re-breakage and allowing, at the same time, some use of the injured muscle before the healing process is complete (Kääriänen et al., 2001; 2002). It appears very interesting the fact of how mechanical stress is a pre-requisite for the process of lateral adherence, as recently some studies have suggested that they show how the phenomena does not come about in absence of the latter (Kääriänen et al., 2001). In a more advanced phase of the repair process a strong terminal adherence at the end of each stump is stabilized, which consists in the same type of molecule associated with integrin and distrofin that we can observe in a normal MJT (Song et al.., 1992; Kääriänen et al., 2000a; 2000b; 2001; 2002) (Figure9). Contextually, the original (prelesion) unit "tendon-myofiber-tendon, is replaced by two consecutive units of "tendon-myofiber-mini MTJ " type separated by the scar. These two consecutive units contract at the same time, thanks to the fact that both are re-innerved by the same nerve (Rantanen et al., 1995). In the ECM, on a level of the place of the new MTJs, elastic and adhesive molecules are profusely expressed, whose role is to absorb the strength created by the muscular contractions (Hurmea and Kalimo, 1992; Järvinen et al., 2000). At this point of the repair process, having re-established solid terminal adhesions through these mini MTJs, the myofibers no longer need lateral adhesions of strengthening and, consequently, the strong expression of integrin decreases on a level of the lateral sarcolemma (Kääriänen et al., 2000a). The scar gradually diminishes in dimension, in such a way the stumps come close to each other and in the end the myofibers become intertwined, even though, not fully reunited (Kääriänen et al., 1998; 2000a; Vaittinen et al., 2002) (figure9 box C).

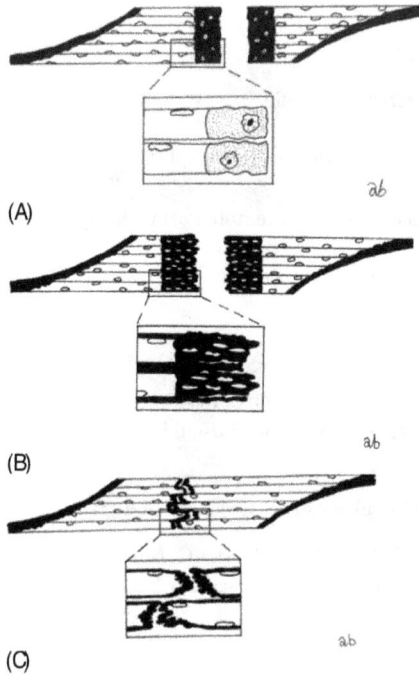

(A)

(B)

(C)

Figure 9. At the beginning of the healing process of the injured skeletal muscle (Box A) the expression of cellular adhesion of the integrin α7β1 molecules is enriched in the terminal part of the fibers of the damaged muscle in regeneration phase, whereas only a small amount of the latter are present in the lateral profile of the myofiber. A dramatic increase in the expression of integrin α7β1 happens along the lateral aspect of the plasmatic membrane (Box B), both in the intact part and in the part in growth phase of the injured myofibers, at the moment in which the muscular fibers in repair phase penetrate the injured tissue. In such a way, the integrin α7β1 supplies stability to the muscular fibers in growth phase which are missing in adhesion in their terminal part. The expression of the integrin α7β1 returns to normal levels in the lateral sarcolemma (Box C) contextually to the normality of the re-distribution of the integrin α7β1 in the terminal part of the fibers in repair, when the latter form new myotendon junctions and adhere to the scar.

28. Conclusions

Today there are only a few clinical studies concerning the treatment of muscular lesions, for this reason the principles of current treatments are mainly based on experimental studies or only on empirical evidence. The experimental studies have shown that the biological basis of the processes that occur during muscle repair are identical regardless of the primary cause of the injury (contusion, elongation or tear). This emphasizes the importance of understanding the basic principles of muscle repair, which represent the essential pre-requisite for a correct approach to the treatment of muscle injuries.

Author details

Gian Nicola Bisciotti[1] and Cristiano Eirale[1,2]

1 Qatar Orthopaedic and Sport Medicine Hospital, FIFA Center of Excellence, Doha, Qatar

2 Kinemove Rehabilitation Centers, Pontremoli, Parma, La Spezia, Italy

References

[1] Äärima V., Kääriäinen M., Vaittinen S. Restoration of myofiber continuity after transection injury in the rat soleus. Neuromuscul Disord. 14: 421-428, 2004.

[2] Abbot BC. Aubert XM. Changes of energy in a muscle during very slow stretches. Proceedings of the Royal Society B 139: 104-117, 1951

[3] Aldridge R, Cady EB, Jones DA, Obletter G. Muscle pain after exercise is linked with an inorganic phosphate increase as shown by 31P NMR. Biosci Rep.Jul;6(7):663-7, 1986.

[4] Allikian MJ., Hack AA., Mewborn S., Mayer U., McNalli EM. Genetic compensation for sarcoglycan loss by integrin α 7β1 in muscle. J Cell Sci. 117:3821-3830, 2004.

[5] Anitua E, Sanchez M, Nurden AT., Zalduendo M., De La Fuente M., Azofra J., Andia I. Reciprocal actions of platelet-secreted TGF-beta1 on the production of VEGF and HGF by human tendon cells. Plast Reconstr. 119(3):950-959, 2007.

[6] Anitua E., Sanchez M., Nurden AT., Orive G., Zalduendo M., De La Fuente M., Azofra J., Andia I. Autologous fibrin matrices: a potential source of biological mediators that modulate tendon cell activities. J Biomed Mat Res. 77: 285-93, 2006.

[7] Arieli D, Nahmany G, Casap N, Ad-El D, Samuni Y. The effect of a nitroxide antioxidant on ischemia-reperfusion injury in the rat in vivo hind limb model. Free Radic Res. Feb;42(2):114-23, 2008.

[8] Arkhipenko IuV, Pisarev VA, Kagan VE. Modification of an enzymic system of Ca2+ transport in sarcoplasmic reticulum membranes during lipid peroxidation. Induction and regulation systems of lipid peroxidation in skeletal and heart muscles Biokhimiia. Aug;48(8):1261-70, 1983

[9] Armstrong RB, Laughlin MH, Rome L, Taylor CR. Metabolism of rats running up and down an incline. Journal of Applied Physiology 55: 518-521, 1983a.

[10] Armstrong RB, Ogilvie RW, Schwane JA. Eccentric exercise-induced injury to rat skeletal muscle. Journal of Applied Physiology 54: 80-93, 1983b

[11] Armstrong RB, Warren GL, Warren JA. Mechanisms of exercise-induced muscle fibre injury. Sports Med. Sep;12(3):184-207, 1991.

[12] Armstrong RB. Initial events in exercise induced muscular injury. Med. Sci. Sports Exerc. 22: 429- 437, 1991a.

[13] Armstrong RB. Initial events in exercise-induced muscular injury. Medicine and Science in Sports and Exercise 22: 429-435, 1990.

[14] Armstrong RB. Mechanisms of exercise-induced delayed onset muscular soreness: a brief review. Medicine and Science in Sports and Exercise 16: 529-538, 1984.

[15] Armstrong RB., Warren GL., Warren A. Mechanism of exercise induced fiber injury. Sports Med. 12: 184-207, 1991b.

[16] Arroyo CM, Kramer JH, Dickens BF, Weglicki WB. Identification of free radicals in myocardial ischemia/reperfusion by spin trapping with nitrone DMPO. FEBS Lett. 1987

[17] Asmussen E. Observations on experimental muscular soreness. Acts Rheumatologica Scandinavica 2: 109-116, 1956.

[18] Aspenberg P., Virchenko O. Platelet concentrate injection improves Achilles tendon repair in rats. Acta Orthopaed Scand 75:93–9, 2004.

[19] Banfi G., Corsi MM., Volpi P. Could platelet rich plasma have effects on systemic circulating growth factors and cytokine release in orthopaedic applications? Br J Sports Med. 40:816, 2006.

[20] Bao ZZ., Iakonishok M., Kaufman S., Horwitz AF. $\alpha7\beta1$ integrin is a component of the myotendinous junction on skeletal muscle. J Cell Sci. 106: 579-590, 1993.

[21] Baracos VE, Wilson EJ, Goldberg AL. Effects of temperature on protein turnover in isolated rat skeletal muscle. Am J Physiol. 1984 Jan;246(1 Pt 1):C125-30

[22] Barrett S., Erredge S. Growth factors for chronic plantar fascitis. Podiatry Today. 17:37–42, 2004.

[23] Best TM., Hunter KD. Muscle injury and repair. Phys Med Rehabil Clin N Am. 11: 251-266, 2001.

[24] Bhattacharya SK. Crawford AJ, Thakar 1H, Johnson PL Path genetic roles of intracellular calcium and magnesium in membrane-mediated progressive muscle degeneration. In Duchenne muscular dystrophy. In Fiskum G tEd.) Cell calcium metaholism. pp. 513-525, Plenum. New York. 1989.

[25] Bonde-Petersen F. Knuttgen HG, Henriksson J. Muscle metabolism during exercise with concentric and eccentric contractions. Journal of Applied Physiology 33: 792-795, 1972

[26] Boobis AR, Murray S, Hampden CE, Davies DS. Genetic polymorphism in drug oxidation: in vitro studies of human debrisoquine 4-hydroxylase and bufuralol 1'-hydroxylase activities. Biochem Pharmacol. Jan 1;34(1):65-71, 1985.

[27] Brand MD, Lehninger AL. Superstoichiometric Ca2+ uptake supported by hydrolysis of endogenous ATP in rat liver mitochondria. J Biol Chem. Oct 10;250(19):7958-60, 1975.

[28] Braughler JM, Burton PS, Chase RL, Pregenzer JF, Jacobsen EJ, VanDoornik FJ, Tustin JM, Ayer DE, Bundy GL. Novel membrane localized iron chelators as inhibitors of iron-dependent lipid peroxidation. Biochem Pharmacol. Oct 15;37(20):3853-60, 1988.

[29] Brewer BJ. Instructional Lecture American Academy of Orthopaedic Surgeons 17: 354-358, 1960.

[30] Brickson S., Hollander J., Corr DT., Ji LL., best TM. Oxidant production and immune response after stretch injury in skeletal. Med Sci Sport Exerc. 33: 2010-2015, 2001.

[31] Brickson S., Ji LL., Schell K., Olabisi R. St Pierre Schneider B., Best TM. M1/70 attenuates blood-borne neutrophil oxidants, activation and myofiber damage following stretch injury. J Appl Physiol. 95: 969-976, 2003.

[32] Brooks SV, Zerba E, Faulkner JA. Injury to muscle fibres after single stretches of passive and maximally stimulated muscles in mice. J Physiol. Oct 15;488 (Pt 2):459-69, 1995

[33] Brooks SV, Vasilaki A, Larkin LM, McArdle A, Jackson MJ. Repeated bouts of aerobic exercise lead to reductions in skeletal muscle free radical generation and nuclear factor kappa B activation. J Physiol. Aug 15;586(16):3979-90, 2008.

[34] Brown RH. Dystrophin-associated proteins and the muscular dystrophies: a glossary. Brain Pathol. 6: 19-24, 1996.

[35] Burkin DJ., Kaufman SJ. The α7β1 integrin in muscle development and disease. Cell tissue Res. 296: 183-190, 1999.

[36] Bush ME, Alkan SS, Nitecki DE, Goodman JW. Antigen recognition and the immune response. "Self-help" with symmetrical bifunctional antigen molecules. J Exp Med. Dec 1;136(6):1478-83, 1972.

[37] Byrd SK., Bode AK., Klug GA. Effects of exercise of varying duration on sarcoplasmetic reticulum function. J Appl Physiol. 66: 1383-1389, 1989.

[38] Caldwell MD., Shearer J., Morrs A. Evidence for aerobic glycolysis in lambda-carrageenan-wounde skeletal muscle. J Surg Res. 37: 63-68, 1984.

[39] Cannon IP., Pierre BA. Cytokines in exertion-induced skeletal muscle injury. Mol, Cell Biochem. 179: 159-167, 1998.

[40] Carafoli E. The homeostasis of calcium in heart cells. Journal of Molecular and Cell Cardiology 17: 203-212, 1985.

[41] Carda C, Mayordomo E, Enciso M. Structural effects of the application of a preparation rich in growth factors on muscle healing following acute surgical lesion. Poster presentation at the 2nd International Conference on Regenerative Medicine 2005

[42] Carpenter S, Karpati G. Segmental necrosis and its demarcation in experimental micropuncture injury of skeletal muscle fibers. J Neuropathol Exp Neurol. Mar;48(2): 154-70, 1989.

[43] Castilho RF, Carvalho-Alves PC, Vercesi AE, Ferreira ST. Oxidative damage to sarcoplasmic reticulum Ca(2+)-pump induced by Fe2+/H2O2/ascorbate is not mediated by lipid peroxidation or thiol oxidation and leads to protein fragmentation. Mol Cell Biochem. Jun 21;159(2):105-14, 1996.

[44] Castilho RF, Kowaltowski AJ, Vercesi AE. The irreversibility of inner mitochondrial membrane permeabilization by Ca2+ plus prooxidants is determined by the extent of membrane protein thiol cross-linking. J Bioenerg Biomembr. Dec;28(6):523-9, 1996.

[45] Chan YS., Li Y., Foster W. Antifibrotic effects of suramin in injured skeletal muscle after laceration. J Appl Physiol. 95: 771-780, 2003.

[46] Chang J, Musser JH, McGregor H. Phospliolipase A2: function and pharmacological regulation. Biochemical Pharmacology 36: 2429-2436, 1987.

[47] Chang R, Turcotte R, Pearsall D. Hip adductor muscle function in forward skating Sports Biomech. Sep;8(3):212-2222, 2009.

[48] Chargé SBP., Rudnicki MA. Cellular and molecular regulation of muscle regeneration. Physiol Rev. 84: 209-238, 2004.

[49] Chazaud B., Sonnet C., Lafuste P. Satellite cells attract monocytes and use macrophages as a support to escape apoptosis and enhance muscle growth. J Cell Biol. 163: 133-1143, 2003.

[50] Cheah KS, Cheah AM. Malignant hyperthermia: molecular defects in membrane permeability. Experientia. May 15;41(5):656-61, 1985.

[51] Childs A, Jacobs C, Kaminski T, Halliwell B, Leeuwenburgh C. Supplementation with vitamin C and N-acetyl-cysteine increases oxidative stress in humans after an acute muscle injury induced by eccentric exercise. Free Radic Biol Med. Sep 15;31(6): 745-753, 2001.

[52] Chiquet M. How do fibriblast translate mechanical signal into changes in extracellular matrix production? Matrix Biol. 22. 73-80, 2003.

[53] Clanton TL. Hypoxia-induced reactive oxygen species formation in skeletal muscle. J Appl Physiol. Jun;102(6):2379-88, 2007.

[54] Close GL, Ashton T, McArdle A, Maclaren DP. The emerging role of free radicals in delayed onset muscle soreness and contraction-induced muscle injury. Comp Biochem Physiol A Mol Integr Physiol. Nov;142(3):257-66, 2005.

[55] Cohn RD., Capmbell KP. Molecular basis of muscular dystrophies. Muscle Nerve. 23: 1456-1471, 2000.

[56] Colomo F, Lombardi V, Piazzesi G. The mechanisms of force enhancement during constant velocity lengthening in tetanized single fibres of frog muscle. Adv Exp Med Biol. 226:489-502, 1988.

[57] Comstock JP., Udenfriend S. Effect of lactate on collagen proline hydroxilase activity in cultured L-929 fibroblast. Proc Natl Acad Sci USA. 66 : 522-557, 1970.

[58] Corsi A. Xu T., Chen XD. Phenotypic effects of biglycan deficiency are linked to collagen fibril abnormalities, are synergized by decorin deficiency, and mimic Ehlers-Danlos-like changes in bone and other connective tissues. J Bone Miner Res. 17: 1180-1189, 2002.

[59] Creaney L, Hamilton B. Growth factor delivery methods in the management of sport injuries: the state of play. Br J Sports Med. 42:314-320, 2008.

[60] Creaney L., Hamilton B. Growth factor delivery methods in the managements of sports injuries: the state of play. Br J Sports Med. 42: 314-320, 2008.

[61] Cullen MJ, Fulthorpe JJ. Phagocytosis of the A band following Z line, and I band loss. Its significance in skeletal muscle breakdown. J Pathol. Oct;138(2):129-43, 1982.

[62] Davies CT, White MJ. Muscle weakness following eccentric work in man. Pflugers Arch. Dec;392(2):168-71, 1981.

[63] Dayton WR, Goll DE, Zeece MG, Robson RM, Reville WJ. A Ca2+-activated protease possibly involved in myofibrillar protein turnover. Purification from porcine muscle. Biochemistry. May 18;15(10):2150-2158, 1976.

[64] Dayton WR, Schollmeyer JV, Chan AC, Allen CE. Elevated levels of a calcium-activated muscle protease in rapidly atrophying muscles from vitamin E-deficient rabbits. Biochim Biophys Acta. May 1;584(2):216-30, 1979.

[65] De Vos R., Wei A., Van Schie H., Bierma-Zeinstra S., Verhaar J., Tol J. Plateled-rich plasma injection for chronic Achilles tendinopaty. A randomized controlled trial. JAMA. 303(2): 144-149, 2010.

[66] Deal DN., Lipton J., Rosencrance E. Curl WW., Smith Il. Ice reduces edema: a study of microvascular permeability in rats. J Bone Joint Surg Am. 84: 1573-1578, 2002.

[67] Demopoulos HB. Control of free radicals in biologic systems. Fed Proc. Aug;32(8): 1903-1908, 1973a.

[68] Demopoulos HB. The basis of free radical pathology. Fed Proc. Aug;32(8):1859-1861, 1973b.

[69] Dreyfus PA., Chretien F., Chazaud B. Adult bone marrow-derived stem cells in muscle connective tissue and satellite cell niches. Am J Pathol. 164: 773-779, 2004.

[70] Duan C, Delp MD, Hayes DA, Delp PD, Armstrong RB. Rat skeletal muscle mitochondrial [Ca2+] and injury from downhill walking. J Appl Physiol. Mar;68(3): 1241-1251, 1990.

[71] Duchen MR. Effects of metabolic inhibition on the membrane properties of isolated mouse primary sensory neurones. J Physiol. May;424:387-409. 1990.

[72] Duncan CJ, Greenaway HC, Smith JL. 2,4-dinitrophenol, lysosomal breakdown and rapid myofilament degradation in vertebrate skeletal muscle. Naunyn Schmiedebergs Arch Pharmacol.;315(1):77-82, 1980.

[73] Duncan CJ. Role of calcium in triggering rapid ultrastructural damage in muscle: a study with chemically skinned fibres. J Cell Sci. May;87 (Pt 4):581-594, 1987.

[74] Ebbeling CB, Clarkson PM. Exercise-induced muscle damage and adaptation. Sports Med. Apr;7(4):207-34, 1989.

[75] Ekstrand J, Hägglund M, Waldén M . Injury incidence and injury patterns in professional football - the UEFA injury study. Br J Sports Med. 2009 Jun 23, E pub.

[76] Ervasti JM. Costameres: the Achille'hell of Herculean muscle. J Biol Chem. 278: 13591-13594, 2004.

[77] Evans, C. Cytokines and the Role They Play in the Healing of Ligaments and Tendons. Sports Medicine. 28(2): p. 71-76, 1999.

[78] Everts P, Mahoney C, Hoffmann J. Platelet-rich plasma preparation using three devices: Implications for platelet activation and platelet growth factor release. Growth Factors. 24(3):165-171, 2006.

[79] Falanga V., Qian SW., Danielpour D., Katz MH., Roberts AB., Sporn MB. Hypoxia upregulates the synthesis of TGF-beta 1 by human dermal fibroblasts. J Invest Dermatol. 97(4):634-7, 1991.

[80] Farges MC., Balcerzak D., Fisher BD. Increased muscle proteolysis and antifibrosis after local trauma mainly reflets macrophage-associated lysosomial protheolysis. Am J Physiol Endocrinol Metab. 282: E326-E335, 2002.

[81] Faulkner JA, Jones DA, Round JM. Injury to skeletal muscles of mice by forced lengthening during contractions. Q J Exp Physiol. Sep;74(5):661-70, 1989.

[82] Faust KB, Chiantella V, Vinten-Johansen J, Meredith JH. Oxygen-derived free radical scavengers and skeletal muscle ischemic/reperfusion injury. Am Surg. Dec;54(12): 709-719, 1988.

[83] Fisher JW. Pharmacologic modulation of erythropoietin production. Annu Rev Pharmacol Toxicol.;28:101-22, 1988.

[84] Fluk M., Carson JA., Gordan SE., Ziemieeki Booth FW. Focal adhesion proteins FAK and paxillin increase in hypertrophied skeletal muscle. Am J Physiol Cell. 277: 152-C162, 1999.

[85] Foster W., Li Y., Usas A., Somogyi G., Huard G. Gamma interferon as an antifibrosis agent in skeletal muscle. J Orthop Res. 21: 798-804, 2003.

[86] Frank CB., hart DA., Shrive NG. Molecular biology and biomechanics of normal and healing ligaments: a review. Osteoarthritis Cartilage. 7: 130-140, 1999.

[87] Fridén J, Sjöström M, Ekblom B. A morphological study of delayed muscle soreness. Experientia. May 15;37(5):506-507, 1981.

[88] Fridén J., Lieber RL. Structural and mechanical basis of the exercise-induced muscle injury. Med. Sci. Sports Exerc. 24: 521-530, 1992.

[89] Fukudaka S., Miyagoe-Suzuki Y., Tsukihara H. Muscle regeneration by reconstitution with bone marrow or fetal liver cells from green fluorescent protein-gene transgenic mice. J Cell Sci. 115: 1285-1293, 2002.

[90] Fukushima K., Badlani N., Usas A., Riano F., Fu F., Huard J. The use of antifibrosis agent to improve muscle recovery after laceration. Am J Sports Med. 29: 394-402, 2001.

[91] Ganote CE, Humphrey SM. Effects of anoxic or oxygenated reperfusion in globally ischemic, isovolumic, perfused rat hearts. Am J Pathol. Jul;120(1):129-145, 1985.

[92] Garret WE. Jr., Califf JC., Basset FH. Histochemical correlates of hamstring injuries. Am. J. Sports Med. 12: 98-103, 1984.

[93] Garret WE. Muscle strain injury: clinical and basic aspects. Med. Sci. Sports Exerc. 22: 439-443, 1990.

[94] Garrett WE., Safran MR., Seaber AV. Biomechanical comparison of stimulated and
      non stimulated skeletal muscle pulled to failure. Am. J. Sports Med. 15: 448-454, 1987.

[95] Giancotti FG., Rouslathi E. Integrin signaling. Science. 285: 1028-1032, 1999.

[96] Gigante A, Del Torto M, Alberto B. Platelet-Rich Plasma in Muscle Healing. In:
      EFOST; 2008; Antalya, Turkeyp. 41-42, 2008.

[97] Gillis JM. Relaxation of vertebrate skeletal muscle. A synthesis of the biochemical
      and physiological approaches. Biochim Biophys Acta. Jun 3; 811(2):97-145, 1985.

[98] Goetsch SC., Hawke TJ., Gallardo TD., Richardson JA., Garry DJ. Transcriptional
      profiling and regulation of the extracellular matrix during muscle regeneration.
      Physiol Genomics. 14: 261-271, 2003.

[99] Goodman MN. Differential effects of acute changes in cell Ca2+ concentration on my-
      ofibrillar and non-myofibrillar protein breakdown in the rat extensor digitorum lon-
      gus muscle in vitro. Assessment by production of tyrosine and N tau-
      methylhistidine. Biochem J. Jan 1;241(1):121-127, 1987.

[100] Graham TE., Barklay JK., Wilason BA. Skeletal muscle lactate release and glycolytic
      intermediates during hypercapnia. J Appl Physiol. 60 : 568-575, 1986.

[101] Green H., Goldberg B. Collagen and cell protein synthesis by an established mamma-
      lian fibroblast line. Nature. 204 : 347-349, 1963.

[102] Griffiths HR, Lunec J, Jefferis R, Blake DR, Willson RL. A study of ROS induced de-
      naturation of IgG3 using monoclonal antibodies; implications for inflammatory joint
      disease. Basic Life Sci.;49:361-364, 1988.

[103] Grounds MD. Towards understanding skeletal muscle regeneration. Pathol Res
      Pract. 187: 1-22, 1991.

[104] Grounds MD., White JD., Rosenthal N., Bogoyevitch MA. The role of stem cells in
      skeletal and cardiac muscle repair. J Histochem Cytochem. 50: 589-610, 2002.

[105] Hall-Craggs EC. Early ultrastructural changes in skeletal muscle exposed to the local
      anaesthetic bupivacaine (Marcaine). Br J Exp Pathol. Apr;61(2):139-49, 1980.

[106] Hamilton B. Therapeutic use of autologus blood products in track and field. IAAF
      World Antidoping Symposium 2006.

[107] Hammond JW, Hinton RY, Curl LA, Muriel JM, Lovering RM. Use of autologous pla-
      telet-rich plasma to treat muscle strain injuries. Am J Sports Med. Jun;37(6):1135-42,
      2009.

[108] Hansford RG. Relation between mitochondrial calcium transport and control of ener-
      gy metabolism. Rev Physiol Biochem Pharmacol. 102:1-72, 1985.

[109] Harris AJ, Duxson MJ, Fitzsimons RB, Rieger F. Myonuclear birthdates distinguish the origins of primary and secondary myotubes in embryonic mammalian skeletal muscles. Development. Dec;107(4):771-84, 1989.

[110] Hess ML, Manson NH, Okabe E. Involvement of free radicals in the pathophysiology of ischemic heart disease. Can J Physiol Pharmacol. Nov;60(11):1382-1389, 1982.

[111] Hidebrand K, Woo S, Smith D. The effect of platelet derivedgrowth factors-BB on healing of the rabbit medial collateral ligament. An in vivo study. Am J Sports 26: 549-54, 1998.

[112] Higuchi H, Umazume Y. Lattice shrinkage with increasing resting tension in stretched, single skinned fibers of frog muscle. Biophys J. Sep;50(3):385-389, 1986.

[113] Hildebrand A., Romaris M., Rasmussen LM. Interaction of the small interstitial proteoglycans byglican, decorin, and fibromodulin with transforming growth factor β. Biochem J. 302: 527-534, 1994.

[114] Hirata A., Matsuda S., Tamura T. Expression profiling of cytokines and related genes in regeneration skeletal muscle after cardiotoxin injection : a role for osteopontin. Am J Pathol. 163: 203-215, 2003.

[115] Hoffmann EP. Clinical and histopathological features of abnormalities of the distrophin-based membrane cytoskeleton. Brain Pathol. 163: 203-215, 1996.

[116] Hofmann WW. Musculotrophic effects of insulin receptors before and after denervation. Brain Res. Jan 20;401(2):312-321, 1987.

[117] Horáková L, Strosová M, Skuciová M. Antioxidants prevented oxidative injury of SR induced by $Fe2+/H2O2$/ascorbate system but failed to prevent $Ca2+$-ATPase activity decrease. Biofactors.;24(1-4):105-109, 2005.

[118] Huard J., Li Y., Fu FH. Muscle injury and repair: current trends in research . J Bone Joint Surg Am. 84: 822-832, 2002.

[119] Hunt TK., Connoly WB., Aronson B. Anaerobic metabolism and woud healing. An hypothesis for the initiation and cessation of collagen synthesis in wound. Am J Surg. 135. 328-332, 1978.

[120] Hunt TK., Hussain Z. Can wound healing be a paradigm for tissue repair? Med Sci Sport Exerc. 25(6): 755-788, 1993.

[121] Hunt TK., Twomey P., Zederfeldt B. Respiratory gas tensions in healing wounds. Am J Surg. 114: 302-307, 1967.

[122] Hurme T., Kalimo H. Activation of myogenic precursor cells after muscle injury. Med Sci Sport Exerc. 24: 197-205, 1992.

[123] Hurme T., Kalimo H. Adhesion in skeletal muscle regeneration. Muscle Nerve. 15: 482-489, 1992.

[124] Hurme T., Kalimo H., Lehto M., Järvinen M. Healing of skeletal muscle injury: an ultrastructural and immunohistochemical study. Med Sci Sport Exerc. 23: 801-810,
1991a.

[125] Hurme T., Kalimo H., Sandemberg M., Lehto M., Vuorio E. Localization of type I and
III collagen and fibronectin production in injure gastrocnemius muscle. Lab Invest.
64: 76-84, 1991c.

[126] Hurme T., Lehto M., Falck B., Taino H., Kalimo H. Electromyography and morphology during regeneration of muscle injury in rat. Acta Physiol Scand. 142: 443-456,
1991b.

[127] Huxley AF., Peachey LD. The maximum length for contraction in vertebrate striated
muscle. J Physiol. 156: 150-166, 1961.

[128] Im MJC., Hoopes JE. Energy metabolism in healing skin wounds. J Surg Res. 10:
459-464, 1970.

[129] Im MJC., Hoopes JE. Glycolysis in healing skin wounds. J Surg Res. 10: 173-179,
1970a.

[130] Infante AA., Klaupiks D., Davies RE. Length, tension and metabolism during short
isometric contractions of frog Sartorius muscles Biochim Biophys Acta. Jul
29;88:215-217, 1964.

[131] Ishiura S, Sugita H, Nonaka I, Imahori K. Calcium-activated neutral protease. Its localization in the myofibril, especially at the Z-band. J Biochem. Jan;87(1):343-346,
1980.

[132] Jankowski RJ., Deasy BM., Cao B., Gates C., Huard J. The role of CD34 expression
and cellular fusion in the regeneration capacity of myogenic progenitor cells. J Cell
Sci. 115: 4361-4374, 2002.

[133] Järvinen M, Lehto M, Sorvari T. Effect of some anti-inflammatory agents on the healing of ruptured muscle: an experimental study in rats. J Sports Traumatol Rel Res.
14:19-28, 1992.

[134] Järvinen M. Sorvari T. A histochemical study of the effect of mobilisation and immobilisation on the metabolism of healing muscle injury. In: Landry E ed. Sport Medicine. Miami, Fla: Symposia Specialist, Orban WAR: 177-181, 1978.

[135] Järvinen M. Healing of a crush injury in rat striated muscle, 2: a histological study of
the effect of early mobilization and immobilization on capillary ingrowth. Acta Pathol Microbiol Scand. 84A: 269-282, 1975.

[136] Järvinen M. Healing of a crush injury in rat striated muscle, 3: a microangiographical
study of the effect of early mobilisation and immobilisation an capillary ingrowth.
Acta Phatol Microbiol Scand. 84A: 85-94, 1976.

[137] Järvinen M. Healing of a crush injury in rat striated muscle, 3: a microangiographical study of the effect of early mobilization and immobilization on capillary ingrowth. Acta Pathol Microbiol Scand. 84A:85-94, 1976.

[138] Järvinen M. Healing of a crush injury in rat striated muscle, 4: effect of early mobilisation an immobilisation on the tensile properties of gastrocnemius muscle. Acta Chir Scan. 142: 47-56, 1976.

[139] Järvinen M., Aho Aj., Lehto M., Toivonen H. Age dependent repair of muscle rupture: qa histological and microangiographical study in rats. Acta Orthop Scand. 54: 64-74, 1983.

[140] Järvinen M., Sorvari T. Healing of a crush injury in rat striated muscle, 1: description and testing of a new method of inducing a standard injury to the calf muscles. Acta Pathol Microbiol Scand. 83A: 259-265, 1975.

[141] Järvinen MJ., Einola SA., Virtanen EO. Effect of the position of immobilisation upon the tensile properties of the rat gastrocnemius muscle. Arch Phys med Rehabil. 73: 253-257, 1992.

[142] Järvinen MJ. Immobilization effect on the tensile properties of striated muscle: an experimental study in the rat. Arch Phys Med Rehabil. 58: 123-127, 1977.

[143] Järvinen TAH., Kannus P., Järvinen TLN., Jósza L., Kalimo H., Järvinen M. Tenascin-C in the patobiology and healing process of musculoskeletal tissue injury. Scan J Med Sci Sports. 10: 367-382, 2000.

[144] Järvinen TAH., Järvinen TLN., Kääriänen M., Kalimo H., Järvinen M. Muscle injury. Biology and treatment. Am J Sports Med. 33(5): 745-764, 2005.

[145] Järvinen TAH., Järvinen TLN., kannus P., Kalimo H. Ectopic expression of tenascin-C. J Cell Sci. 116: 3851-3853, 2003.

[146] Järvinen TAH., Jósza L., Kannus P. Mechanical loading regulates the expression of tenascin-C in the myotendinous junction and tendon but does not induce de novo-syntesis in the skeletal muscle. J Cell Sci. 116: 857-866, 2003.

[147] Järvinen TAH., Józsa L:, Kannus P., Järvinen TL., Järvinen M. Organization and distribution of intramuscular connective tissue in normal and immobilized skeletal muscle: an immunohistochemical polarization and scanning electron microscopic study. J Muscle Res cell Motil. 23.245-254, 2002.

[148] Jenkins RR Free radical chemistry. Relationship to exercise. Sports Med. Mar;5(3): 156-170, 1988.

[149] Józsa L., Reffy A., Demel Z. Alterations of oxygen and carbon dioxide tension in crush-injured cal muscle of rat. A Exp Chir. 13: 91-94, 1980.

[150] Julian FJ, Morgan DL. The effect on tension of non-uniform distribution of length changes applied to frog muscle fibres. J Physiol. Aug;293:379-392, 1979.

[151] Kääriäinen M, Kääriäinen J, Järvinen TLN, Sievanen H, Kalimo H, Järvinen M. Correlation between biomechanical and structural changes during the regeneration of skeletal muscle after laceration injury. J Orthop Res. 16:197-206, 1998.

[152] Kääriäinen M., Järvinen TAH., Järvinen M., kalimo H. Adhesion and regeneration of myofibers in injured skeletal muscle. Scan J Med Sci Sport. 10. 332-337, 2000a.

[153] Kääriäinen M., Kääriäinen J. Järvinen TNL., Sievanen H., Kalimo H., Järvinen M. Correlation between biomechanical and structural changes during the regeneration of skeletal muscle after laceration injury. J Orthop Res. 16: 197-206, 1998.

[154] Kääriäinen M., Kääriäinen J., Järvinen TLN. Integrin and dystrophin associated adhesion protein complexes during regenerating of shearing-type muscle injury. Neuromuscul Disord. 10: 121-134, 2000.

[155] Kääriänen M., Liljamo T., Pelto-Huikko M., Heino J., Järvinen M., Kalimo H. Regulation of α 7 integrin by mechanical stress during skeletal muscle regeneration. Neuromuscul Disord. 11: 360-369, 2001.

[156] Kääriänen M., Nissinen L., Kaufman S. Expression of α 7 β1 integrin splicing variants during skeletal muscle regeneration. Am J Pathol. 161: 1023-1031, 2002.

[157] Kajikawa Y, Morihara T, Sakamoto H, Matsuda K, Oshima Y, Yoshida A. Platelet-rich plasma enhances the initial mobilization of circulation-derived cells for tendon healing. J Cell Physiol. 215(3):837–45, 2008.

[158] Kalimo H., Rantanen J., Järvinen M. Muscle injuries in sports. Baillieres Clin Orthop. 2: 1-24, 1997.

[159] Kameyama T, Etlinger JD. Calcium-dependent regulation of protein synthesis and degradation in muscle. Nature. May 24;279(5711):344-346, 1979.

[160] Kano Y, Masuda K, Furukawa H, Sudo M, Mito K, Sakamoto K. Histological skeletal muscle damage and surface EMG relationships following eccentric contractions. J Physiol Sci. Oct;58(5):349-355, 2008.

[161] Kärkkäinen AM., Kotimaa A., Huusko J., Heinon SE et al. Vascular endothelial growth factor-D transgenic mice show enhanced blood capillary density, improved postischemic muscle regeneration, and increased susceptibility to tumor formation. Blood 113:4468–4475, 2009.

[162] Katz B. The relation between force and speed in muscular contraction. J Physiol. Jun 14;96(1):45-64, 1939.

[163] Kerkweg U, Petrat F, Korth HG, de Groot H. Disruption of skeletal myocytes initiates superoxide release: contribution of NADPH oxidase. Shock. May;27(5):552-558, 2007.

[164] Kerkweg U, Petrat F, Korth HG, de Groot H. Disruption of skeletal myocytes initiates superoxide release: contribution of NADPH oxidase. Shock. May;27(5):552-558, 2007.

[165] Koh TJ, Escobedo J. Cytoskeletal disruption and small heat shock protein translocation immediately after lengthening contractions. Am J Physiol Cell Physiol. Mar;
286(3):C713-22, 2004.

[166] Klug GA, Tibbits GF The effect of activity on calcium-mediated events in striated
muscle. Exerc Sport Sci Rev.16:1-59, 1988.

[167] Koh TJ. Do small heat shock proteins protect skeletal muscle from injury? Exerc
Sport Sci Rev. 2002 Jul;30(3):117-21, 2002.

[168] Koh ESC., McNally EG. Ultrasound of skeletal muscle injury. Semin Musculoskeletal
Radiol. 11: 162-173, 2007.

[169] Kon M, Kimura F, Akimoto T, Tanabe K, Murase Y, Ikemune S, Kono I. Effect of
Coenzyme Q10 supplementation on exercise-induced muscular injury of rats. Exerc
Immunol Rev. 13:76-88, 2007.

[170] Kon M, Tanabe K, Akimoto T, Kimura F, Tanimura Y, Shimizu K, Okamoto T, Kono
I. Reducing exercise-induced muscular injury in kendo athletes with supplementation of coenzyme Q10. Br J Nutr. Oct;100(4):903-909, 2008.

[171] Krisanda JM, Paul RJ. Dependence of force, velocity, and O2 consumption on
[Ca2+]o in porcine carotid artery. Am J Physiol. Sep;255(3 Pt 1):C393-400, 1988.

[172] Kuipers H, Drukker J, Frederik PM, Geurten P, van Kranenburg G. Muscle degeneration after exercise in rats. Int J Sports Med. Feb;4(1):45-51, 1983.

[173] Labarge MA., Blau HM. Biological progression from adult bone marrow to mononu-
cleate muscle stem cell to multinucleate muscle fiber in response to injury. Cell.
589-601, 2002.

[174] Lee JC. Calcium ion and cellular function Sheng Li Ke Xue Jin Zhan. 11(1):55-64,
1980.

[175] Lee TC., Chow KL., Pang P., Schwartz RJ. Activation of skeletal a-actine gene transcription: the cooperative formation of serum response factor-binding complexes
over positive cis-actin promoter serum response elements displaces a negative-actin
nuclear factor enriched in replicating myoblast and nonmyogenic cells. Mol Cell Biol.
11: 5090-5100, 1991.

[176] Lehto M., Duance VC. Restall D. Collagen and fibronectin in a healing skeletal muscle injury: o immunohistochemical study of the effects of physical activity on the repair of injured gastrocnemius muscle in the rat. J Bone Joint Surg Br. 67: 820-828,
1985.

[177] Lehto M., Järvinen., Nelimarkka O. Scar formation after skeletal muscle injury: a histological and autoradiographical study in rats. Arch Orthop Trauma Surg. 104:
366-370, 1986.

[178] Lehto M., Sims TJ., Bailey AJ. Skeletal muscle injury: molecular changes in the collagen durin healing. Res Exp med (Berl). 185. 95-106, 1985b.

[179] Leitner G, Gruber R, Neumuller J. Platelet content and growth factor release in platelet-rich plasma: a comparison of four different systems. Vox Sanguinis. 91:135-139. 2006.

[180] Leonard JP, Salpeter MM. Agonist-induced myopathy at the neuromuscular junction is mediated by calcium. J Cell Biol. Sep;82(3):811-819, 1979.

[181] Levine CJ., Bates CJ. The effect of hypoxia on collagen synthesis in cultured 3T6 fibroblasts and its relationship to the mode of action of ascorbate. Biochim Biophys Acta. 444: 446-452, 1976.

[182] Li Y., Huard J. Differentiation of muscle-derived cells into myofibroblast in injured skeletal muscle. Am J Pathol. 161: 895-907, 2002.

[183] Lieber RL, Fridén J. Selective damage of fast glycolytic muscle fibres with eccentric contraction of the rabbit tibialis anterior. Acta Physiol Scand. Aug;133(4):587-588, 1988.

[184] Lieber RL., Woodburn TM., Fridén J. Muscle damage induced by eccentric contractions of 25% strain. J. Appl. Physiol. 70: 2498-2507, 1991.

[185] López JR, Alamo L, Caputo C, Wikinski J, Ledezma D. Intracellular ionized calcium concentration in muscles from humans with malignant hyperthermia. Muscle Nerve. Jun;8(5):355-358, 1985.

[186] Lovering RM, De Deyne PG. Contractile function, sarcolemma integrity, and the loss of dystrophin after skeletal muscle eccentric contraction-induced injury Am J Physiol Cell Physiol. Feb;286(2):C230-8, 2004.

[187] Lyras DN, Kazakos K, Verettas D, Botaitis S, Agrogiannis G, Kokka A, Pitiakoudis M, Kotzakaris A. The effect of platelet-rich plasma gel in the early phase of patellar tendon healing. Arch Orthop Trauma Surg. 2009.

[188] Malis CD, Bonventre JV. Susceptibility of mitochondrial membranes to calcium and reactive oxygen species: implications for ischemic and toxic tissue damage. Prog Clin Biol Res. 1988;282:235-59

[189] Marx RE. Platelet-rich plasma: evidence to support its use. J Oral Maxillofac Surgery 62:489–96, 2004.

[190] Massagué J. TGFbeta in cancer. Cell. Jul 25;134(2):215-30, 2008.

[191] Matsunaga M, Ohtaki H, Takaki A, Iwai Y, Yin L, Mizuguchi H, Miyake T, Usumi K, Shioda S. Nucleoprotamine diet derived from salmon soft roe protects mouse hippocampal neurons from delayed cell death after transient forebrain ischemia. Neurosci Res. Nov;47(3):269-267, 2003.

[192] Matsunaga S, Inashima S, Yamada T, Watanabe H, Hazama T, Wada M. Oxidation of sarcoplasmic reticulum Ca(2+)-ATPase induced by high-intensity exercise. Pflugers Arch. Jun;446(3):394-399, 2003.

[193] Mayers U. Integrins: redundant or important players in skeletal muscle? J Biol Chem. 278: 14587-14590, 2003.

[194] McCully KK, Faulkner JA. Characteristics of lengthening contractions associated with injury to skeletal muscle fibers. Journal of Applied Physiology 61: 293-299. 1986.

[195] McCully KK, Faulkner JA. Injury to skeletal muscle fibers of mice following lengthening contractions. J Appl Physiol. Jul;59(1):119-126, 1985.

[196] McMahon T.A. Muscles, reflexes, and locomotion. Princeton University. Press. 1984

[197] McMillin JB, Madden MC. The role of calcium in the control of respiration by muscle mitochondria. Med Sci Sports Exerc. Aug;21(4):406-410, 1989.

[198] McNeil PL. Repairing a torn cell surface: make way, lysosomes to the rescue. J cell Sci. 115: 873-879, 2002.

[199] McNeil PL., Khakee R. Disruption of muscle fiber plasma membranes. Role in exercise-induced damage. Am J Pathol. 140(5): 1097-1099, 1992.

[200] Menetrey J, Kasemkijwattana C, Fu FH, Moreland MS, Huard J. Suturing versus immobilization of a muscle laceration: a morphological and functional study in a mouse model. Am J Sports Med. 27:222-229, 1999.

[201] Messina S., Mazzeo A., Bitto A, Migliorato A., De Pasquale MG et al. VEGF overexpression via adeno-associated virus gene transfer promotes skeletal muscle regeneration and enhances muscle function in mdx mice. FASEB J 21:3737–3746, 2007.

[202] Michele DE., Campbell KP. Dystrophin-glycoprotein complex: post-transational processing and dystroglycan function. J Biol Chem. 278: 15457-15460, 2003.

[203] Middleton WD Ultrasonography of rotator cuff pathology. Top Magn Reson Imaging. Spring;6(2):133-138, 1994.

[204] Mishra A, Pavelko T. Treatment of chronic elbow tendinosis with buffered platelet rich plasma. Am J Sports Med. 34:1774–1778. 2006.

[205] Mishra DK, Fridén J, Schmitz MC, Lieber RL. Anti-inflammatory medication after muscle injury: a treatment resulting in short-term improvement but subsequent loss of muscle function. J Bone Joint Surg Am. 77:1510-1519. 1995.

[206] Mishra DK., Fridèn J., Schmitz MC., Lieber RL. Anti-inflammatory medication after muscle injury; a treatment resulting in short-term improvement but subsequent loss of muscle function. J Bone Joint Sur Am. 77: 1510-1519, 1995.

[207] Miyake K., McNeil PL., Suzuki K., Tsunoda R., Sugai N. An actin barrier to realising. J Cell Sci . 114: 3487-3494, 2001.

[208] Molloy, T., Y. Wang, and G.A. Murrell. The Roles of Growth Factors in Tendon and Ligament Healing. Sports Medicine. 33(5): p. 381-394, 2003.

[209] Morgan DL New insights into the behaviour of muscle during active lengthening Biophys J. Jul;60(1):290-2, 1991.

[210] Morgan DL. New insights into the behavior of muscle during active lengthening. Biophysical Journal 57: 209-221, 1990.

[211] Morla A., Zhang Z., Rioslathi E. Superfibronectin is a functionally distinct form of fibronectin. Nature. 367: 193-196, 1994.

[212] Murachi S, Nogami H, Oki T, Ogino T. Familial tricho-rhino-phalangeal syndrome Type II. Clin Genet. Mar;19(3):149-155, 1981

[213] Musaro A, Giacinti C, Borsellino G. Stem cell-mediated muscle regeneration is enhanced by local isoform of insulin-like growth factor 1. Proc Natl Acad Sci USA. 101:1206-1210, 2004.

[214] Nadel ER, Bergh U, Saltin B. Body temperature during negative work. Journal of Applied Physiology 33: 553-558, 1972

[215] Nakamura N., hart DA., Boorman RS. Decorin antisense gene therapy improves functional healing of early rabbit ligament scar with enhanced collagen fibrillogenesis in vivo. J Orthoped Res. 18: 517-523, 2000.

[216] Newham DJ, Jones DA, Ghosh G, Aurora P. Muscle fatigue and pain after ecceninc contractions at long and short length. Clinical Science 74: 553-557, 1988

[217] Newham DJ. Mills KR. Quigley BM, Edwards RHT. Pain and fatigue after concentric and eccentric muscle contractions. Clinical Science 64: 55-62, 1983.

[218] Nielsen B. Thermoregulation in rest and exercise. Acta Physiologica Scandinavica (Suppl.) 323: 1-74, 1969.

[219] Ogilvie RW, Armstrong RB, Baird KE, Bottoms CL. Lesions in the rat soleus muscle following eccentrically biased exercise. Am J Anat. Aug;182(4):335-346, 1988.

[220] Ogilvie RW, Hoppeler H, Armstrong RB. Decreased muscle function following eccentric exercise in the rat. Medicine and Science in Sports and Exercise 17: 195, 1985.

[221] Orrenius S, McConkey DJ, Bellomo G, Nicotera P. Role of Ca2+ in toxic cell killing. Trends Pharmacol Sci. Jul;10(7):281-285, 1989.

[222] Otey CA., Pavalko FM., Burridge K. An interaction between α-actinin and β-integrin subunit in vitro. J cell Biol. 111: 721-729, 1990.

[223] Pahud P, Ravussin E, Acheson KJ, Jequier E. Energy expenditure during oxygen deficit of submaximal concentric and eccentric exercise. Journal of Applied Physiology 49: 16-21. 1980.

[224] Pahud P, Ravussin E, Acheson KJ, Jequier E. Energy expenditure during oxygen defi-
       cit of submaximal concentric and eccentric exercise. Journal of Applied Physiology
       49: 16-21. 1980.

[225] Patel TJ., Das R., Fridén J., Lutz GJ., Lieber RL. Sarcomere strain and heterogeneity
       correlate with injury to frog skeletal muscle fiber bundles. J Appl Pysiol. 97:
       1803-1813, 2004.

[226] Patel TJ, Cuizon D, Mathieu-Costello O, Fridén J, Lieber RL. Increased oxidative ca-
       pacity does not protect skeletal muscle fibers from eccentric contraction-induced in-
       jury. Am J Physiol. May;274(5 Pt 2):R1300-8, 1998.

[227] Perrone CE., Fenwich-Smith D., Vanderburgh HH. Collagen and stretch modulate
       autocrine secretion of insulin-like growth factor-1 and insulin growth factor binding
       proteins from the differentiated skeletal muscle cells. J Biol Chem. 270: 2099-2106,
       1995.

[228] Perrone CE., Fenwich-Smith D., Vanderburgh HH. Collagen and stretch modulate
       autocrine secretion of insulin-like growth factor-1 and insulin growth factor binding
       proteins from the differentiated skeletal muscle cells. J Biol Chem. 270: 2099-2106,
       1995.

[229] Pomeranz SJ., Heidt RS Jr. MR imaging in the prognostication of hamstring injury.
       Work in progress. Radiology. Dec, 189(3): 897-900, 1993.

[230] Pontremoli S, Melloni E Extralysosomal protein degradation. Annu Rev Biochem.
       55:455-81, 1986.

[231] Popov EP. Engineering mechanics of solids, Prentice Hall, 1990 Publicover SJ, Dun-
       can Si, Smith JL The use of A23187 to demonstrate the role of intracellular calcium in
       causing uluastructural damage in mammalian muscle. Journal of Neuropathology
       and Experimental Neurology 37: 554-557. 1978.

[232] Potvin JR. Effects of muscle kinematics on surface amplitude and frequency during
       fatiguing dynamic contractions J Appl Physiol. Jan;82(1):144-51, 1997.

[233] Publicover SJ, Duncan CJ, Smith JL. The use of A23187 to demonstrate the role of in-
       tracellular calcium in causing ultrastructural damage in mammalian muscle. J Neu-
       ropathol Exp Neurol. Sep;37(5):554-557, 1978.

[234] Qu- Petersen Z., Deasy B., Jankowski R. Identification of a novel population of mus-
       cle stem cells in mice: potential for muscle regeneration. J Cell Biol. 157: 851-864,
       2002.

[235] Quintanilha AT, Packer L, Davies JM, Racanelli TL, Davies KJ. Membrane effects of
       vitamin E deficiency: bioenergetic and surface charge density studies of skeletal mus-
       cle and liver mitochondria. Ann N Y Acad Sci. 393:32-47, 1982.

[236]   Radin EL., Simon SR., Rose RM., Paul IL. Practical biomechanics for the orthopaedic
        surgeon. New York: A Wiley Medical Publication. 1979, pp 165.

[237]   Rak J., Kerbel RS. bFGF and tumor angiogenesis: bach in the lime-light? Nat Med.
        1083-1084, 1997.

[238]   Rantanen J, Thorsson O, Wollmer P, Hurme T, Kalimo H. Effects of therapeutic ultra-
        sound on the regeneration of skeletal muscle myofibers after experimental muscle in-
        jury. Am J Sports Med. 27:54-59, 1999.

[239]   Rantanen J., Hurme T., Lukka R., Heino J., Kalimo H. Satellite cell proliferation and
        expression of myogenin and desmin in regenerating skeletal muscle: evidence for
        two different population of satellite cells. Lab Invest. 72: 341-347, 1995.

[240]   Rantanen J., Ranne J., Hurme T., Kalimo H. Denervated segments of injured skeletal
        muscle fibres are reinnervated by newly formed neuromuscular junctions. J Neuro-
        pathol Exp Neurol. 54: 188-194, 1995.

[241]   Rapoport SI. Mechanical properties of the sarcolemma and myoplasma in frog mus-
        cle as a function of sarcomere length. Journal of General Physiology 59: 559-585. 1972.

[242]   Research Committee of the AOSSM. Hyperbaric oxygen therapy in sports. Am J
        Sports Med. 26:489-490, 1998.

[243]   Richardson TP., Peters MC., Ennett AB., Mooney DJ. Polymeric system for dual
        growth factor delivery. Nat Biotechnol 19:1029–1034, 2001.

[244]   Robertson SP, Johnson JD, Potter JD. The time-course of Ca2+ exchange with calmo-
        dulin, troponin, parvalbumin, and myosin in response to transient increases in Ca2+.
        Biophys J. Jun;34(3):559-569, 1981.

[245]   Rodemann HP, Waxman L, Goldberg AL. The stimulation of protein degradation in
        muscle by Ca2+ is mediated by prostaglandin E2 and does not require the calcium-
        activated protease. J Biol Chem. Aug 10;257(15):8716-8723, 1982.

[246]   Rouger K., Brault M., Daval N. Muscle satellite cell heterogeneity: in vitro an in vivo
        evidences of population that fuse differently. Cell Tissue res. 317: 319-326, 2004.

[247]   Rouslathi E. Integrin signaling and matrix assembly. Tumor Biol. 17: 117-124, 1996.

[248]   Sacheck JM, Blumberg JB. Role of vitamin E and oxidative stress in exercise. Nutri-
        tion. Oct;17(10):809-814, 2001.

[249]   Sanchez AR, Sheridan PJ, Kupp LI. Is platelet-rich plasma the perfect enhancement
        factor? A current review. Int J Oral Maxillofac Implants 18:93–103, 2003.

[250]   Sanchez M, Anitua E, Andia I. Application of autologous growth factors on skeletal
        muscle healing. Poster Presentation at 2nd International Conference on Regenerative
        Medicine 2005.

[251] Sanchez M, Anitua E, Azofra J. Comparison of surgically repaired Achilles tendon tears using platelet-rich fibrin matrices. Am J Sports Med 35:245–51, 2007.

[252] Sanchez M, Anitua E, Gorka O, Mujika I, Andia I. Platelet Rich Therapies in the Treatment of Orthopedic Sport Injuries. Sports Med 39 (5); 345-354, 2009.

[253] Sanchez M, Azofra J, Anitua E, et al Use of a preparation rich in growth factors in the operative treatment of ruptured Achilles tendon. Poster Presentation at 2nd International Conference on Regenerative Medicine 2005.

[254] Schache AG, Wrigley TV, Baker R, Pandy MG. Biomechanical response to hamstring muscle strain injury. Gait Posture. Feb;29(2):332-338, 2009.

[255] Schneider BS., Sannes H., Fine J., Best T. Desmin characteristics of CD11b-positive fibers after eccentric contractions. Med Sci Sports Exerc. 34: 274-281, 2002.

[256] Schraufstätter I, Hyslop PA, Jackson JH, Cochrane CG. Oxidant-induced DNA damage of target cells. J Clin Invest. Sep;82(3):1040-1045, 1988.

[257] Schwane JA. Armstrong RB. Effect of training on skeletal muscle injury from downhill running in rats. Journal of Applied Physiology 55: 969-975, 1983

[258] Schwartz W, Bird JW. Degradation of myofibrillar proteins by cathepsins B and D. Biochem J. Dec 1;167(3):811-20, 1977.

[259] Schwarz A. A promising Treatment for Athletes, in the Blood. New York Times February 16, 1009, 2009.

[260] Sembrowich WL, Quintinskie JJ, Li G. Calcium uptake in mitochondria from different skeletal muscle types. J Appl Physiol. Jul;59(1):137-141, 1985.

[261] Snow MH. Metabolic activity during the degenerative and early regenerative stages on skeletal muscle. Anat rec. 176: 185-204, 1973.

[262] Song WK., Wang W., Foster RF., Biesler DA., Kaugman SJ. H36-α7 is a novel integrin α chain that is developmentally regulated during skeletal myogenesis. J Cell Biol. 117: 643-657, 1992.

[263] Sorokin LM., Maley Mal., Moch H. Laminin α 4 and integrin α 6 are upregulated in regenerating dy/dy skeletal muscle: comparative expression of laminin and integrin isoform in muscle regenerating after crush injury. Exp cell res. 256: 500-514, 2000.

[264] Statham HE, Duncan CJ, Smith JL. The effect of the ionophore A23187 on the ultrastructure and electrophysiological properties of frog skeletal muscle. Cell Tissue Res. Oct 6;173(2):193-209, 1976.

[265] Statham HE, Duncan CJ, Smith JL. The effect of the ionophore A23187 on the ultrastructure and electrophysiological properties of frog skeletal muscle. Cell Tissue Res. Oct 6;173(2):193-209, 1976.

[266]   Stauber WT. Eccentric action of muscles: physiology, injury and adaptation. Exerc. Sport Sci. Rev. 17: 157-185, 1989.

[267]   Steenbergen C, Hill ML, Jennings RB. Cytoskeletal damage during myocardial ischemia: changes in vinculin immunofluorescence staining during total in vitro ischemia in canine heart. Circ Res. Apr;60(4):478-486, 1987.

[268]   Steer JH, Mastaglia FL, Papadimitriou JM, Van Bruggen I. Bupivacaine-induced muscle injury. The role of extracellular calcium. J Neurol Sci. Apr;73(2):205-217, 1986.

[269]   Steer JH., Mastaglia FL. Protein degradation in bupivacaine-treated muscles. The role of extracellular calcium. J Neutol Sci. Oct; (75): 343-351, 1986.

[270]   Strosová M, Skuciová M, Horáková L. Oxidative damage to Ca2+-ATPase sarcoplasmic reticulum by HOCl and protective effect of some antioxidants. Biofactors. 24(1-4):111-6, 2005.

[271]   Sunada Y., Campbell KP. Dystrophin-glycoprotein complex: molecular organisation and critical roles in skeletal muscle. Curr Opin Neurol. 8: 379-384, 1995.

[272]   Suresh SPS, Ali KE, Jones H. Medial epicondylitis: is ultrasound guided autologous blood injection an effective treatment? Br J Sports Med 40: 935-9 Surg 2007; 119: 950-959, 2006.

[273]   Talbot JA, Morgan DL. The effects of stretch parameters on eccentric exercise-induced damage to toad skeletal muscle. J Muscle Res Cell Motil. Apr;19(3):237-45, 1998.

[274]   Takala TE, Virtanen P. Biochemical composition of muscle extracellular matrix: the effect of loading. Scand J Med Sci Sports. 10:321-325, 2000.

[275]   Tappel AL. Lipidoperoxidation damage to cell components. Fed Proc. Aug;32(8): 1870-1874, 1973.

[276]   Taylor M, Norman T, Clovis N, Blaha D. The response of rabbit patellar tendons after autologous blood injection. Med Sci Sports Exerc. 34(1):70–3, 2002.

[277]   Thorsson O, Rantanen J, Hurme T, Kalimo H. Effects of nonsteroidal antiinflammatory medication on satellite cell proliferation during muscle regeneration. Am J Sports Med. 26:172-176, 1998.

[278]   Tidball JG. Force transmission across muscle membrane. J Biomech. 24 (supp 1): 43-52, 1991.

[279]   Tidball JG., Daniel TL. Myotendinous junctions of tonic muscle cells: structure and loading. Cell Tissue Res. 245: 315-322, 1986.

[280]   Tidball JG, Daniel TL. Elastic energy storage in rigored skeletal muscle cells under physiological loading conditions. American Journal of Physiology 250: R54-R64,.1986

[281] Tiidus PM., Ianuzzo CD. Effects of intensity and duration of muscular exercise on delayed muscular soreness. Med Sci Sport Exerc. 15: 461-465, 1973.

[282] Timball JG. Inflammatory cell response to acute muscle injury. Med Sci Sport Exerc. 27: 1022-1032, 18995.

[283] Turner JD, Rotwein P, Novakofski J, Bechtel PJ. Induction of mRNA for IGF-I and -II during growth hormone-stimulated muscle hypertrophy. Am J Physiol. Oct;255(4 Pt 1):E513-517, 1988.

[284] Uchiyama A, Kim JS, Kon K, Jaeschke H, Ikejima K, Watanabe S, Lemasters JJ. Translocation of iron from lysosomes into mitochondria is a key event during oxidative stress-induced hepatocellular injury. Hepatology. Nov;48(5):1644-54, 2008.

[285] Vaittinen S., Hurme T. Rantanen J., Kalimo H. Transected myofibers may remain permanently divided in two parts. Neuromuscular Disord. 12: 584-587, 2002.

[286] Vaittinen S., Lukka R., Sahlgren C. Specific and innervation-regulated expression of the intermediate filament protein nestin at neuromuscular and myotendinous junctions in skeletal muscle. Am J Pathol. 154: 591-600, 1999.

[287] Vaittinen S., Lukka R., Sahlgren C. The expression of intermediate filament protein nestin as related to vimentin and desmin in regenerating skeletal muscle. J Neuropathol Exp Neurol. 60: 588-597, 2001.

[288] Van Der Vusse GJ, Janssen GM, Coumans WA, Kuipers H, Does RJ, Hoor F. Effect of training and 15-, 25-, and 42-km contests on the skeletal muscle content of adenine and guanine nucleotides, creatine phosphate, and glycogen. Int J Sports Med. Oct;10 Suppl 3:S146-152, 1989.

[289] Van Kuijk FJ, Dratz EA. Detection of phospholipid peroxides in biological samples. Free Radic Biol Med. 1987;3(5):349-54.

[290] Vane J, Botting R. Inflammation and the mechanism of action of anti-inflammatory drugs. FASEB J. Aug;1(2):89-96, 1987.

[291] Vihko V, Salminen A, Rantamäki J. Acid hydrolase activity in red and white skeletal muscle of mice during a two-week period following exhausting exercise. Pflugers Arch. 1978 Dec 28;378(2):99-106

[292] Virchenko O, Aspenberg P. How can one platelet injection after tendon injury lead to a stronger tendon after 4 weeks? Interplay between early regeneration and mechanical stimulation. Acta Orthop 77 (5): 806-812, 2006;

[293] Voss P, Engels M, Strosova M, Grune T, Horakova L. Protective effect of antioxidants against sarcoplasmic reticulum (SR) oxidation by Fenton reaction, however without prevention of Ca-pump activity. Toxicol In Vitro. Oct;22(7):1726-1733, 2008.

[294] Warren GL., Hulderman T., Jensen N. Physiological role of tumor necrosis factor α in traumatic muscle injury. FASEB J. 16: 1630-1632, 2002.

[295] Warren JS, Johnson KJ, Ward PA. PAF and immune complex-induced injury. J Lipid Mediat. 2 Suppl:S229-37, 1990.

[296] Wasserman K., Beaver WL., Whipp BJ. Gas exange theory and lactic acidosis (anaerobic) threshold. Circulation. 81: 1114-1130, 1990.

[297] Wierzbika-Patynowski I., Schwarzbauer JE. The ins and outs of fibronectin matrix assembly. J Cell Sci. 116: 3269-3276, 2003.

[298] Woledge RC, Curtin NA, Homsher E Energetic aspects of muscle contraction. Monogr Physiol Soc. 41:1-357, 1985.

[299] Wrogemann K, Pena SD. Mitochondrial calcium overload: A general mechanism for cell-necrosis in muscle diseases. Lancet. Mar 27;1(7961):672-674, 1976.

[300] Xu KY, Zweier JL, Becker LC. Hydroxyl radical inhibits sarcoplasmic reticulum Ca(2+)-ATPase function by direct attack on the ATP binding site. Circ Res. Jan;80(1): 76-81, 1997.

[301] Xu KY, Zweier JL, Becker LC. Oxygen-free radicals directly attack the ATP binding site of the cardiac Na+,K+-ATPase. Ann N Y Acad Sci. Nov 3;834:680-683, 1997.

[302] Yamaguchi Y., Mann DM., Ruoslahti E. Negative regulation of transforming growth factor –β the proteoglycan decorin. Nature. 346: 281-284, 1990.

[303] Yan Z., Choi S Liu X. Highly coordinated gene regulation in mouse skeletal muscle regeneration. J Biol Chem. 278: 8826-8836, 2003.

[304] Yao C., Ziober BL., Squillace RM., Kramer RH. α7 integrin mediates cell adhesion and migration on specific lamin isoforms. J Biol Chem. 271: 25598-25603, 1996.

[305] Zammit PS., Golding JP., Nagata Y., Hudon V., Partridge TA., Beauchamp JR. Muscle satellite cells adopt divergent fates: a mechanism for self-renewal? J Cell Biol. 166: 347-357, 2004.

[306] Zerba E, Komorowski TE, Faulkner JA. Free radical injury to skeletal muscles of young, adult, and old mice. Am J Physiol. Mar;258(3 Pt 1):C429-435, 1990.

Imaging and Clinical Evaluation

Chapter 3

Diagnostic Imaging in Muscle Injury

Massimo Manara, Danilo Manari and Giulio Pasta

Additional information is available at the end of the chapter

1. Introduction

It might be strange to begin a chapter on diagnostics in the 21st century by highlighting doubts. Yet, the structure and physiology of muscles still escape our full understanding as the muscular system is a heterogeneous structure able to adapt to numerous functional demands, linked to physiological needs or pathologies. Indeed, the muscle is a complex mechanism, in which the phenotypical and morphological profile of the fibres varies between the double insertions and from surface to depth, and it adapts depending on stressors and stimuli which, independently of age, gender and physical activity, give rise to different responses within the same muscle. For these reasons the muscle appears to be a complex and not fully explored world.

This aspect is mainly concerned with physiopathology, and diagnostics nowadays has reached levels which perhaps were unimaginable 20 years ago. The development of electronic engineering has led to the construction of diagnostic machinery able to identify the finest details of the muscle. As history has proved, the continuous development of Ultrasound and MRI equipment, not to mention TAC, has changed the doctors' modus operandi over a period starting from the first musculoskeletal ultrasound image in 1972 by Leopold and McDonald to current 3D images, or from the first MRI image developed in the '70s to the current 3 Tesla MRI equipment.

The use of these devices in muscular injury diagnostics has acquired fundamental importance in Sports Medicine as regards diagnosis, prognosis and rehabilitation. The choice of using either Ultrasound or MRI is still subject to debate as it is influenced by several factors, such as type of injury, availability of the devices, the Radiologist's knowledge of Sport injuries, and the cost-benefit ratio, all of which the Sports Physician must evaluate carefully.

As the clinical cases shown prove, the difference in quality and accuracy of the images is well defined in favour of the MRI, but the decision still remains subject to a multifaceted vision.

2. Current uses of Ultrasound and MRI

Acute muscular strain injuries are frequently found in sports, at both amateur and competitive level, so much so that diagnostic imaging has acquired primary importance in identifying the trauma, assessing the damage, estimating possible complications and predicting recovery. Ultrasound and MRI play an important role in the study of muscle injuries owing to their ability to identify lesions effectively, which is closely related to the presence of oedema in the damaged muscle. [1]

The aim of our work is to analyse and compare the diagnostic value of ultrasound and MRI in terms of sensitivity, and recommend the best route to follow when studying muscular injuries.

First and foremost, advances in technology have dramatically improved image quality and nowadays a physician can easily prescribe either an MRI or an echography.

Although ultrasound has been used to evaluate the musculoskeletal system for approximately 25 years and despite the increasingly frequent use of MRI, there has been a renewed interest in Ultrasound for several reasons. The spatial resolution of Ultrasound exceeds the resolution obtainable with magnetic resonance (MR) imaging without the use of small surface coils and specific imaging parameters. For example, commercially available transducers with frequencies of 9 MHz to 15 MHz produce in-plane resolutions of 200 mm to 450 mm and section thicknesses of 0.5 mm to 1 mm. The resolution of sonographic imaging with standard high-frequency transducers allows visualization of individual neuronal fascicles in peripheral nerves.

Another reason for the increased interest in musculoskeletal Ultrasound is an understanding of its role in connection with MR imaging. MR imaging is valuable when the global assessment of a joint requires evaluation of the muscles, tendons, cartilage, and bone marrow. Ultrasound, however, can produce similar results when a focused evaluation of muscle, tendon, and joint recesses is needed. Frequently this can be performed at a lower cost and with less delay when compared with MR imaging.

More importantly, however, there are several applications where Ultrasound outperforms MR imaging. One deserving emphasis is the use of dynamic imaging with musculoskeletal Ultrasound.

Dynamic imaging is very helpful when differentiating full-thickness from partial-thickness tendon tears because tendon retraction indicates full-thickness tear. Additionally, there are several conditions where muscle, tendon, and nerve subluxation or dislocation only occur with specific extremity positions or movements. These abnormal subluxations or dislocations reduce in neutral position and remain undetected with routine MR imaging.

One last advantage of Ultrasound over MR imaging is the ability to focus the examination precisely at the region of symptoms and obtain imaging which is directly correlated to the patient's complaints. This correspondence is invaluable for a physician from a diagnostic perspective. [2]

US and MRI play an important role in the study of muscle injuries owing to their ability to identify lesions effectively, which is closely related to the presence of oedema in the damaged muscle. [1]

MRI is regarded as the gold standard. [3]

Literature contains no generally accepted classification of muscle traumas, and classification of minor traumas, in which imaging patterns are often identical, is even more complex.

In our experience, only a combination of imaging and accurate clinical examination makes it possible to achieve a correct diagnosis.

In our study, we observed only 26 minor traumas out of a total of 81 traumas (32%). The small number of minor traumas observed reflects the vagueness of their clinical symptoms rather than their rarity. Ultrasound sensitivity to minor traumas is much lower than that obtained for major traumas (76.92% vs. 92.72%). This is because Ultrasound findings in minor traumas are vague and indistinct if the oedema is small. In our study, the lowest Ultrasound sensitivity values were recorded for DOMS. [4]

Studying 40 patients with DOMS, Dierking et al. observed that ultrasound had low sensitivity in detecting the complaint. [5]

Although MRI correctly detected the muscle oedema in seven of our patients with DOMS, the pattern was non-specific and the correct diagnosis required integration with laboratory findings such as creatine-kinase assay.

De Smet states that MRI is reliable only if it is preceded by a thorough clinical assessment that enables selection of the most appropriate sequences and scan planes, and observed specificity and sensitivity values of 80% and 83%, respectively, for diagnosis of contractures and length-ening. This may also be correlated to the presence of considerable muscle oedema, which facilitates lesion identification. In such cases, Ultrasound demonstrates diffuse hypoechoge-nicity with displacement of the tertiary bundles. [6]

Hashimoto et al. suggest the use of very-high-frequency transducers to detect minor le-sions.Ultrasound sensitivity increases slightly in mild contusions. In these cases, as the trauma has an external origin, the sonographer is guided by knowledge of the site of impact.

In our experience, the Ultrasound imaging pattern of small contusions does not differ much from that of other minor traumas; in all cases, it shows muscle oedema without interruption of the continuity of muscle fibres. Differentiation was only possible on the basis of the patient's history.

As regards major traumas, Ultrasound had 84% sensitivity in identifying muscle strain. The extent of tissue alterations affects the Ultrasound pattern.

Significant differences were observed between third-degree muscle strains (which are readily detected) and first-degree muscle strains. In two cases of false negative results, Ultrasound underestimated lesions subsequently classified as second-degree injuries by MRI. The reason for such underestimation was that both lesions were located deep in the femoral quadriceps and therefore less amenable to Ultrasound.

Ultrasound examination enables identification of typical lesions of muscle strains: discontinuity of tertiary bundles, reactive oedema and haematoma. In first-degree strains, the involvement of a small number of myofibrils can make it difficult to recognise the lesion with Ultrasound so the use of MRI is necessary. More-severe lesions (second and third degree) with involvement of a larger number of myofibrils, will exhibit a hypoechoic or anechoic haematoma, which can remain localised or extend along the bundles. Immediately after a trauma, the true extent of a lesion may be masked by a hyperechoichaemorrhage whereas Ultrasound done after 48–72 hours will reveal the evolution of the haematoma and the extent of the area affected. [7]

In cases of complete tears of the muscle belly, the retracted muscle bundles have the typical Ultrasound appearance of a bell clapper surrounded by a hypoechoichaematoma. In cases of complete tears of the muscle belly, the retracted muscle bundles have the typical Ultrasound appearance of a bell clapper surrounded by a hypoechoichaematoma. As previously emphasised, a dynamic examination is fundamental in all cases and particularly in first-degree strains, as it enables detection of the separation and dislocation of tertiary bundles and evaluation of the effective extent of the lesion. [8]

Muscle strains are recognisable at MRI due to changes in muscle volume and composition, variations in signal intensity and pathological alterations of surrounding tissues. [9]

Axial scans allow for comparative examination to detect changes in muscle volume and signal intensity. Coronal or sagittal images along the muscle belly axis make it possible to define the extent of the lesion. [6]

An important finding by Megliola et al. was that in all patients with severe contusion, the haematoma was detected with both Ultrasound and MRI, leading to a sensitivity of 100% for Ultrasound. According to Peetrons, a sonographic classification of major muscle lesions into four different types may be made on the basis of the percentage of muscle involved, but it is essential to distinguish lesions giving rise to haematomas from those causing tearing of muscle fibres only.

Megliola et al. studied 29 patients with severe contusion, and Ultrasound was able not only to locate the haematoma but also to evaluate its extent in total agreement with MRI. Ultrasound has far higher sensitivity for major traumas than for minor traumas.

This is because the ability of Ultrasound to evaluate minor traumas is related to the presence of severe muscle oedema. In major traumas, it can accurately evaluate the extent of the lesion, the percentage of muscle affected, the size of the scar and possible complications. [4]

Bianchi et al. examined 17 patients with acute injury of the rectus femoris with both MRI and Ultrasound. There was concordance between the two techniques in identifying the lesions and evaluating lesion extent. The authors therefore concluded that for lesions of the rectus femoris, a very superficial muscle, Ultrasound should be considered the first-line technique. [10]

In contrast, in the study of deeper muscles, Kolouris and Connell identified a discrepancy between Ultrasound and MRI in the evaluation of hamstring injuries and observed that MRI is more accurate in assessing the extent of injury.These studies confirm that Ultrasound is limited in the study of muscle injury in that its resolution is limited to the tertiary bundle, it is unable to identify pathological alterations to the secondary and primary bundles and myofibrils, and cannot evaluate deep muscle planes. [11]

But Ultrasound (US) technologies are rapidly advancing, offering several refined transducer technologies as well as soft and hardware facilities to improve the potential clinical impact in the field of musculoskeletal (MSK) imaging.

Nowadays when using B-mode ultrasound, compound imaging and beam-steering are of help in decreasing anisotropy in tendons and ligaments, which are less well depicted due to their oblique course.

Doppler imaging has become sensitive in the detection of flow in small vessels and the use of US micro bubble contrast agents (Contrast-enhanced ultrasound –CEUS) improves detection of low-volume blood flow in smaller vessels, by increasing the signal-to-noise ratio and thereby facilitating detection of angiogenetic vessels in inflammatory conditions as for muscular lesion.

The use of US blood pool contrast agents enables molecular imaging in real-time, and thus the diagnostic potential of US is expanded, opening up a new field of US applications. Objective quantification of altered tissue (e.g., synovial proliferation) needs further development and might be improved by the use of three-dimensional imaging and software tools such as parametric evaluation.

Real-time sonoelastography (EUS) is a new development for visualization of tissue elasticity by measurement of tissue displacement in terms of stiffness changes, promising new insights into tendon disorders.

Image fusion is an exciting development that enables superimposition of CT/MRI data sets on real-time US scanning.

This technique might be helpful in guiding injections under real-time conditions even in regions less easily accessible by US as, for instance, the axial skeleton, and can additionally provide an interesting tool for teaching MSK imaging and ways to guide interventions. [12]

But, as described, MRI has very good sensitivity for the depiction of muscle lesions. Various MRI patterns of muscle injury have been described, usually including oedema-like signal alterations within torn muscle bundles. [1]

The importance of the STIR technique in detection of muscle injuries has been stressed by Greco et al., who recognized that subtle abnormalities, not easily seen on long echo T2-weighted images, are highlighted with the STIR technique as the short T1 induces suppression of fat signal and makes the effects of prolonged T1 and T2 on signal intensity additive. [13]

Imaging of muscular lesions has been greatly improved with the use of the contrast medium (Gadolinium), which grants a better definition of the muscular strain. A proof of this was provided by El-Noueam KI, Schweitzer ME, Bhatia, who described how muscle strain injury was demonstrated only in the post contrast MR scans, a pattern that we believe was not previously reported.

This pattern may be explained on the basis of the clinical spectrum of muscle strain injury described by O'Donoghue, as well as by considering the histological changes occurring at the miotendon junction in cases of muscle strain. O'Donoghue classified muscle strain injury as being mild, moderate, and severe. In the mild (first degree) strain, there is no appreciable tissue disruption, with neither discernible loss of strength nor any restriction of motion; the pathological changes observed at this stage are confined to low grade inflammatory process. In a moderate (second degree) strain, there is actual tissue damage that compromises the strength of the muscle tendon unit.

A severe (third degree) strain denotes complete disruption of some portion of the unit. A possible correlation is that the mild (first degree) muscle strain injury is the one detectable only on the post contrast MR scans and that the moderate and severe strain muscle injuries are readily recognized in the non contrast T2 and STIR MR sequences.However, these injuries limited the athletes' competitive participation for significant periods of time, suggesting that they were not minor injuries; so a perhaps more plausible explanation for this phenomenon is that the proliferation of MRI sites as well as the high level of medical care required by professional athletes usually mandate rapid imaging after injury. Therefore, if a longer delay in imaging had occurred, more oedema might have been present, allowing depiction of the muscle injury in the non enhanced MR study.Thus, the possibility of false negative non enhanced early MR images should be considered. A number of limitations are associated with this study but despite these limitations, they suggest the consideration of intravenous gadolinium in the setting of clinically suspected muscle injuries not visualized on T2 or STIR sequences. [14]

However, MRI remains the gold standard for detecting changes in muscle tissue. In some cases, MRI examinations can take the place of muscle biopsy for diagnosis. New advances in MRI include diffusion-weighted imaging, which permits assessment of fluid motion in muscles, and blood-oxygen-level-dependent imaging to evaluate tissue oxygenation. [15]

3. Images

In this paragraph we have used several images in order to emphasise the characteristics of muscular lesion diagnosed over the years in professional athletes.

We do not wish to provide a new classification but rather definitions which may help better understand the type of injury and choose the best diagnostic tool.

3.1. Indirect muscular injuries

3.1.1. D.O.M.S.

D.O.M.S. stands for DELAYED ONSET of MUSCULAR SORENESS.This refers to the pain felt several hours or even days after hard training and is caused by structural damage to the microscopic contracting functional units present in muscular fibres, with metabolic changes which lead to an alteration of the muscular tone, but does not reveal macroscopic damage to the fibres.

All that appears with Ultrasound, despite inconsistently is greater echogenicity of the whole muscle and a slight enlargement of the muscle due to oedema.

MRI instead reveals slight diffuse signal hyperintensity with undefined edges due to interstitial and perifascialoedema.

This proves MRI to be the gold standard in diagnosing D.O.M.S..

Indeed several articles have shown that the small number of minor injuries observed in clinical practice is not due to their frequency but rather to ill-defined symptoms and to the fact that Ultrasound appears to be unreliable in identifying such small alterations.

Actually Ultrasound sensitivity in identifying minor injuries is much lower compared to greater ones (70% vs 90%), as previously highlighted. MRI instead accurately identifies even minimal muscular oedemas such as D.O.M.S. thanks to adequate sequences which grant approximately 90% sensitivity.

Case 1

Example of a professional runner

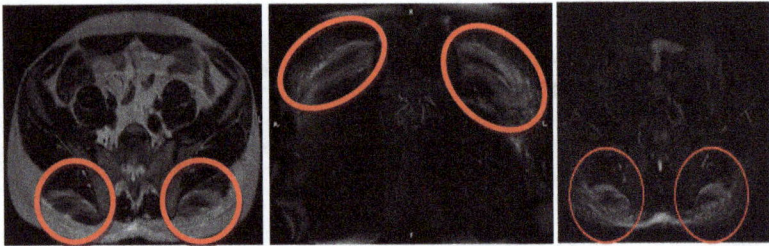

Figure 1. Example of RMN with DOMS in a professional runner

D.O.M.S. of glutei maximi of a runner who had carried out long traning for the New York marathon a few days. Diffused oedema is shown by signal hyperintensity (Fig.1)

3.2. Contracture

No macroscopic anatomical injury of the fibres is shown by Ultrasound, but rather alteration of the muscular tone due to fatigue with metabolic changes, revealed by greater echogenicity of the muscle

MRI shows minimal inconsistent increase in the size of the muscle due to diffused oedema and slight signal hyperintensity with ill-defined edges because of interstitial and perifascialoedema

Case 1

Example of a professional footballer

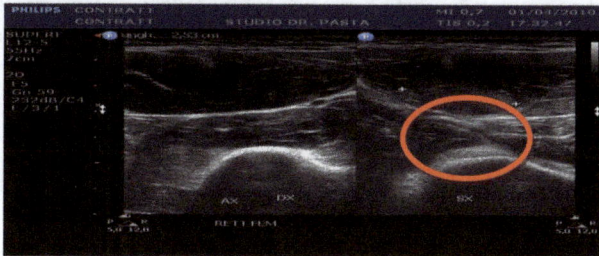

Figure 2. US image of Contracture in a professional footballer

This athlete had no problem finishing the match but the following day complained of slight undefined pain in his quadriceps femoris involving a large area of the muscle. Two days after the match Ultrasound showed slight hyperechogenicity in an area with ill-defined edges in the rectus femoris. (Fig.2)

3.3. Strain (Elongation)

No macroscopic anatomical injury of the fibres is shown by Ultrasound, rather microscopic alteration which in the acute stage are revealed by slight hyperechogenicity due to oedema and affected muscle and by a hypoechoic blurred area in the sub acutestage.MRI reveals slight focal signal hyperintesity

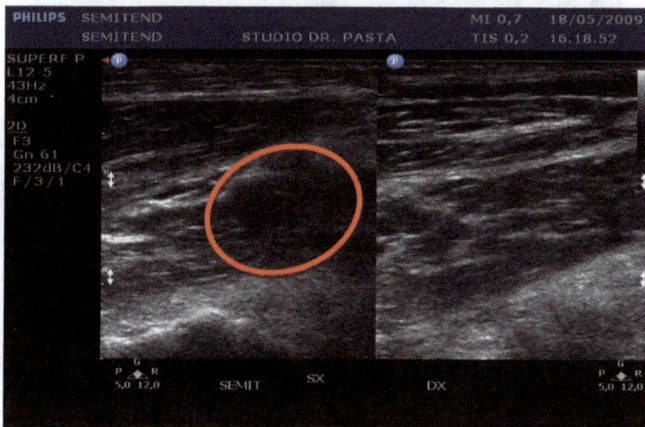

Figure 3. US image of Elongation in a professional footballer

Case 1

Example of a professional footballer

This athlete had no problem finishing the match but the following day complained of undefined pain and slight functional impotence in his Hamstrings involving a large area. Two days after the match Ultrasound showed slight hypoechogenicity, due to slight oedema, in an area with ill-defined edges in the Semitendinosus. (Fig.3)

Case 2

Example of a professional footballer

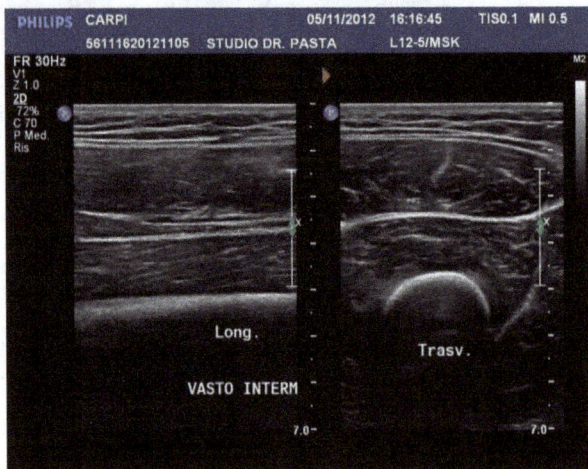

Figure 4. US image of Elongation in a professional footballer

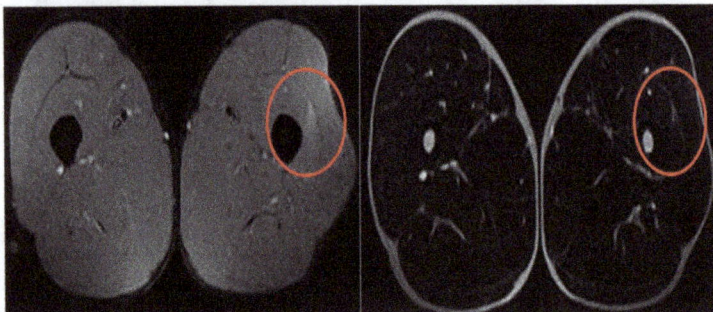

Figure 5. Example of Elongation in an RMN of a professional footballer

The ultrasound of this athlete was negative (Fig.4), yet the MRI carried out because of the symptoms highlighted an oedema of VastusIntermedius, shown by a minimal area of hyper-intensity due to minimal myofascial elongation (Fig.5)

3.4. First degree injuries

First degree injuries are characterized by the tear of fibres in the muscle (<5%) with oedema and small haemorrhage because of the vascularisation of connective tissue.

In the acute stage the Ultrasound highlighted a slightly hypoechoic area whilst in the sub-acute phase a dishomogeneoushypoechoic focal area was revealed with initial modification showing a small anaechoic inter or intramuscular area (usually<1cm) depending of the size of the muscle.

MRI instead showed an increase in muscle size due to oedema with slight dishomogeneous signal hyperintensity due to interstitial and perifascialoedematogheter with small focal signal hyperintensity due to small haemorrhage

Case 1

Example of a professional rugby player

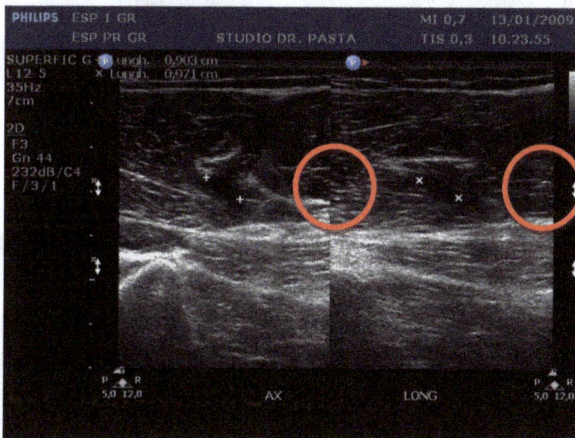

Figure 6. US image of First degree lesion in a professional rugby player

The player came for a check two days after a match when after a sharp movement in a tackle he started felling pain in a precise point of his thigh.

Ultrasound highlighted an anaechoic area due to haemorrage as from first degree injury of the Hamstrings (Fig.6)

Case 2

Example of a professional rugby player

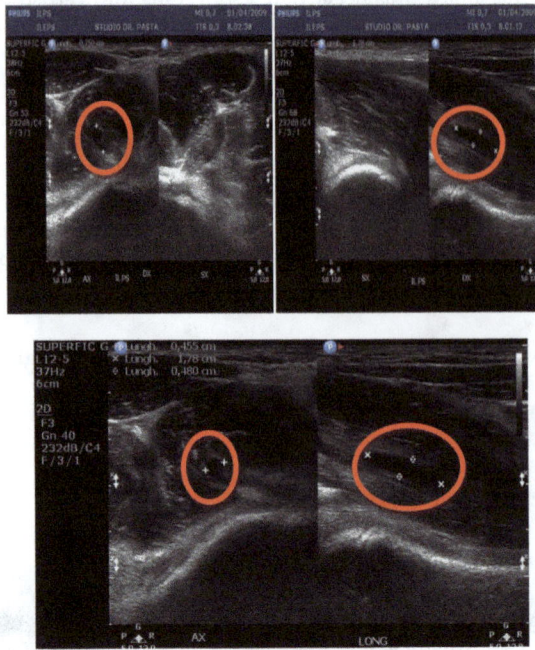

Figure 7. US images of First degree lesion in a professional rugby player

The player came for a check three days after a match when after a sharp movement in a tackle he complained of hyperextention of the pelvis followed by sharp pain in the lower abdomen.

Ultrasound highlighted an anaechoic area due to haemorrage as from first degree injury of the Abdominal external obliquemuscle. (Fig.7)

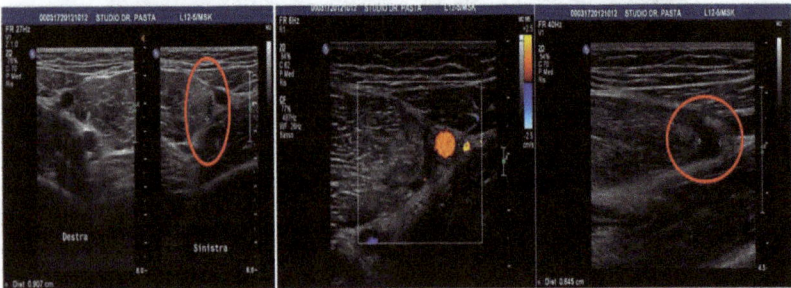

Figure 8. US images of First degree lesion in a professional footballer

Case 3

Example of a professional footballer (Fig.8-Fig.9)

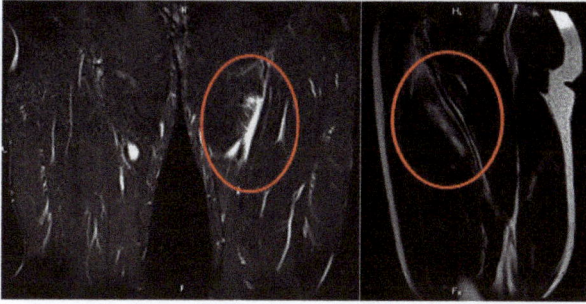

Figure 9. RMN images of First degree lesion in a professional footballer

A professional footballer felt a slight pain in the distal section of the adductor muscle while playing a match but felt no further symptoms.

He therefore started a rehabilitation program but when he started more intense activity he complained of the same pain.

The ultrasound showed an anaechoic area due to haemorrhage. (Fig.8)

The MRI was therefore essential to assess the real extension of the injury and highlight mio tendon retraction. (Fig.9)

The analysis was carried out the following day and showed changes in muscle volume and structure and signal hyperintensity when using axial imaging in comparative assessment for volume and variations, whilst coronal and sagital images defined the extension of the injury, i.e. a first degree myofascial injury of longus adductor.

Case 4

Example of a professional swimmer

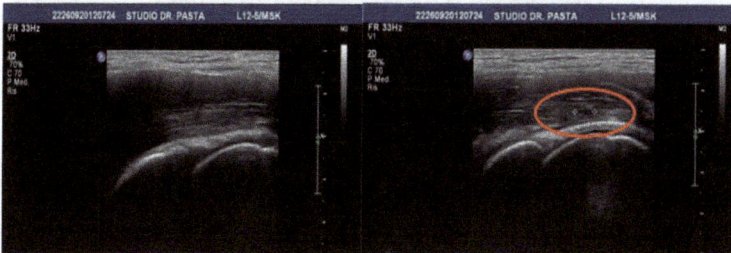

Figure 10. US images of First degree lesion in a professional swimmer

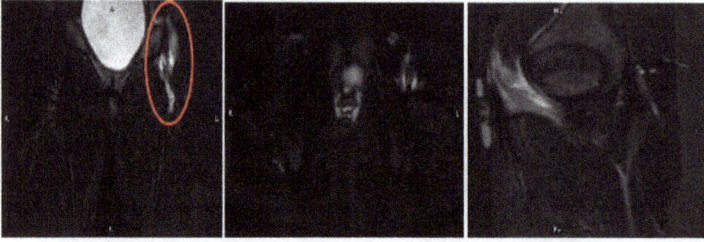

Figure 11. RMN images of First degree lesion in a professional swimmer

This is the case of a professional swimmer who complained of left groin pain for two days after diving but was able to compete.

Ultrasound highlighted a small thin hypoechoic area due to oedema along the ileo-psoas. (Fig. 10)

Due to the mismatch between the symptoms and diagnostics an MRI was carried out

This showed changes in muscle volume and structure and signal hyperintensity when using axial imaging in comparative assessment for volume and variations as for oedema and haemorrhage from ileo-psoas injury linked to tendon partial tear. (Fig.11)

Case 5

Example of a professional runner

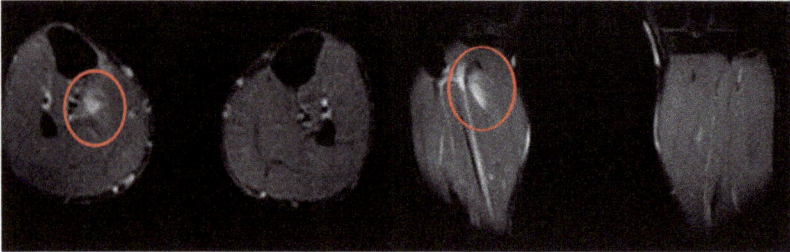

Figure 12. RMN images of First degree lesion in a professional runner

Example of a runner complaining of a sharp pain in the calf

The Ultrasound showed a small thin oedema along the flexor hallucislongusmuscle.Due to the mismatch between the symptoms and diagnostics an MRI was carried out.

This showed changes in muscle volume and structure and signal hyperintensity when using axial imaging in comparative assessment for volume and variations as for oedema and haemorrhage from first degree injury of the flexor hallucislongus muscle. (Fig.12)

Case 6

Example of a professional footballer

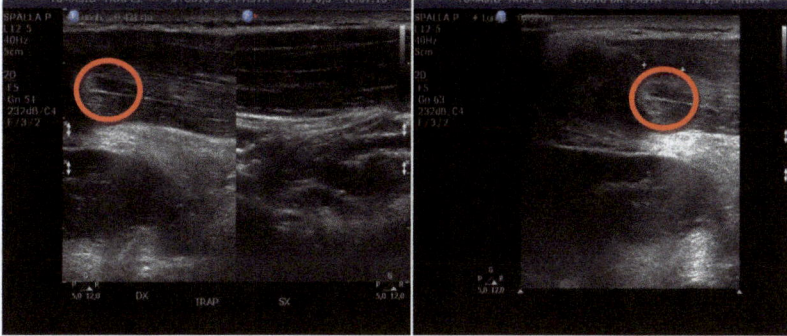

Figure 13. US image of First degree lesion in a professional footballer

This is the case of a goalkeeper who felt a slight pain in his shoulder during a save.The Ultrasound showed a small thin hypoechoic area due to oedema along the Trapezius muscle as for first degree injury. (Fig.13)

3.5. Second degree injury

Second degree injuries are characterized by the tear of a higher number of fibres in the muscle (<70%, < 2/3 of the muscle) with greater oedema and haemorrhage due to the wider involvement of the connective tissue.

Because of the wide range they are divided into initial and advanced second degree injuries.

It is sometimes difficult to define the injury degree precisely as the muscles affected can be very long, so injuries which are first degree should be classified as second degree and this leads to a simple description without a real classification.

In the acute stage the Ultrasound highlighted an iso-hyperechoic area whilst in the sub-acute phase a large, clearly dishomogeneousanaechoic area was revealed with structural change showing a large anaechoic inter or intramuscular area (usually<3cm) depending of the size of the muscle.

MRI instead showed an increase in muscle size due to oedema with dishomogeneous signal hyperintensity due to interstitial and perifascialoedema together with a mass of fluid with focal signal hyperintensity due to haemorrhage

Case 1

Example of a professional footballer

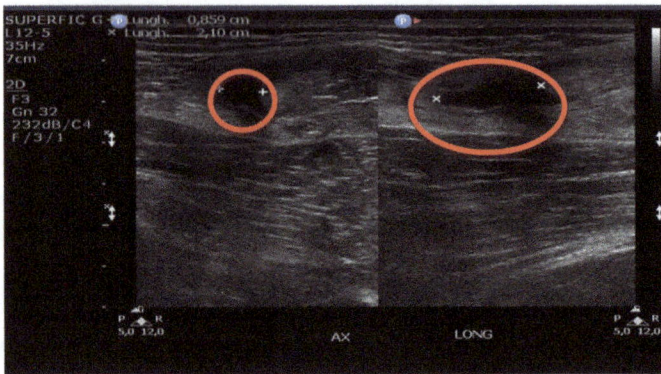

Figure 14. US image of Second degree lesion in a professional footballer

Major League footballer who on the previous day felt a very sharp pain in a sprint and left the match

Ultrasound highlighted a clearly dishomogeneous area with marked structural change showing a large intramuscular anaechoic area (<3cm), as from second degree injury of the Biceps Femoris. (Fig.14)

Case 2

Example of a professional volleyball player

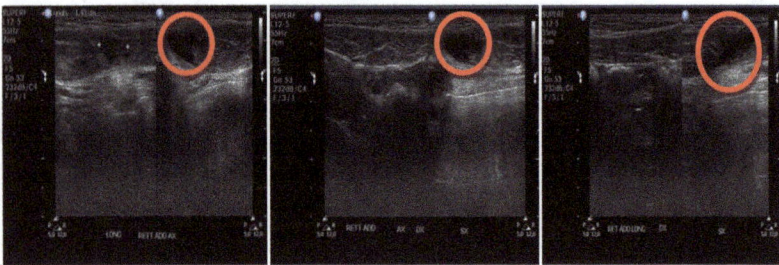

Figure 15. US image of First degree lesion in a professional volleyball player

Example of a volleyball player who, following the movement of the arm in spiking during a match, felt a sharp pain in the abdomen

Ultrasound highlighted a clearly dishomogeneous area with marked structural change showing a large intramuscular anaechoic area (>3cm), as from second degree injury of the Rectus Abdominis. (Fig.15)

Case 3

Example of a professional footballer

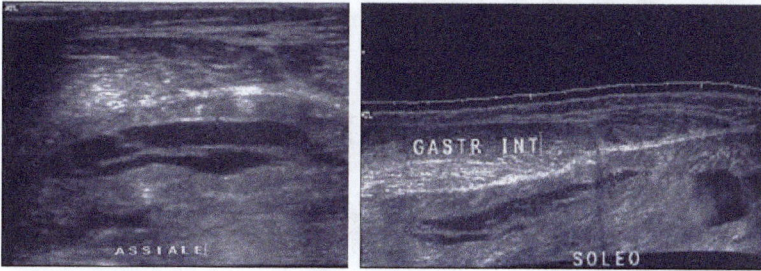

Figure 16. US images of Second degree lesion in a professional footballer

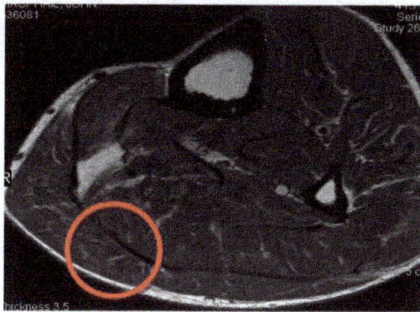

Figure 17. RMN images of Second degree lesion in a professional footballer

Example of a footballer who during pre-match warm-up felt a sharp pain in the calf which did not prevent him from playing up to the second half

Ultrasound highlighted a clearly dishomogeneous area with marked structural change showing a large intramuscular anaechoic area (>5 cm) with large haemorrage, as from second degree injury. (Fig.16)

MRI instead showed an increase in muscle size due to oedemawith dishomogeneous signal hyperintensity due to interstitial and perifascialoedema together with a mass of fluid with focal signal hyperintensity due to haemorrhage. (Fig.17)

These images are typical of a second degree injury of Soleus mucle

Case 4

Example of a professional footballer

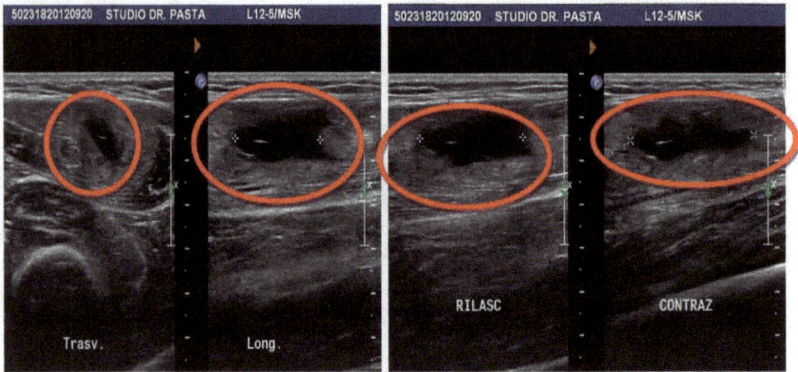

Figure 18. US images of Second degree lesion in a professional footballer

Example of a goalkeeper who during a kick felt a very sharp pain in the quadriceps

Ultrasound highlighted a clearly dishomogeneous area with marked structural change showing a large intramuscular anaechoic area (>5 cm) with large haemorrhage.

MRI instead showed an increase in muscle size due to oedema with dishomogeneous signal hyperintensity due to interstitial and perifascialoedema together with a mass of fluid with focal signal hyperintensity due to haemorrhage.

These images are typical of a second degree injury of RectusFemoris

Case 5

Example of a professional footballer

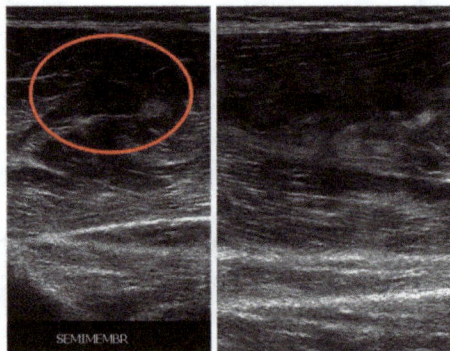

Figure 19. US images of Second degree lesion in a professional footballer

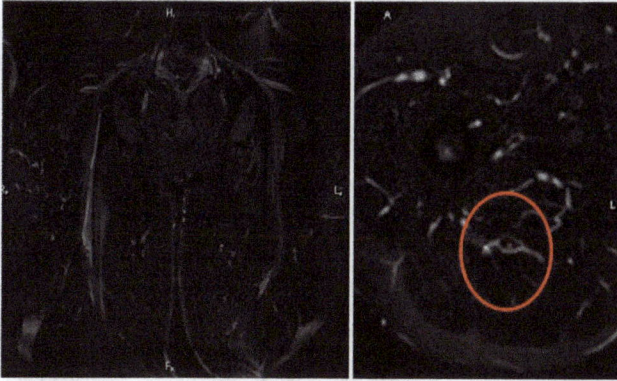

Figure 20. RMN images of Second degree lesion in a professional footballer

Major League footballer who felt a very sharp pain in a sprint on 29 September.

The first Ultrasound on 1October highlighted a large anaechoic area as from second degree miotendon injury of the Semimembranosus. (Fig.19)

MRI on 15 October highlighted a wide area with signal hyperintensity confirming the mio-tendon injury and intratendon tear too. (Fig.20)

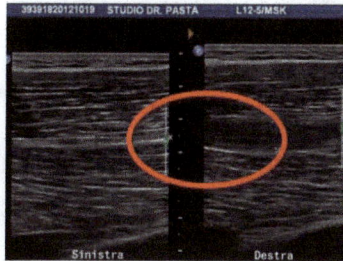

Figure 21. US image of Second degree lesion in a professional footballer

Follow-up analyses, i.e. Ultrasound on 19 October (Fig.21), MRI on 24 October and MRI on 2 November show the development of the pathology up to the disappearance of the modified signal in MRI as from recovery. (Fig.22)

Case 6

Example of a professional footballer

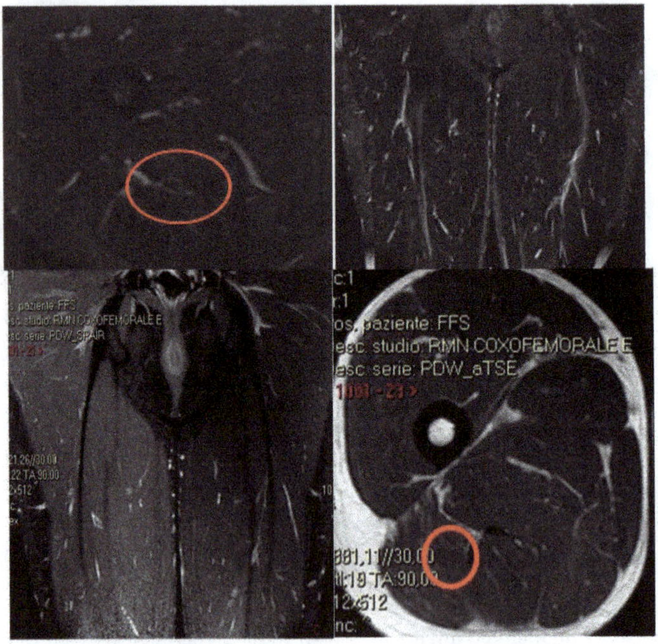

Figure 22. RMN images of Second degree lesion in a professional footballer

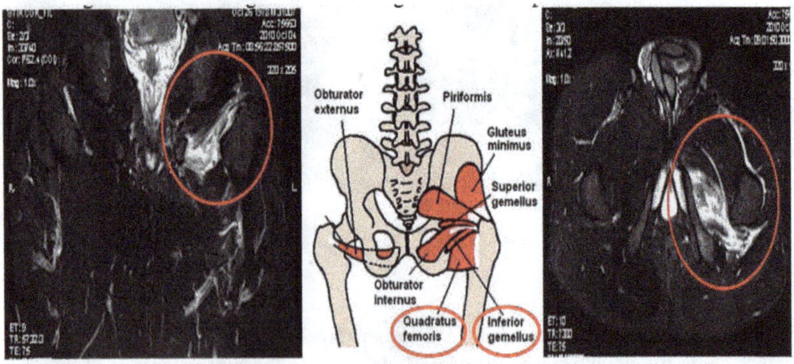

Figure 23. RMN images of Second degree lesion in a professional footballer

Professional footballer who felt a harp pain in the groin after a match but was able despite the pain to carry out differentiated training for four-five days.

The pain persisted so after a negative Ultrasound MRI was carried

This highlighted a large serum-haemorragic area characterized by clear signal hyperintensity as from second degree injury of the QuadratusFemoris and of the Inferior Gemellus. (Fig.23)

Case 7

Example of a professional footballer

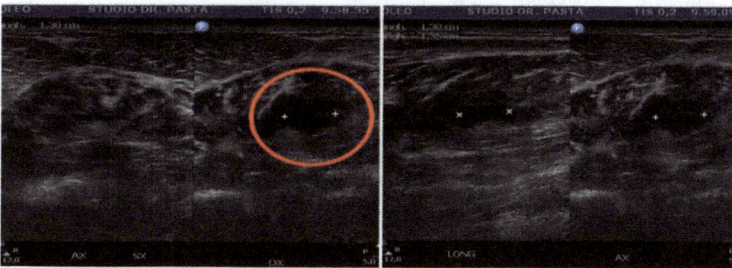

Figure 24. US images of Second degree lesion in a professional footballer

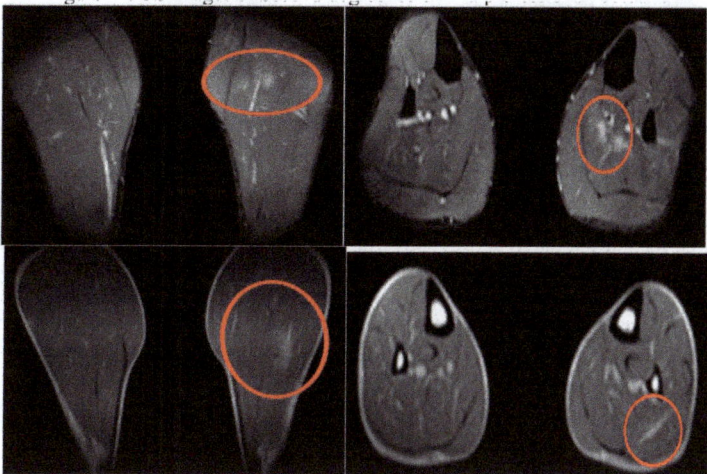

Figure 25. RMN images of Second degree lesion in a professional footballer

Example of a professional footballer who felt sharp pain in the calf during pre-match warm up.

Ultrasound highlighted a single intramuscular anaechoic area (>5 cm) with large haemorrhage as from isolated second degree injury of the Soleus muscle. (Fig.24)

Because of an unclear diagnosi MRI was carried out which showed a double area with dishomogeneous signal hyperintensity due to interstitial and perifascialoedema together with haemorrhage as from a double second degree injury of the Soleus muscle. (Fig.25)

These images are typical of a complex second degree injury

Case 8

Example of a professional football player

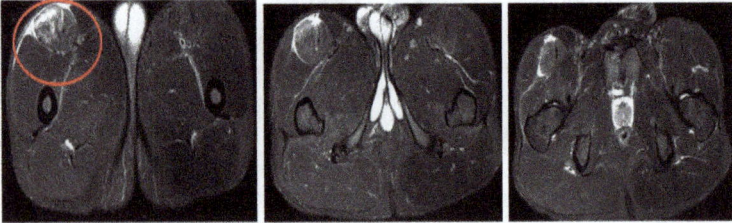

Figure 26. RMN images of Second degree lesion in a professional footballer

Professional footballer who felt a sharp pain during pre-season camp.

An initial Ultrasound (not published here) highlighted a large anaechoic area (>5 cm) as from miotendon second degree injury of the Rectus Femoris muscle.

MRI showed relevant signal hyperintensity due to oedema together with haemorrhage as from second degree injury of the Anterior or Straight Tendon of RectusFemoris muscle. (Fig.26)

Follow-up MRIs show the development of the pathology up to the disappearance of the modified signal in MRI as from recovery. (Fig.27)

Caso 9

Example of a professional footballer

Professional footballer who came for Ultrasound a few days after kicking a goal and feeling a sharp pain in the quadriceps.

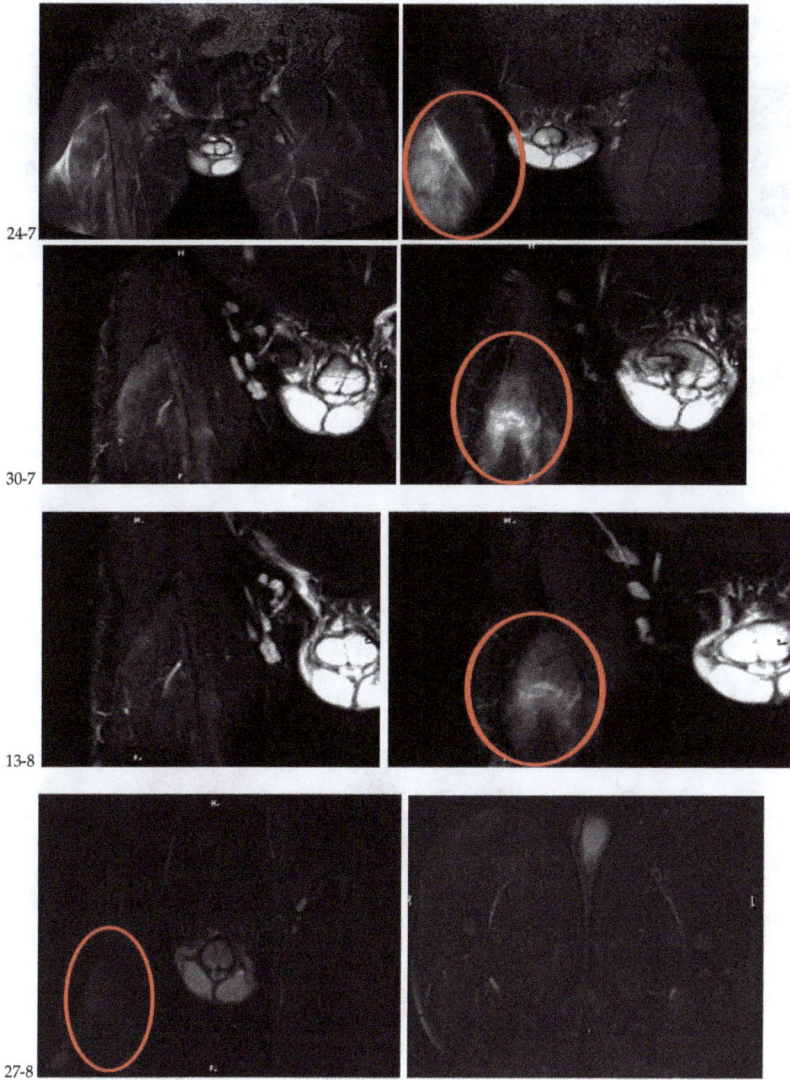

Figure 27. RMN images of Second degree lesion in a professional footballer

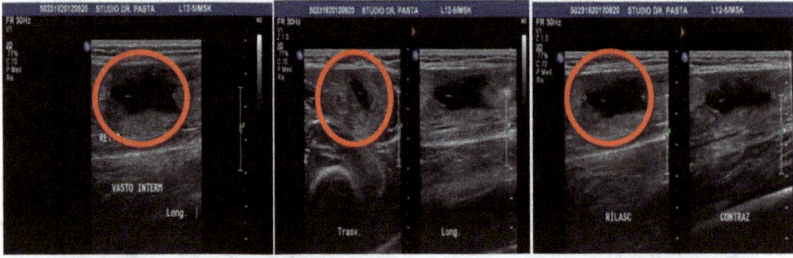

Figure 28. US images of Second degree lesion in a professional footballer

Ultrasound showed a large anechoic area of structural alteration due to haemorrhage with distancing of muscular extremities as from second degree injury of Posterior or Reflected Tendon. (Fig.28)

Subsequent MRI (Fig.29-30-31) and Ultrasound (Fig.32) show the development of the pathology up to disappearance of the modified signal in MRI as from recovery.

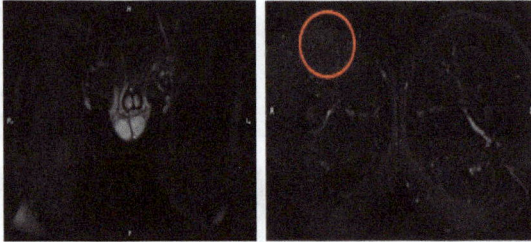

Figure 29. Rmn 11-11 in stir without Gadolinium

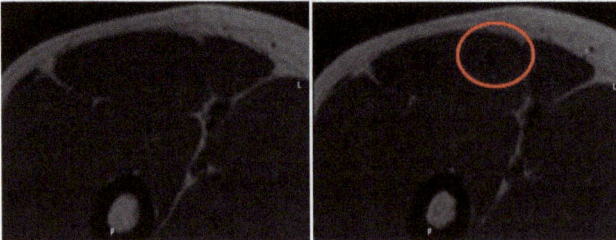

Figure 30. Rmn 11-11 in T1 without Gadolinium

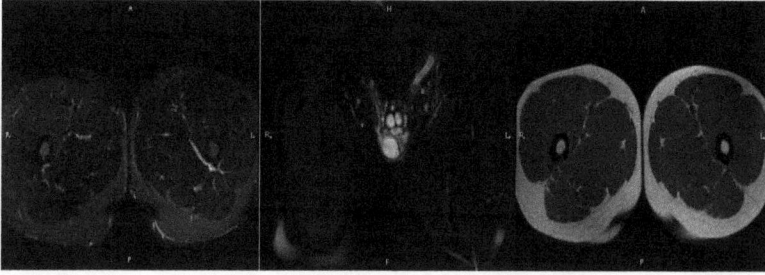

Figure 31. Rmn 3-12

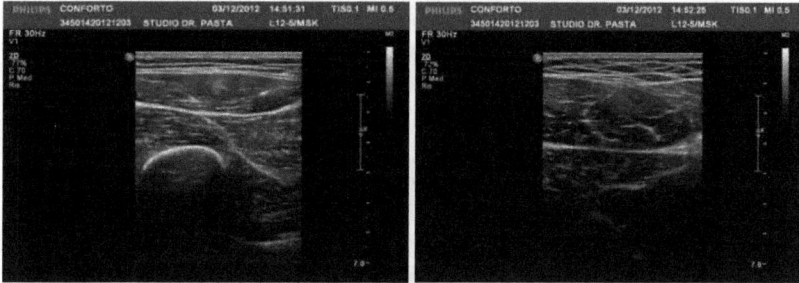

Figure 32. US 3-12

3.6. Third degree injury

Third degree injuries are defined as Subtotal with a tear of a higher number of fibres in the muscle (>70%, > 2/3 of the muscle belly) or Total with a tear of the whole muscle belly.

In the acute stage the Ultrasound highlighted a clearly dishomogeneous and disorganized iso-hyperechoic area, whilst in the sub-acute stage a clearly dishomogeneous area with marked structural change was revealed together with retraction of the stumps and a large anaechoic inter or intramuscular area (usually>3cm) depending of the size of the muscle.

MRI instead revealed a retraction of the stumps which showed irregular, wavy edges and hyperintense mass of fluid due to the haemorrhage between the two stumps.

Case 1

Example of a professional rugby player

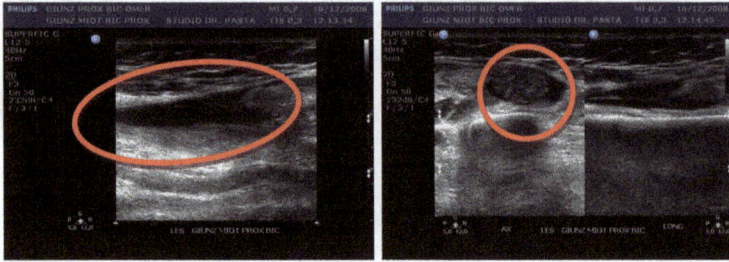

Figure 33. US images of Third degree lesion in a professional rugby player

Example of a professional rugby player who came for Ultrasound to his arm after prolonged tackle. A large anechoic area was revealed due to haematoma associated to retraction of the muscle head as from a complete tear of the Proximal Biceps Brachii. (Fig.33)

Case 2

Example of a professional footballer

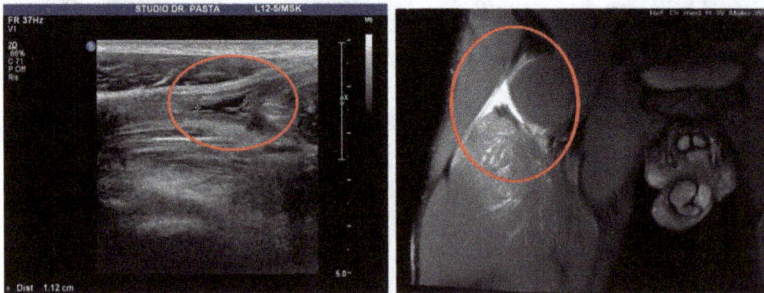

Figure 34. US images of Third degree lesion in a professional footballer

Example of a young goalkeeper who after a kick felt a sharp pain in the upper thigh as if from hip dislocation.

Ultrasound showed a small haemorrage as from miotend injury.

However symptoms led to a more severe injury.

MRI highlighted a haematoma shown by a hyperintense area associated to miotendon retraction as from sub-total tear of the Rectus Femoris Tendon. (Fig.34)

Case 3

Example of a professional footballer

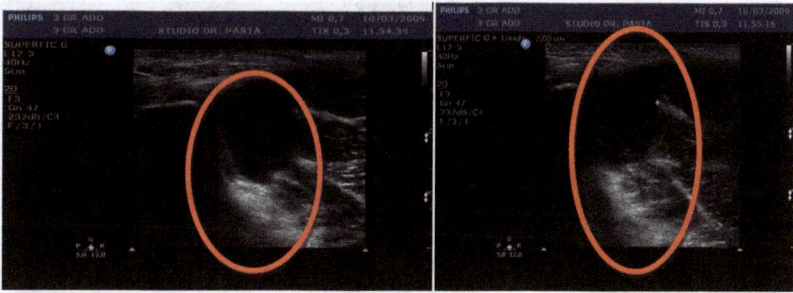

Figure 35. US images of Third degree lesion in a professional footballer

Example of a footballer who after a kick felt a very sharp pain in the groin.

Ultrasound showed a large anaechoic area due to haematoma with retraction of the muscle head as from complete third degree tear of the Adductor Longus muscle. (Fig.35)

Case 4

Example of a professional footballer

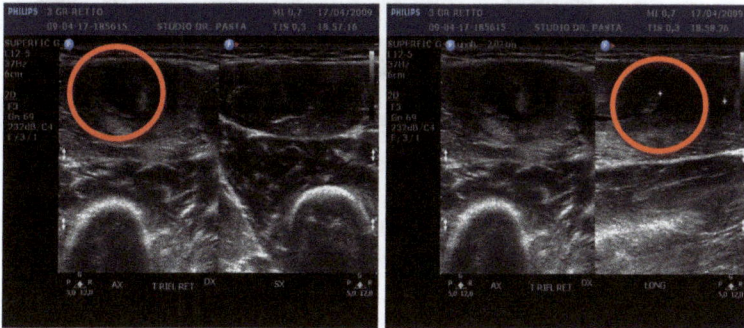

Figure 36. US images of Third degree lesion in a professional footballer

Example of a footballer who after a kick felt a very sharp pain in the upper thigh.

Ultrasound showed a large haematoma with retraction of the muscle head as from complete third degree tear of the Rectus Femoris. (Fig.36)

Case 5

Example of a professional rugby player

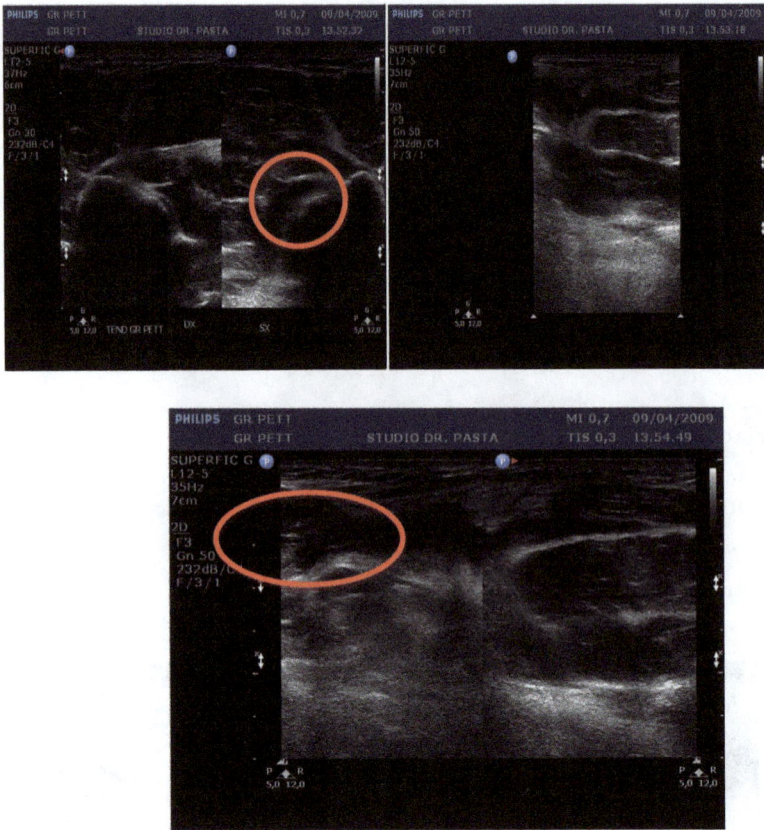

Figure 37. US images of Third degree lesion in a professional rugby player

Example of a professional rugby player who came for Ultrasound to his arm after prolonged tackle.

A large anechoic area was revealed due to haematoma associated to retraction of the muscle head as from a complete tear of the Tendon of the Pectorali Major muscle. (Fig.37)

3.7. Direct muscular injuries

This typically are injuries by contusion followed by hoematoma which by ultrasound revealed no difference from intrinsic hoematoma

Only a correct history of the injury can help in understanding the stages in the level of the fluid.

Case 1

Example of a professional footballer

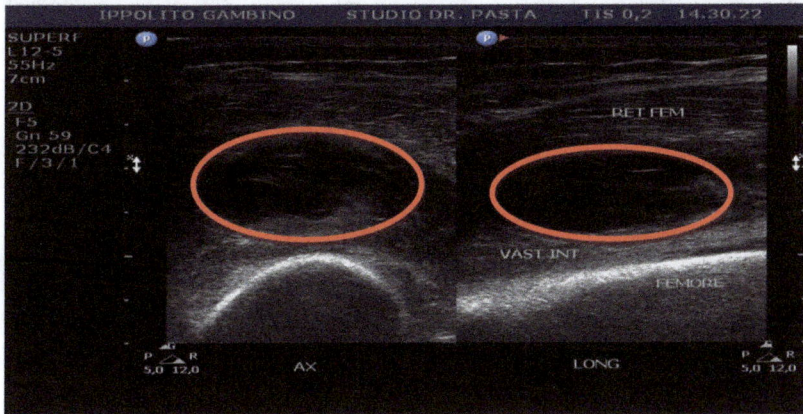

Figure 38. US image of lesion due to a contusion in a professional footballer

Example of a goalkeeper who during jump was hit with a knee on his thigh receving a contusion and subsuequent injury of the VastusIntermedius muscle

The Ultrasound revealed a large anaechoic area. (Fig.38)

Case 2

Example of a professional footballer

Example of a goalkeeper who during jump was kicked in the side of his abdomen receiving a contusion and subsuequent injury of the ObliquusAbdominis Muscle

The Ultrasound revealed a large anaechoic area of the ObliquusAbdominis Muscle. (Fig.39)

4. Chronic lesions in muscle injuries

When a muscle is subject to a trauma (either direct or indirect) the subsequent inflammation is meant to repair the damage tissue in order to allow its complete recovery.

Sometimes, however, the complete recovery does not take place giving raise to complication and conditions which for an athlete can be a serious problem as the performance can be severely limited.

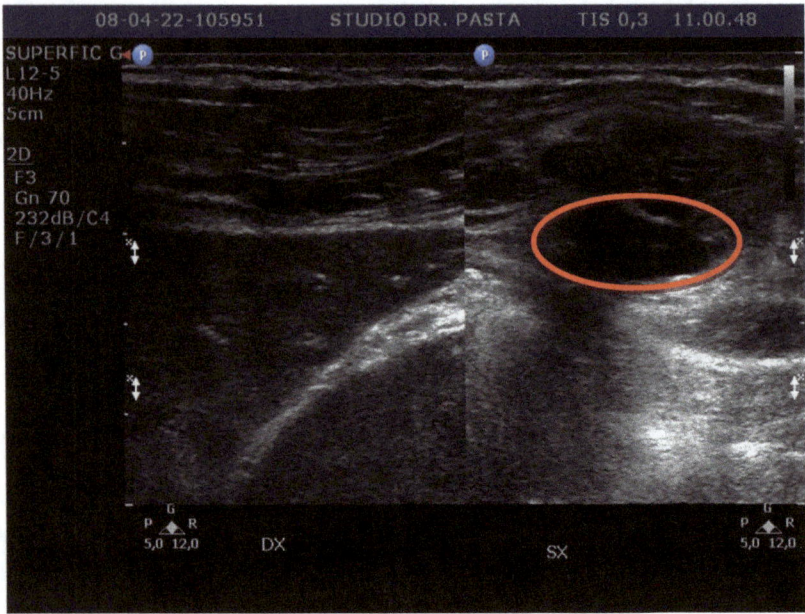

Figure 39. US image of lesion due to a contusion in a professional footballer

Differently from the classification above a definition of muscle injury complication appears to be universally recognized and more simple.

These include:

- Fibrosis

- Intermuscular fluid collection

- Cyst sero-sanguineus

- Ossific myositis

- Muscular atrophia

4.1. Fibrosis

It is the most frequent complication.

It reduces the muscle elastic and functional capacities (the capacity to develop strength) as it replaces the normal tissue.

It is usually caused by early mobilisation or prolonged immobilisation with excessive formation of abnormal, hypertrophic retracting fibrous tissue which affect the functionality of the muscular area involved.

The Ultrasound reveals a hyperechoic area which represents fibrous tissue in the injured muscle

Case 1

Example of a professional footballer

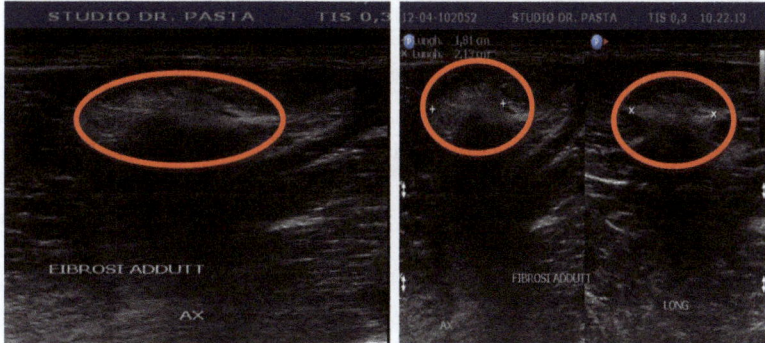

Figure 40. US images of Fibrosis in a professional footballer

Example of a professional footballer with a fibrosis of the Adductor muscle approximately two months after a severe injury

Ultrasound reveals a large hyperechoic area in the previously injured muscle from reparation of the muscular injury with formation of abnormal, hypertrophic retracting fibrous tissue which affect the functionality of the muscular area involved. (Fig.40)

Case 2

Example of a professional footballer

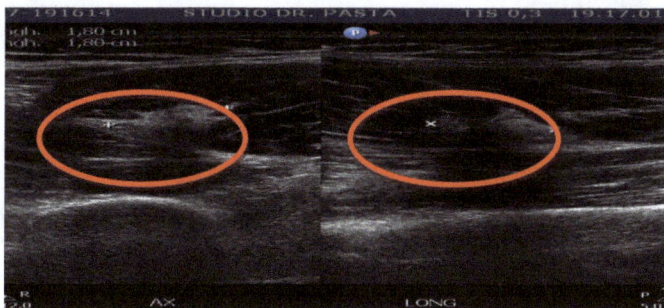

Figure 41. US images of Fibrosis in a professional footballer

Example of a professional footballer with a fibrosis of the Rectus Femoris muscle approximately two months after a severe injury

Ultrasound reveals a large hyperechoic area in the previously injured muscle from reparation of the muscular injury with formation of abnormal, hypertrophic retracting fibrous tissue which affect the functionality of the muscular area involved. (Fig.41)

4.2. Intermuscular fluid collection

It is a reaction process with formation of sero-sanguineus fluid between two muscular fasciae detectable by Ultrasound as a long plate with totally anaechoic or hypoechoisc or echoic structure.

Case 1

Example of a professional footballer

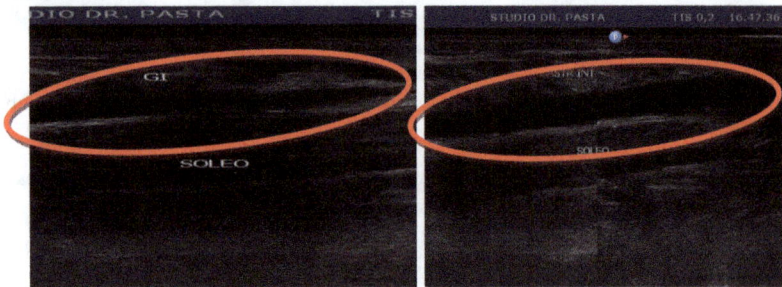

Figure 42. US images of a Fluid Collection in a professional footballer

Example of a footballer with residual and totally colliquative fluid collection between Gastrocnemius and Soleus muscles detectable by Ultrasound as a completely anaechoic long plate. (Fig.42)

Case 2

Example of a professional footballer

Example of a footballer with residual fluid collection partially colliquative and partially structured detectable by Ultrasound as a completely hypoechoic long plate. (Fig.43)

Case 3

Example of a professional footballer

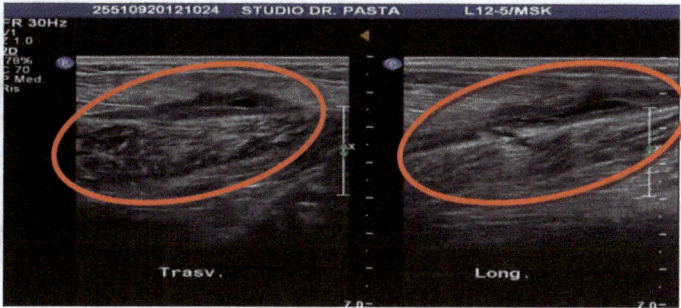

Figure 43. US images of a Fluid Collection in a professional footballer

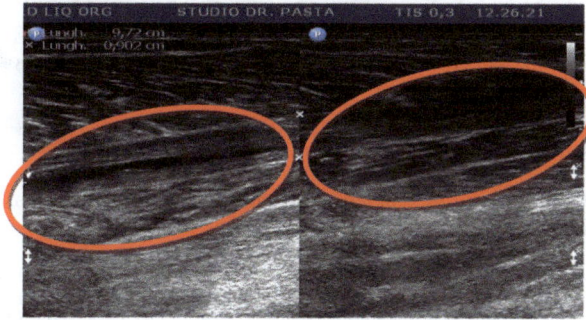

Figure 44. images of a Fluid Collection in a professional footballer

Example of a footballer with totally structured fluid collection between Gastrocnemius and Soleus muscles detectable by Ultrasound as a completely anaechoic long plate. (Fig.44)

4.3. Cyst sero-sanguineus

It is the consequence of a badly treated hoematoma which is not completely absorbed and which is encapsuled by newly formed fibrous tissue which separates it from the surrounding muscular tissue.

It originates from reaction process of the badly treated hoematoma which leads to the formation of sero-sanguineus fluid structured as a cyst capsuled in newly formed fibrous tissue.

Ultrasound reveals a completely anaechoic round shaped structure with posterior acoustic enhancement.

Case 1

Example of professional footballer

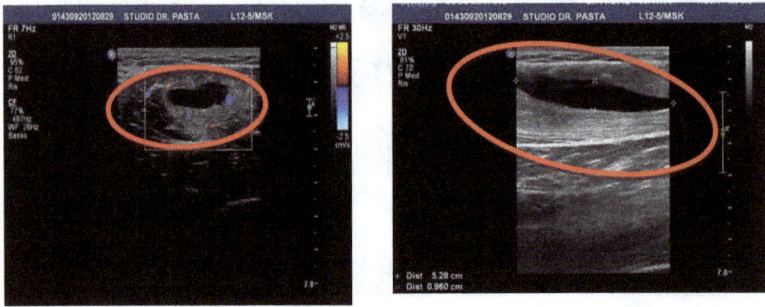

Figure 45. US images of a Sero-sanguineus cyst in a professional footballer

Example of a professional footballer with sero-sanguineus cyst of the Rectus Femoris Muscle approximately three weeks after muscular injury.

Ultrasound reveals a completely anaechoic round shaped structure with posterior acoustic enhancement. (Fig.45)

4.4. Ossific myositis

Badly treated inflammatory process of the injured muscle usually after contusion of large limb muscles close to the bones which leads to calcium deposit.

Two stages can be identified, a pre-calcific stage which is revealed as a pseudo solid mass in Ultrasound with Doppler signal along the edges and a calcific stage represented by a hetero-geneous mass with linear hyperechoich imaging showing posterior acoustic shadows and both central and peripheral vessels

Case 1

Example of a professionale rugby player

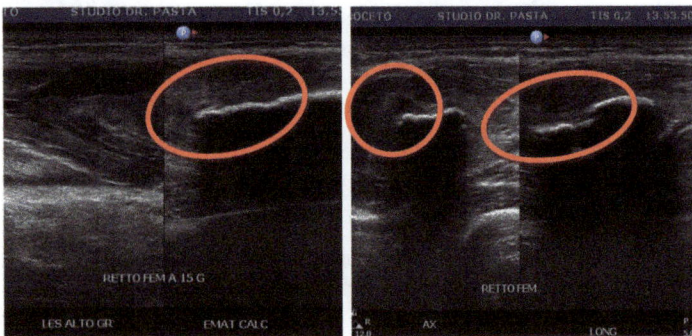

Figure 46. US images of a calcification in a professional rugby player

Post contusion injury of the Rectus Femoris muscle approximately two weeks after the injury with hoematoma linked to calcification easily detectable by Ultrasound as a heterogeneous mass with linear hyperechoich imaging showing posterior acoustic shadows. (Fig.46)

Case 2

Example of a professionale rugby player

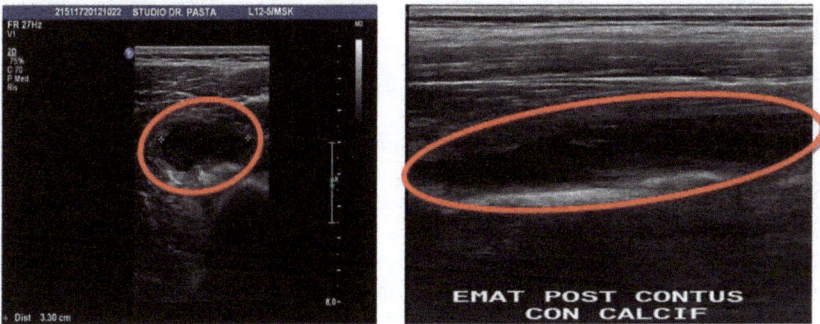

Figure 47. US images of a calcification in a professional rugby player

Example of a post contusion injury approximately seven days after the trauma which shows a pseudo solid mass in Ultrasound. (Fig.47)

4.5. Muscular atrofia

This complication originates from a chronic tendon tear or nerve implication with subsequent muscular adipose infiltration linked to reduction of the muscle volume.

Ultrasound shows a reduced hyperechoic muscle

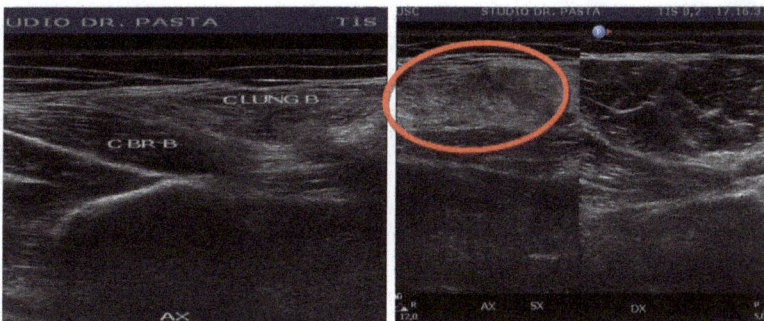

Figure 48. US images of reduced hyperechoic muscle in a professional volleyball player

Case 1

Example of a professional volleyball player (Fig.48)

Example of volleyball player after a severe miotendon injury of the long head of the Biceps Femoris muscle

Ultrasound shows a reduced hyperechoic muscle. (Fig.48)

5. Conclusions

Ultrasound is the first-line technique in the study of muscle traumas, as it is readily available, has a good cost-benefit profile, enables assessment of muscle dynamics and provides reliable assessment of the extent of damage. Musculoskeletal Ultrasound has been shown to be effective for many applications related to sports medicine and has proved itself as one of several imaging methods invaluable to the diagnosis of sport medicine–related abnormalities. Some advantages of Ultrasound over MR imaging include portability, accessibility, high resolution, and relative lower cost. More importantly, dynamic imaging under Ultrasound visualization allows diagnoses that cannot be made with routine MR imaging. Additionally, direct imaging correlation with patient symptoms provides important information to the referring clinicians.

There however some disadvantages.

Among these is the fact that its resolution is limited to the tertiary bundle, it is unable to identify alterations to secondary and primary bundles and myofibrils, and cannot visualise deep muscle planes. For these reasons, Ultrasound may yield negative results in lesions with only slight muscle alterations, such as contracture, lengthening and DOMS. [4]

Other disadvantages of Ultrasound include operator dependence and long learning curve. This can be minimized, however, with proper training and standardized technique.

Musculoskeletal Ultrasound has recently experienced an increase in popularity for several reasons. Advances in technology including the advent of high-frequency transducers have markedly improved image resolution. [2]

Additionally, the relative low expense of Ultrasound compared with MR imaging has made this an attractive alternative imaging method for many indications. Ultrasound does have several potential advantages over MR imaging. Evaluation of a soft tissue process near metal orthopaedic hardware is possible with Ultrasound without the artefact that limits MR imaging. Additionally, Ultrasound can immediately guide percutaneous procedures when an abnormality, such as a joint effusion, is identified. Ultrasound also allows a dynamic evaluation of joints detecting abnormalities that may not be present during MR imaging positioning. Lastly, the improved resolution of superficial structures demonstrates subtle abnormalities that may be difficult to visualize with MR imaging. Current ultrasound technology produces in-plane resolutions of 200 to 450 bm and section thicknesses of 0.5 to 1 mm. For these reasons musculoskeletal Ultrasound has proved to be one of the most valuable imaging methods in the diagnosis of anomalies in sports medicine.

Before it gains universal acceptance in evaluation of the musculoskeletal system, however, Ultrasound must be able to produce results similar to those of MR imaging.

MR imaging is essentially the standard of care for the evaluation of the musculoskeletal system at most centres worldwide.

There exist several advantages of MR imaging over Ultrasound.

The primary advantage is relative lack of operator dependence. This is achieved through the use of standardized MR imaging protocols.

Other advantages include multiplanar capabilities, panoramic views, ability to evaluate deep muscle planes and to detect lesions missed by Ultrasound.

Another advantage is the ability of MR imaging to evaluate globally and thoroughly an anatomic area including deep soft tissues, bone marrow, and joint cartilage with high sensitivity.

Advanced technology has resulted in improved image resolution and shortened imaging times. Images may be acquired at all times of the day at various physical sites. Interpretation of images can also be accomplished promptly with data transfer to computer workstations.

Controversy exists when Ultrasound and MR imaging are compared. Unlike the research results using MR imaging, those pertaining to Ultrasound are usually more variable. Although this can be partially explained by the inherent operator dependence of this imaging method.

Additionally, there are relatively few blinded research studies that directly compare Ultrasound with MR imaging. Many sonographic studies are limited to small subject groups without a gold standard. Additional research is needed to determine Ultrasound's true effectiveness in evaluating the musculoskeletal system relative to MR imaging.

Clinical studies, however, are demonstrating the potential of Ultrasound for several indications and interest in this imaging method continues to grow.

It is obvious that MR imaging will remain the most common advanced imaging method of the musculoskeletal system until research demonstrates that Ultrasound can produce similar results. It is clear, however, that there are several areas where musculoskeletal Ultrasound has been proved effective. Each of these points has allowed MR imaging to become widely accepted for evaluating the musculoskeletal system in sports medicine. [14]

As the images of the cases presented have shown, we too believe that MRI is to be considered the Gold Standard in muscular injuries, but we still consider Ultrasound the first choice because of its specific characteristics.

Further developments will extend applications of Ultrasound and MRI within muscularskeletal diagnostics, granting many more advantages in real-time performance, high tissue resolution and cost-benefit ratio.

Author details

Massimo Manara[1], Danilo Manari[2] and Giulio Pasta[3]

1 Association of Parma, Italy

2 FC Parma, Italy

3 Pasta Associate Clinic for Imaging Diagnostics, Italy

References

[1] Rubin, S. J, Feldman, F, Staron, R. B, et al. (1995). Magnetic resonance of muscleinjury. Clin Imaging , 19, 263-269.

[2] Ultrasound in sports medicineJon AJacobson, MDRadiolClin N Am (2002). , 40(2002), 363-386.

[3] Takebayashi, S, & Takasawa, H. Banzai Yet al ((1995). Sonographic findings inmuscle strain injury: clinical and MRimaging correlation. J Ultrasound Med, 14, 899-905.

[4] A. Megliola, F. Eutropi, A. Scorzelli, D. Gambacorta, A. De Marchi, M. De Filippo, C. Faletti & F.S. Ferrari. Ultrasound and magnetic resonance imaging in sports-related muscle injuries. Ruolo dell'ecografia e della risonanza magnetica nello studio delle lesioni muscolari. Radiol med (2006) 111; DOI 10.1007/s11547-006-0077-5

[5] Dierking, J. K, & Bemben, M. G. Bemben DAet al ((2000). Validity of diagnosticultrasound as a measure of delayed onsetmuscle soreness. J Orthop Sports PhysTher , 30, 116-122.

[6] De Smet, A. A. (1993). Magnetic resonancefindings in skeletal muscle tears.Skeletal Radiol , 22, 479-484.

[7] Hashimoto, B. E, Kramer, D. J, & Wiitala, L. (1999). Applications of musculoskeletalUltrasound. J Clin Ultrasound, 27, 293-318.

[8] Fornage, B. D. (1995). Muscular trauma.ClinDiagn Ultrasound , 30, 1-10.

[9] Garrett WE Jr ((1996). Muscle straininjuriesAm J Sports Med 24: SS8, 2.

[10] Bianchi, S, Martinoli, C, Waser, N. P, et al. (2002). Central aponeurosis tears of therectus femoris: sonographic findings.Skeletal Radiol , 31, 581-586.

[11] Kolouris, G, & Connell, D. (2003). Evaluation of the hamstring musclecomplex following acute injury. SkeletalRadiol , 32, 582-589.

[12] Developments in musculoskeletal ultrasound and clinical applicationsKlauser AS, Peetrons P. Skeletal Radiol. (2009). Sep 3.

[13] Greco, A, Mcnamara, M. T, Escher, M. B, et al. (1991). Spin-Echo and STIR MRImaging of sports-related muscleinjuries at 1.5 T. J Comput AssistTomogr , 15, 994-999.

[14] El-Noueam, KI, Schweitzer, ME, & Bhatia, . (1997) The utility of contrastenhancedMRI in diagnosis of muscleinjures occult to conventional MRI.J Comput Assist Tomogr 21:965-968

[15] Imaging and skeletal muscle diseaseNancy JOlsen MD, Jing Qi MD, Jane H. Park PhDCurrent Rheumatology Reports (2005). , 7(2), 106-114.

Chapter 4

Overview of Different Location of Muscle Strain

Francisco Arroyo

Additional information is available at the end of the chapter

1. Introduction

Up to 30% or more of all the sports injuries that we deal with in our daily medical practice, including contusions and bruises [1] are injuries to muscle.

Muscular injuries can occur anywhere on our whole body. The treatment methods available to us today are of such a wide variety that the athlete can to return to physical activity as soon as possible (in most of the cases) without any permanent damage or secondary reactions.

Many of these injuries are not properly treated due to several factors, for example, physician inexperience or that athletes minimize the injury in their quest to stay in the competition; athletes hide (especially during the clinical evaluation) their pain, which is very important information for the medical doctors to set the guidelines on how to treat the pathology.

Unfortunately, now we have these injuries in children and adolescent athletes because of the availability of high level of competition in all sports even at those ages.

So having the knowledge to make the correct diagnosis in these pathologies is essential for physicians who treat athletes every day.

2. Injury

2.1. Pectoral strains

A strained pectoral muscle is actually a slight tear in the chest muscles named pectoral muscles and these two muscles are located at the front of the chest. One is the largest (pectoralis major) and originates from the sternum, ribs and collar bone and goes to the upper part of the humerus and the smallest is the pectoralis minor that finish in the front of the shoulder blade.

An injury happens when the muscle is stretched too far and the pain can be felt at the same moment or in some cases latter during the cooling down phase after the exercise and sometimes the pain radiates to the upper arm or neck [2].

Diagnosis.- During the physical examination some patients show an obvious swelling and bruising area that is tender under digital palpation and others just have pain when you ask them to move the arms backwards, (Fig. 1) in some others you can ask them to try to do a push up and the patients refers pain over the affected area.

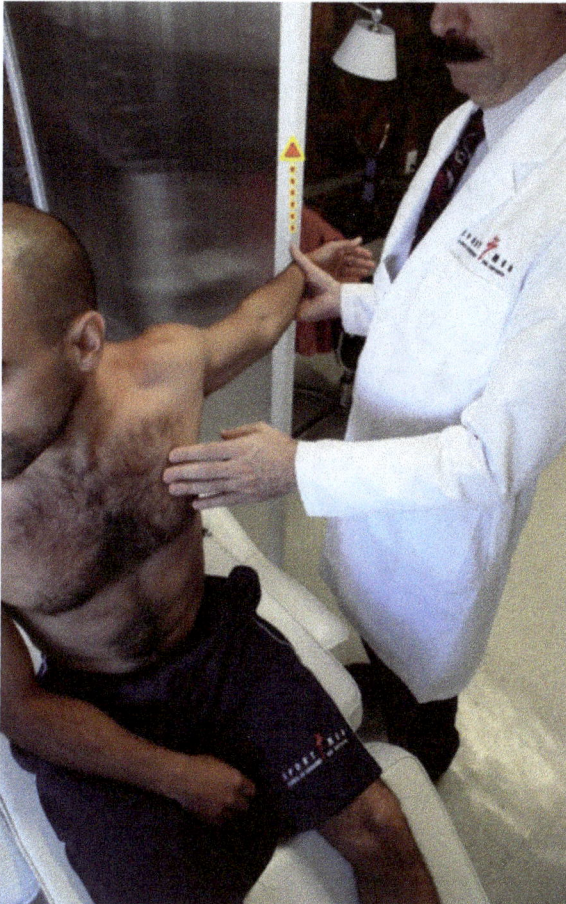

Figure 1. With the arm in lateral extension ask the patient to move forward against resistance

Another way to make the diagnosis is to ask the athlete that with the arms extended try to get together the hands and you put your fist between the hands for not allow him to do it (fig. 2)

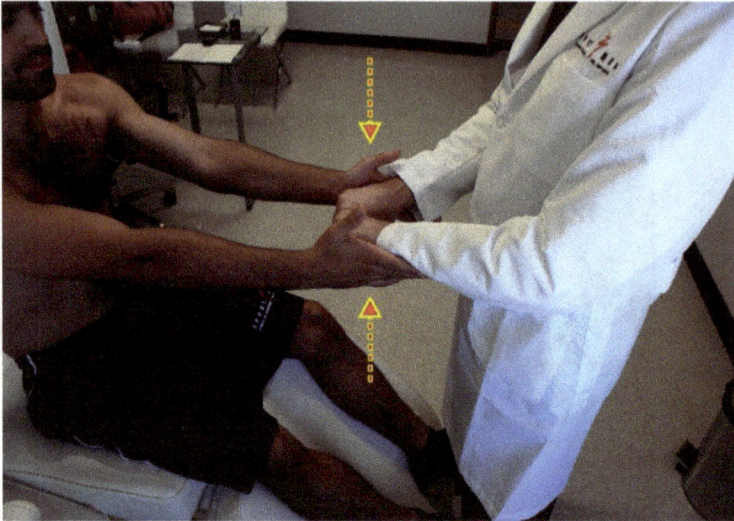

Figure 2. With both arms straighten at front ask the patient to put their hand together against resistance

To assess the severity of the injury an Ultrasound, CT scan or MRI scan may be required.

2.2. Biceps strains

The biceps is located in the front of the upper arm and it is attached to the elbow and the shoulder. When we flex the elbow most of this movement is done by the biceps.

Symptoms of a biceps strain include sudden and severe pain at the front of the shoulder and also the athlete can experience swelling, deformity of the muscle and loss of strength, presence of a bruise over the affected area, depending on the severity.

In the physical evaluation with the elbow straighten palpate all along the biceps (fig. 3) ask the patient to flex the elbow with the palm up and tell him not to let you push it toward the floor (fig. 4) an ultrasound study is very useful to assess the severity of the injury because some tears at the level of the elbow more often require surgical repair [3].

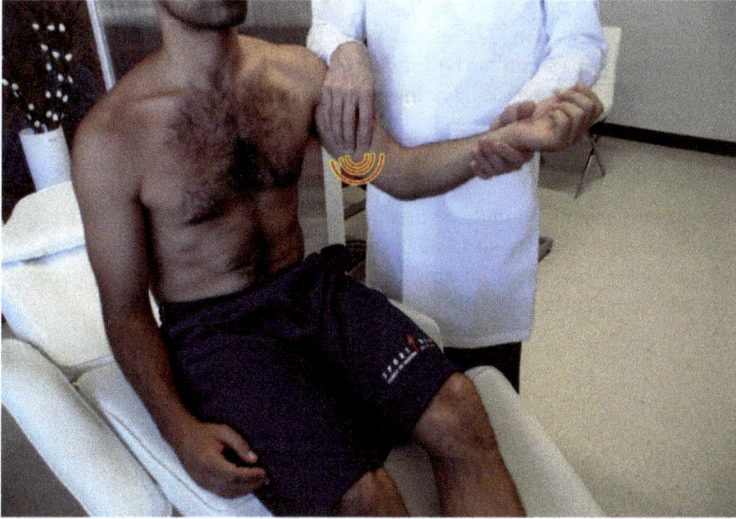

Figure 3. With the elbow flex at 90° palpate the biceps all along

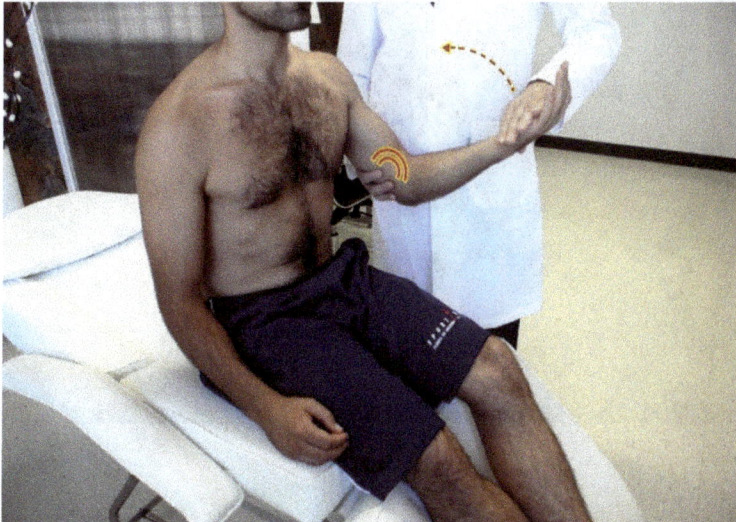

Figure 4. A With the elbow flex at 90° ask the patient to flex it against resistance

3. Triceps strains

The triceps muscle is located in the back side of the upper arm and its main action is straightening the elbow. A triceps strain can be a simple overstretch to a partial or complete tear. This pathology may result from overusing or in a single boost of force.

When this occurred the symptoms are pain, stiffness, tenderness, edema, in some cases bruising and loss of strength.

During the physical examination the patient refers pain over the area and the palpation can be done with the elbow in flexion to relax the muscle (fig. 5), also if we ask the athlete to straighten the elbow with the palm down against resistance (fig. 6). Some patients require surgical treatment depends on the site and the severity of the injury. [4]

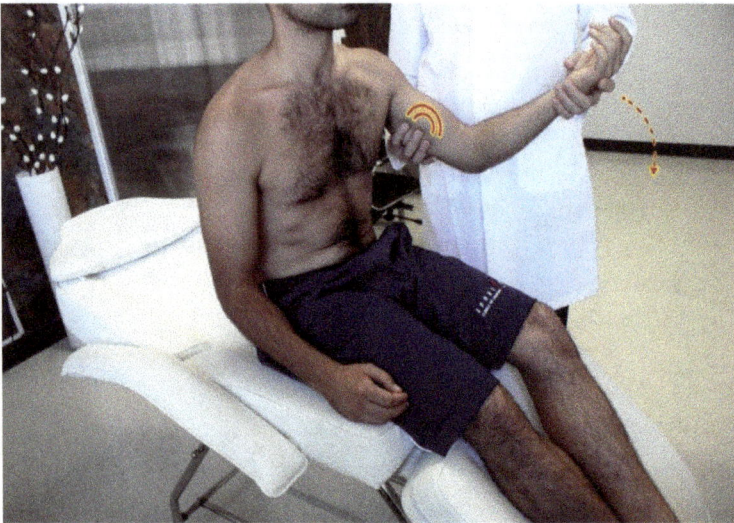

Figure 5. With the elbow flex at 90° palpate the triceps all along

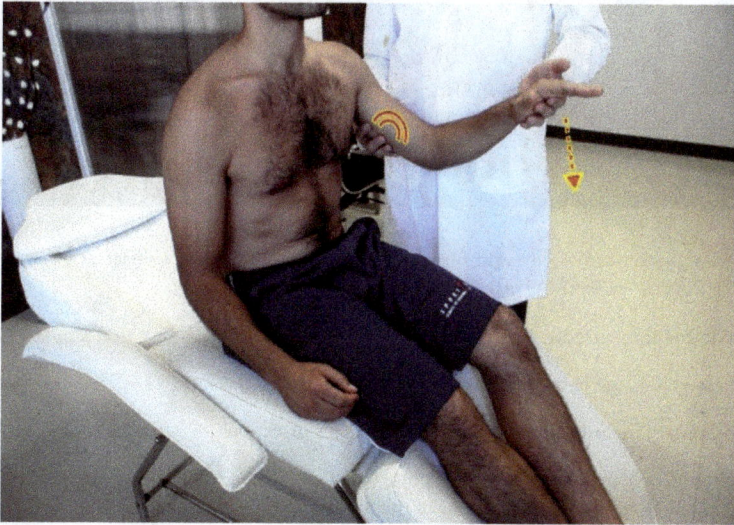

Figure 6. With the elbow at 90° and the palm facing down ask the patient straighten the elbow against resistance

4. Medial flexor pronator muscles strain) medial flexor pronator strain

This is an injury that occurs on the inside of the elbow after either direct trauma as in wrestling or baseball or from valgus strain in golf or football soccer.

The injury occurs to the forearm muscles that attach to the inside (medial) aspect of the elbow; the first indication of injury is pain, swelling, or even in an acute hematoma may be present.

Physical examination should determine the exact location of the injury according to pain (using digital palpation). The maneuvers to be performed include:

Ask patient to perform wrist flexion and pronation. Pain is often referred into the affected area (figure 7a).

With the elbow at 45° of flexion, movements of flexion, extension, pronation, and valgus stress are carried to determine the location and magnitude of the injury.(figure 7c)

These maneuvers should be done on the contralateral elbow as well to see how great is the difference in pain intensity and location as well as motion between the two joints.

Another maneuver that can be used to assess pain is forced flexion of the wrist against resistance (figure 7b).

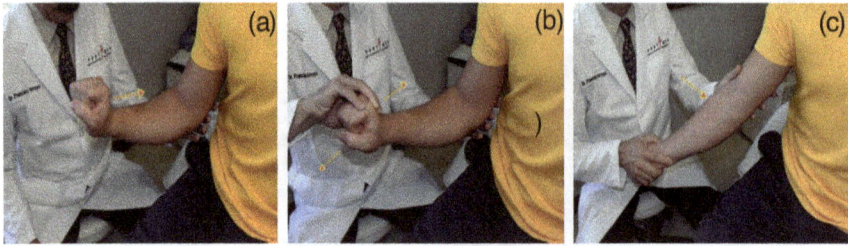

Figure 7. a) Ask the patient to flex the wrist; b) Ask the patient flex the wrist against resistance; c) Apply force to the lateral side of the elbow to take it to a valgus position

You can define three grades of injury:

First.-There is damage to a small fraction of muscle fibers.

Second.-This can include an avulsion of the muscles insertion

Third.-There is a broader breakdown of muscle fibers. There may also be the presence of an avulsion fracture cause by detachment of the tendon in the affected area.

One complication may be an injury to the ulnar nerve. If this happens the sensitivity of the little finger and the ring finger are affected [5] to be sure to perform a small sensitivity neurological examination (figure 8).

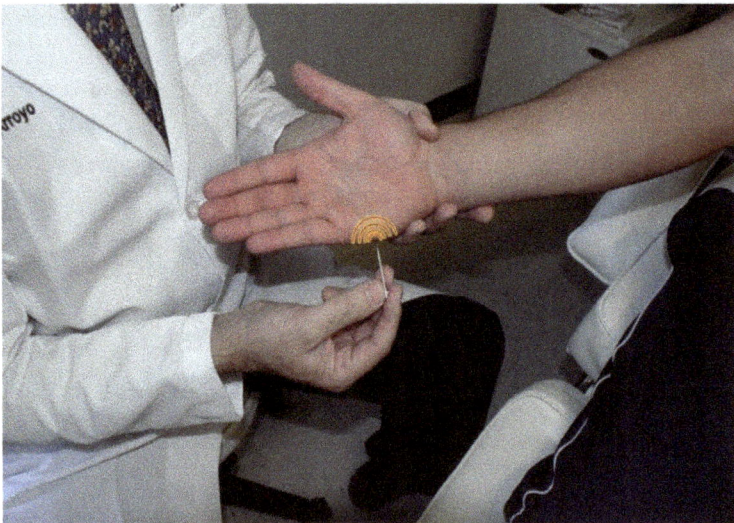

Figure 8. Test the sensitivity neurological area of the little finger using a small needle

5. Flexor muscle strain

Another common injury is the forearm flexor injury.

For example in sports requiring abduction and external rotation after a sudden adduction internal rotation of the can cause forearm flexor muscles to be injured (e.g., baseball, swimming, etc.)

Once injured, there will be tenderness around over the forearm flexor muscles.

The pain from this injury can be provoked by asking the athlete to flex the wrist against resistance; pain should arise in the medial side (figure 9).

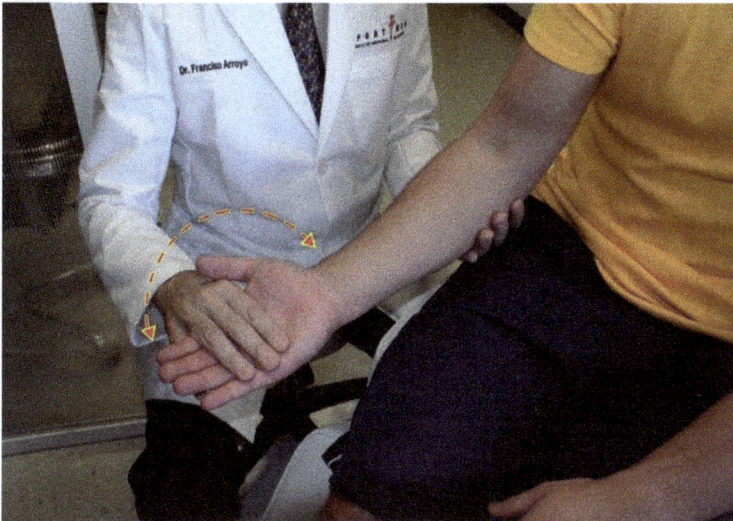

Figure 9. With the wrist straighten ask the patient to flex it against resistance

In some athletes (those with a pronator injury) a hematoma can be present. Pain can be provoked with pressure on the lateral side of the elbow joint forcing the elbow into valgus.

6. Abdominal muscle strain

Several muscles converge in the abdomen: rectus, internal and external obliques and also the transverse and the pyramid

On physical examination is difficult to establish the diagnosis because beneath these muscles is the abdominal cavity that contains different organs that also can cause pain.

Not all the abdominal pain has an muscle origin and it is our challenge to know what signs or symptoms differentiates the different pathologies.

Whenever an athlete refers abdominal pain, we should start the physical examination away from the zone of pain and gradually get closer to the area that the athlete describes as being the most annoying in appearance, swelling, deformity, tumors, etc.

If we suspect a muscular abdominal tear [6], part of the physical examination would be to ask the athlete to do a sit up and putting an effort on the abdominal area. There will be patients in which you have to ask the athlete to contract the abs against resistance in order to get a painful response (figure 10).

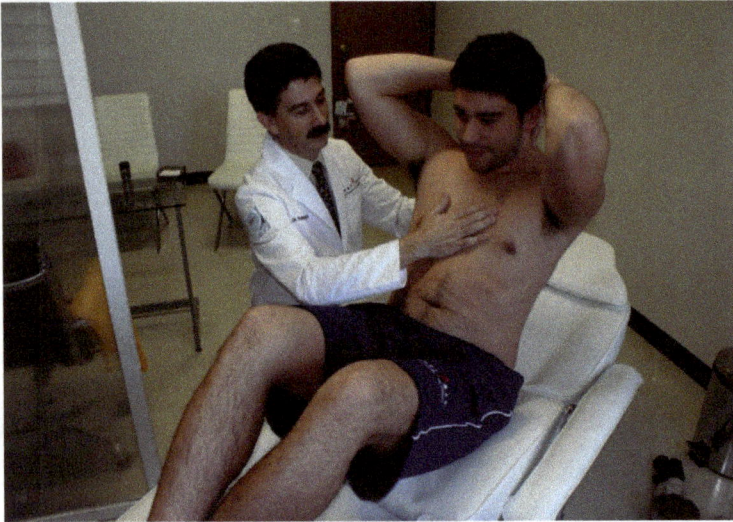

Figure 10. In a sit up position ask the patient to hold it against resistance

Other conditions to rule out are:

Apendicitis.- IPain localized to the bottom and right side of the patient, this is called McBurney's point. (Right lower quadrant). Pain may also be around the navel and usually is accompanied by nausea and vomiting and will likely have evidence of malaise and in some cases fever (figure 11).

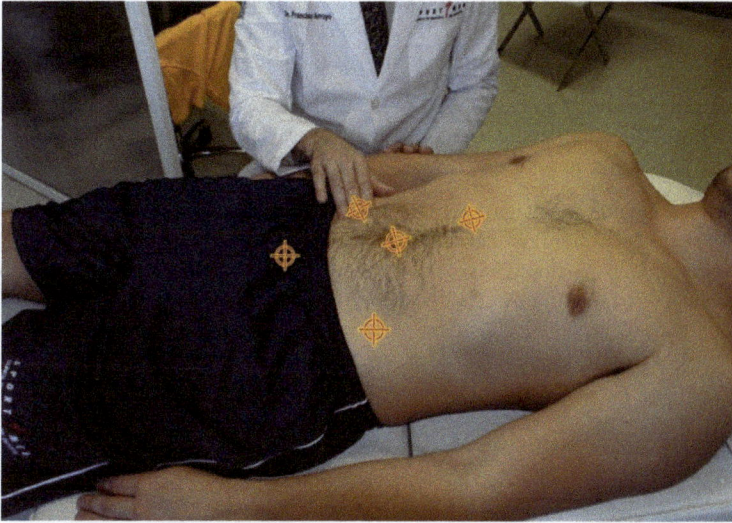

Figure 11. The doctor´s hand is palpating the Mc Burney´s point which is painful at the pressure in appendicitis, all the other target points usually are just related to pelvic inflammation.

PELVIC INFLAMMATORY DISEASE.-This disease occurs mostly in women who may have a pelvic infection. Pain may be related to both iliac fossae.

GASTRITIS, COLITIS, ULCER.- Pain may have been present for many hours of duration coincident with swelling, presence of abdominal gas, bloating, and burning over the stomach area. Pain can also be referred from the colon.

In abdominal pathologies unrelated to the muscle and if we have any doubt, it is best to refer the athlete to a specialist and not cause more damage by waiting and see if the symptoms disappear. This is a very valuable time if the cause is pain comes from an organ of the abdominal cavity.

7. Groin muscle strain

For example in soccer players the incidence of groin injury is approximately 5% to 6.2%, [7].

If we talk about the local anatomy, there are four muscles that converge at the same point and any of them could be torn or stretched so even though the symptoms may be closely related the source, pain could be localized to any of these muscles: rectus femoris, adductors, psoas major or sartorius.

Remember that these muscles are involved in hip flexion so in the physical examination, we must look for pain when the athlete is flexing the hip.

The athlete may have exacerbation and decrease in symptoms while in some cases the pain is only present when there are changes in the speed or change of direction. It is not unusual for the athlete to have no pain when running forward without changing direction.

The symptoms can be vague and often undefined because of the convergence of various anatomical structures. Pain could be due to a sport's hernia, osteitis pubis, nerve pain (neurally referred pain), bursitis, tumors, etc.

A physical examination can begin examining the painful area to rule out that pain that could be from a node or an inguinal hernia (in all the cases there is tenderness).If the lesion is muscular in origin, pain should increase when the athlete is asked the patient to perform hip flexion against resistance (figure 12).

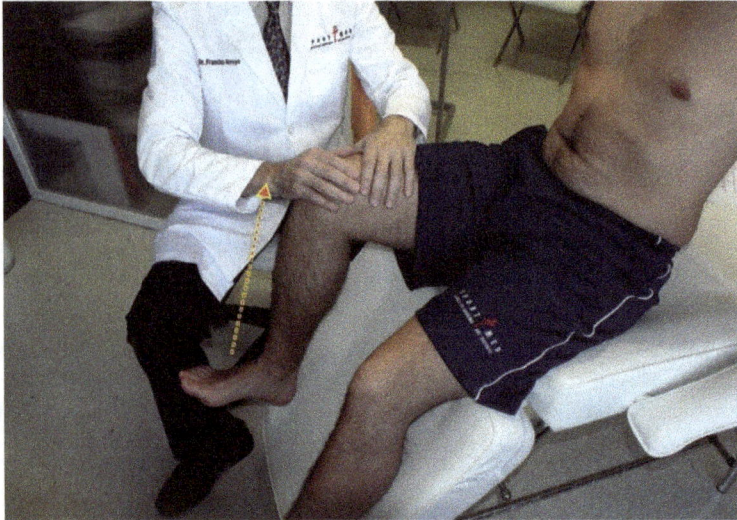

Figure 12. With the knee flex at 90° ask the patient to raise it against resistance

Other provocative maneuvers are to have the athlete lift the leg (with the knee extended) (figure 13a), against resistance or the examiner takes the leg in extension and do some abduction movement (figure 13b, 13c). Si hacemos este movimiento de forma contralateral con la pierna no involucrada podremos ver que el rango de movimiento está limitado en la pierna afectada. Similar tests of the contralateral (uninvolved) leg will show just how much range of motion is limited in the affected leg.

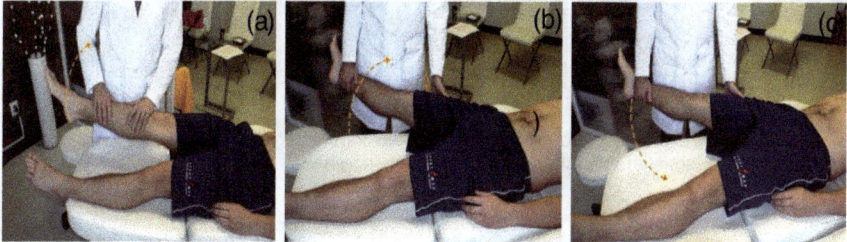

Figure 13. a) Ask the patient to rise the leg straighten against resistance; b) Take the leg straighten to an abduction position till the pain is triggered; c) Ask the patient to move the leg inward (adduction) against resistance

An initial recommendation is for rest to allow time for the symptoms to be minimized. Treatment is based on a good diagnosis and since here we encounter the convergence of various etiologies of pain, any misdiagnosis could lead to chronic pain that can result in limitation of the athlete's sports performance

8. Lumbar strains

Lumbar sprains are the most common causes of low back pain. A low back muscle strain occurs when the muscle fibers are abnormally stretched or torn. The injury can occur because of overuse, improper use, or trauma. It is classified as "acute" if it has been present for days to weeks. If the strain lasts longer than 3 months, it is referred to as "chronic".

Almost all of these low back injuries are due to injuries of the muscle. Certain risk factors, such as excessive lower back curvature, forward-tilted pelvis, weak back and/or abdominal muscles, and tight hamstrings, can increase the risk for this injury.

The symptoms are: Pain around the low back and upper buttocks, Low back muscle spasm, Pain associated with activities, and generally relieved with rest spasms in the lower back that result in more severe pain and lower back feels sore to the touch

Trauma of great force can injure the tendons and muscles in the lower back. Pushing and pulling sports, such as weight lifting or football, can lead to a lumbar strain.

The diagnosis of lumbar strain is based on the history of injury, but in the physical examination we palpate all the back of the patient facing down, to locate the pain (fig.14 a). We also ask him to try to rise the head while we are holding the ankles(fig. 14 b) and another maneuver is ask him to rise the leg with the knee straighten,on at the time, (fig. 14 c).

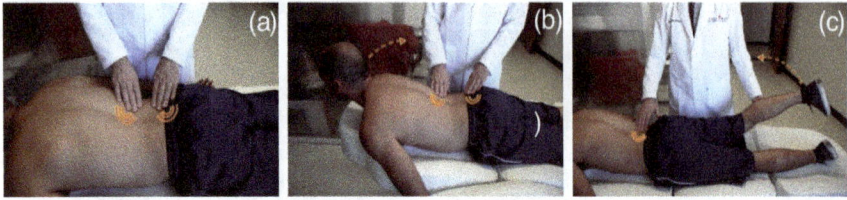

Figure 14. a) With the patient facing down palpate the paravertebral muscles all along; b) Ask the patient to rise the neck to provoke and discomfort; c) Ask the patient to rise the leg straighten

9. Pubic adductor strain

The pubic adductor strain is a very common pathology in runners. Attached to the pubis are three muscle that converge: the adductor magnus, minimus and longus.

This injury usually occurs suddenly after having made a sharp sprint or change of direction and speed. When this injury happens, the athlete suddenly suspends the exercise and seeks medical help.

In the physical examination, pain is referred to a specific area of the adductor region to the inner and upper part of the leg. Palpation of the area may reveal edema, increased temperature, and in some cases a visible bruise (figure 15).

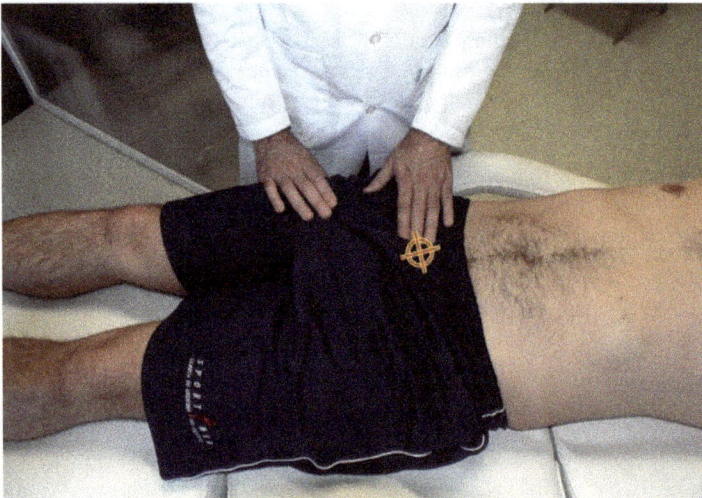

Figure 15. Palpate all over inguinal area searching for pain over the pubic bone

In carrying out exploratory maneuvers, a patient is unable to laterally raise the leg without pain and may require help to perform this movement.

With the athlete lying supine, ask him to to flex the knee and hip to 45° and then ask him to let the leg drop outward to the point of pain., If the injury is minor, the examiner may need to apply some resistance to provoke pain (figure 16a,16b).

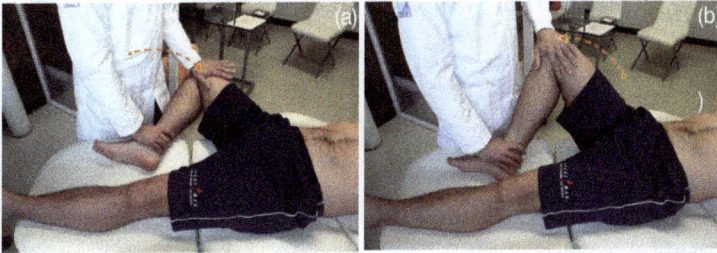

Figure 16. a) With the knee flex at 45° and lying over the lateral side ask the patient to rise it against resistance; b) With the knee flex at 45° ask the patient don´t let you push it out

10. Quadriceps

One of the largest muscles in our body is the one on the front of the thigh. It is called the Quadriceps because it has four distinct beginnings (heads) that form separate muscles (vastus medialis, vastus intermedius, vastus lateralis and rectus femoris) that come together and insert as a single unit to the superior pole of the patella wrapping it and then inserting into the anterior tibial tuberosity.

Functionally, the quadriceps contributes significantly to the knee's stability. The quadriceps is a prime mover of knee extension and assists in hip flexion. The athlete can be injured in two ways. One is by a direct blow to the muscle and a second method is when the extension movement is performed suddenly.

A direct blow can cause blood vessels to break leading to intermuscular or intramuscular hematomas.

Physical examination includes a direct palpation to the injured area that should provoke pain and limping by the patient. This diagnosis is not difficult to determine because the athlete's history leaves no doubt (figure 17).

When there is a torn muscle caused by an overexertion, the examiner can also palpate underlying edema. The athlete will usually be quite uncomfortable in the area of the injury and unable to perform an isometric contraction of the thigh similar to the unaffected leg.

We can check the range of motion of the leg with the athlete lying supine on the edge of the examination table and bending the knee to the limit of pain (figure 18). At this point, stop the

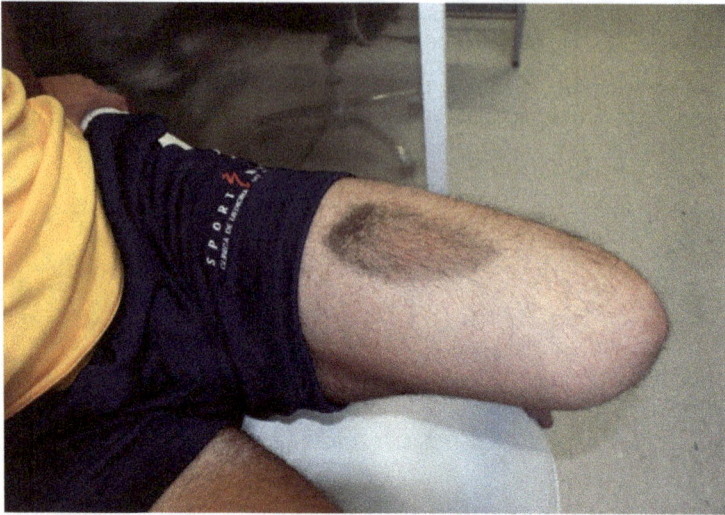

Figure 17. A visible bruise is often seen

movement and measure the hip and knee angles. Repeat the test with the uninvolved leg and determine the difference in the measurements. Treatment should be instituted immediately to prohibit the injury from complicating and increasing the pain as time passes.

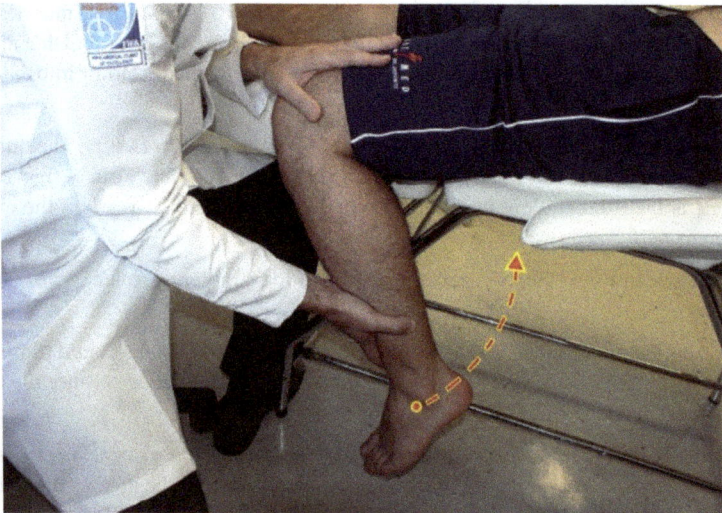

Figure 18. With the injured leg hanging from the lateral of the examination table flex the knee and measure the angle at which the pain is triggered and you can compared it to the contralateral side

Some times in the clinical history we have reports of previous ruptures that left an obvious muscle deformity (such a depression in the rectus femoris), but from the functional point of view the athlete's performance is unaffected even although the defect could be very large and might even need surgery, [8].

11. Hamstring

The hamstring muscles are located on the back of the thigh and function to flex the knee and extend the hip. These muscles form the back and inside out of the thigh (semitendinosus, semimembranosus and biceps femoris (long and short head) the latter being the outermost of these muscles).

When this group of muscles are injured, the athlete reports having felt a "pull" especially when they are doing explosive exercises, and so the athlete stops and suspends all activity immediately.

There are hamstrings injuries that can occur in a slow and chronic manner, so the symptoms are vague and can be confused with pain in the lower back; not all injuries to this muscle group are acute, [9].

The causes of this injury can be very marked imbalance quadriceps strength (muscle imbalance), also often are due to lack of elasticity or warm-up previous to ballistic sports activity [10].

When this injury occurs, pain is widespread, edema occurs quickly and the patient is unable to stand or walk on the injured leg. Moreover, in the course of a few hours a hematoma is present, which can be displaced by gravity towards the back of the knee.

On physical examination (with the patient lying prone) pain in the area of the tear is provoked by palpation and the patient cannot perform an isometric knee flexion or hip extension nor can the athlete perform hip extension (figure 19a).

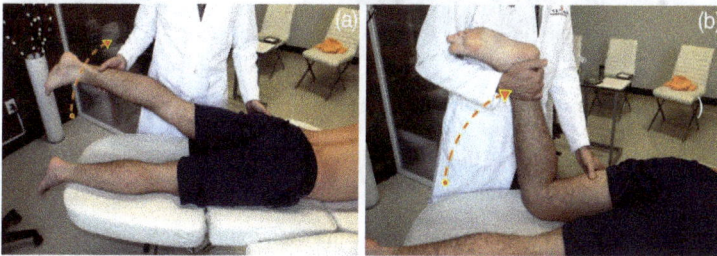

Figure 19. a) With the patient facing down ask to rise the affected leg as high as he can; b) With the knee flex at 90° palpate al the hamstring muscle to locate the exact spot of the muscle injury

When the examiner bends the knee of the affected leg (to relax the hamstrings) palpation of the entire length of the hamstrings can locate the site and of the muscle injury (figure 19b).

12. Gastrocnemius tear

These muscles are the gastrocnemius (medial and lateral head), and soleus and all combine to form the Achilles tendon. Their function is to help flex the knee and the foot (plantar flexion) and also the supination of the foot. Injuries in the calf are often due to lack of adequate warm up, stretching, or by overexertion when the muscle is already fatigued.

Generally speaking, the injury usually occurs acutely and patients say it feels as if someone had stuck in the back of the leg, yet when they turn around nobody is behind them, [11].

Pain is present immediately and the athlete can no longer stand and may have to be removed from the field on a stretcher. On physical examination, the prone patient is examined and the site of injury can be determined by palpation; edema is not always present (figure 20).

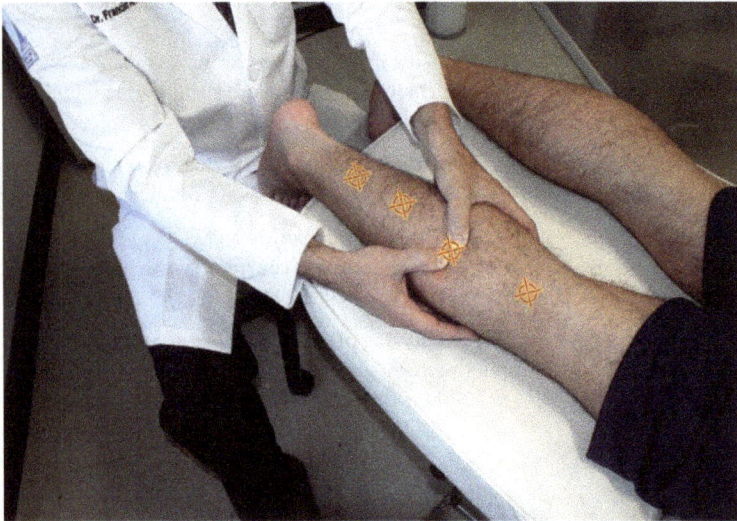

Figure 20. The gastrocnemius with patient prone is palpate all along

With the athlete still lying prone, the knee is flexed to 90°. Pain is triggered when the athlete is asked to perform plantar flexion.

A complication of this condition is when the Achilles tendon ruptures; it is very important to rule out this complication. With the patient in a sitting position, compress the muscles (figure 21) to make the toes goes directly downward (Thompson sign). If this movement does not occur, the tendon could be completely torn and surgical treatment may be necessary.

Standing on the toes causes too much pain and the patient is unable to apply equal force by both legs to remain standing (figure 22).

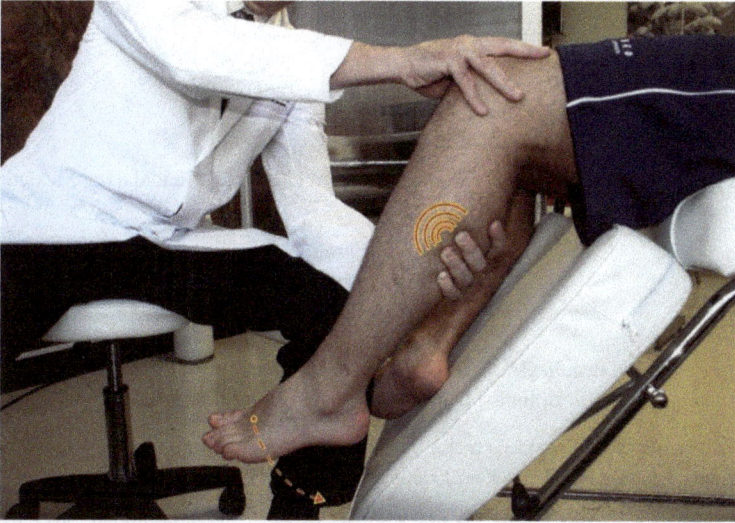

Figure 21. Thompson´s sign. With the knee flex at 90° squeeze the gastrocnemius muscle to provoke a tip toe of the foot

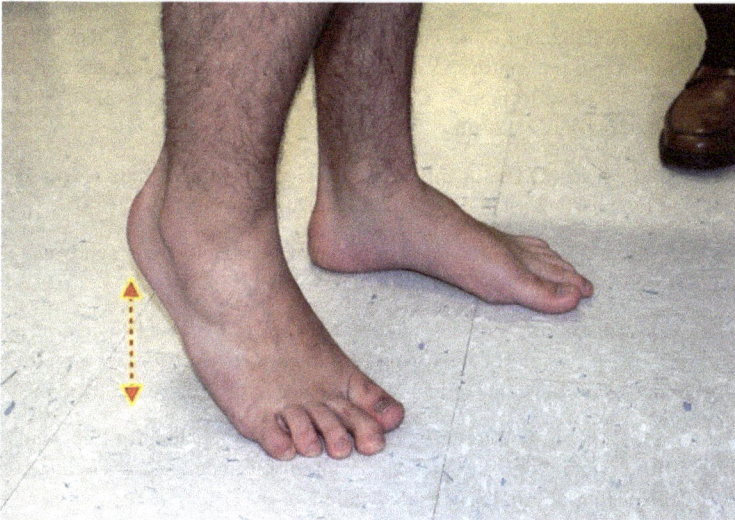

Figure 22. Standing on a tip toe position is painful

Author details

Francisco Arroyo*

Medical Director, Sport Med. FIFA Medical Clinic of Excellence Guadalajara, Mexico

References

[1] Jacobs CL, Hincapié CA, Cassidy JD.Musculoskeletal injuries and pain in dancers: a systematic review update. J Dance Med Sci. 2012;16(2):74-84.

[2] Beloosesky et al.Pectoralis major rupture in elderly patients: a clinical study of 13 patients. Clin Orthop Relat Res. 2003 Aug;(413):164-9.

[3] Sarda et al. Distal biceps tendon rupture: Current concepts Injury. 2013 Apr;44(4): 417-20. doi: 10.1016/j.injury.2012.10.029. Epub 2012 Nov 27.

[4] Kokkalis et al.Distal biceps and triceps ruptures. Injury. 2013 Jan 23. pii: S0020-1383(13)00015-6. doi: 10.1016/j.injury.2013.01.003. [Epub ahead of print].

[5] Giannicola G, Polimanti D, Sacchetti FM, Scacchi M, Gumina S, Greco A, Cinotti G. Soft tissue constraint injuries in complex elbow instability: prevalence, pathoanatomy, and classification. Orthopedics. 2012 Dec;35(12):e1738-45. doi: 10.3928/01477447-20121120-18.

[6] Kulhanek J, Mestak O.Treatment of umbilical hernia and recti muscles diastasis without a periumbilical incision. Hernia. 2013 Jan 20. [Epub ahead of print]

[7] Jankovic S., D.Delimar, and D. Hudetz.2001.The groin pain syndrome (In croatian.Harviv Za Higijenu Rada1 Toksikologiju. 52:421 -428.

[8] Hart ND, Wallace MK, Scovell JF, Krupp RJ, Cook C, Wyland DJ.Quadriceps tendon rupture: a biomechanical comparison of transosseous equivalent double-row suture anchor versus transosseous tunnel repair. J Knee Surg. 2012 Sep;25(4):335-9.

[9] Petersen J, Thorborg K, Nielsen MB, Budtz-Jørgensen E, Hölmich P.Preventive effect of eccentric training on acute hamstring injuries in men's soccer: a cluster-randomized controlled trial. Am J Sports Med. 2011 Nov;39(11):2296-303.

[10] Opar DA, Williams MD, Shield AJ.Hamstring strain injuries: factors that lead to injury and re-injury. Sports Med. 2012 Mar 1;42(3):209-26.

[11] Cheng Y, Yang HL, Sun ZY, Ni L, Zhang HT.Surgical treatment of gastrocnemius muscle ruptures. Orthop Surg. 2012 Nov;4(4):253-7. doi: 10.1111/os.12008.

Treatment

Conservative Treatment of Muscle Injuries: From Scientific Evidence to Clinical Practice

Andrea Foglia, Massimo Bitocchi, Manuela Gervasi, Gianni Secchiari and Angelo Cacchio

Additional information is available at the end of the chapter

1. Introduction

The musculoskeletal injuries, both acute and chronic, are very common in sport activities accounting from 10% to 55% of all injuries and often results in prolonged rehabilitation and time out from competition (Garrett, 1996; Croisier et al.,2002). Their treatment is a challenge for all health care professionals, which are involved in the management of rehabilitation and return sporting activities of the athletes. Usually, skeletal muscle injuries are common in professional and amateur athletes. Muscle injuries often occur with over 90% caused by excessive strain or by contusion (Järvinen et al., 2005) and may result in the inability to train or compete for several weeks and have a high tendency to recur (Verrall et al., 2001; Orchard and Best, 2002). A 5-year study of European soccer players showed that muscle strain represented 30% of injuries. Among these, those of quadriceps (32%), hamstring (28%), adductor (19%), and gastrocnemius (12%) were the most common (Volpi et al., 2004).

It has been showed that injured muscles can initiate regeneration promptly, but the healing process is often inefficient and hindered by the formation of scar tissue, which may contribute to muscle re-injury (Huard et al., 2002).

The first step in the muscle injuries management is to be able to answer questions that are often asked to physician or physical therapist by the injured athlete: "How long will it take to recover?"; "When can I return to the field?". However, answer to these questions is very difficult because it depend on age, activity level of injured athlete, and by pressure of coaches, parents, managers and media, etc. Unfortunately, until today, the answers to these questions are based on personal experience rather than on clinical evidences.

The management of muscle injuries, despite the lack of high quality studies, can be improved with the knowledge of the possible mechanisms that cause muscle injuries (Ekstrand et al., 1983), and with the identification of risk factors associated with injury occurrence (Verrall et al., 2003; Brockett et al., 2004). Acquisition of these knowledge will lead to an improvement of our preventive, therapeutic and rehabilitative strategies (Gibbs et al., 2004; Cross et al., 2004; Orchard and Best, 2002; Sherry and Best, 2004; Cacchio et al, 2006) for a safe return to sport activities.

Although much progress has been made in understanding the pathogenesis of muscle injuries, to date none of the proposed hypotheses can provide a unique explanation of their occurrence, and the multifactorial etiology is frequently evoked (Gleim and McHugh, 1997).

Depending on the trauma mechanism, muscle injuries can be classified as direct and indirect. The direct form is the *contusion*, and the indirect form is the *strain* (Järvinen and Lehto, 1993). A contusion occurs when a muscle is subject to a sudden and heavy compressive force, such as a direct blow provoked by an opposing player or by an object. Muscle strain usually arises from an indirect insult when an application of excessive tensile forces is produced.

The muscle-tendon junction (MTJ) is the most involved site in the acute muscle injuries (Garrett et al., 1988), and bi-articular muscle with a greater percentage of type II fibres and pennate architecture, as rectus femoris, hamstrings, adductor longus and gastrocnemius are the most commonly injured muscles (Hasselman et al., 1995; Hughes et al., 1995; Kasemkijwattana et al., 1998; Volpi et al., 2004).

Sprinting and jumping are the most common activities associated with muscle strains (Crisco et al., 1994).

Additionally, repeated eccentric muscle contractions can result in delayed-onset muscle soreness (DOMS) with symptoms similar to muscle injuries, including decreased function, stiffness, and pain (Warren et al., 2002). DOMS is attributable to a distinct pathophysiological process that includes an inflammatory response and structural changes of the sarcomere, with a consequent reduction of muscular functional ability (Barash et al., 2002; Lieber et al., 2002). In fact, mechanical damage and leukocyte infiltration after intense eccentric exercise are known to coincide with torque reductions (MacIntyre et al., 1996).

Although new classification systems of muscle injuries have been recently proposed (Mueller-Wohlfahrt et al., 2013; Chan et al., 2012), the most widely used system classifies muscle injuries (strain and contusion) according to their severity: amount of pain, weakness, loss of extensibility and reduction of ROM, functional impairment as in the walking or running (Kujala et al., 1997; Mason et al., 2007). A mild (grade I) injury involves damage to a small number of muscle fibers and localized pain without loss of strength. A clear loss of strength coupled with pain reproduced on resistance strength test is indicative of a moderate (grade II) injury. A severe (grade III) injury corresponds with complete rupture of the muscle and loss of strength and function (Verrall et al., 2003).

Generally, the risk factors for injury are divided into intrinsic (athlete related) and extrinsic (environment-related) (Inklaar, 1994; Taimela et al., 1990). Among the intrinsic factors most frequently identified by prospective studies are: age (Gabbe et al., 2006), fatigue (Greig and Siegler, 2009), a history of previous injury (Hagglund et al., 2006; Gabbe et al., 2010), postural and biomechanical deficits (Agre, 1985), lack of extensibility, and imbalance of agonist/antagonist muscular strength and power ratio (Askling et al., 2003; Croisier et al., 2008).

Among the extrinsic factors, importance is attributed to inadequate warm-up, climatic factors, inadequate training, playground surface, inadequate sports equipment (Hawkins and Fuller, 1999).

Orchard and colleagues suggested that intrinsic factors are more predictive of a muscle injury than extrinsic factors. However, a recent systematic review concluded that no single risk factor (intrinsic or extrinsic) showed a significant correlation with hamstring muscles injuries (Foreman et al., 2006). For this reason, as mentioned above the multifactorial etiology of muscle injuries is the predominant one.

The prevention of muscle injuries is an ongoing process where intervention is necessary for as long as participants engage in the physical activities that place them at risk (Goldman and Jones, 2011). This process should be based on the four sequential steps of prevention model introduced by van Mechelen in the early 90s (Van Mechelen et al., 1992):

1. determine the size of the problem sports injuries,

2. establish the etiology and mechanism of onset of sports injuries;

3. insert the preventive measures;

4. evaluate the effectiveness of preventive measures introduced by repeating the analysis in step 1.

Many interventions are widely employed by participants, trainers, coaches and physiotherapists specifically aiming to prevent muscle injuries. Among the most used interventions there are: exercises designed to improve muscle flexibility (Van Mechelen et al., 1993) and strength, in particular by means of eccentric exercises; exercises designed to improve balance, proprioception (Emery et al., 2007), neuromuscular control, and motor skills; education among "training and the risk of injury", functional training exercises and sport-specific activities (Verrall et al., 2005).

Despite the relatively high incidence of sport injuries, evidence of the efficacy of preventive interventions is not well established. In the Systematic Review of Cochrane collaboration Goldman and Jones (2011) assumed that there isn't evidence from randomised controlled trials to draw conclusions on the effectiveness of interventions used to prevent hamstring injuries in people participating in football or other high risk activities for these injuries. Manual therapy interventions aimed to prevention of muscle injuries have produced good results, but they need to be confirmed with further research from RCTs of good quality.

2. Context

Preparing this work we wanted to identify a context characterized by muscle injury in an adult person, skeletally mature, involved in sport activities. The target population was identified in high level professional athletes, but it is obvious that the fallout application in clinical practice involves above all amateur athletes, including different sports from soccer. It seems that the sports involving sprinting, acceleration, deceleration, rapid change of direction and jumping (e.g. soccer, American football, rugby, etc.) may exposed athletes to an increased risk of muscle injuries.

The choice of a conservative treatment program for muscle injuries should be based on its effectiveness, its cost-effectiveness analysis, as well as on the expectations and aims of the athlete.

3. Systematic literature review

3.1. Objectives

The purpose of this study is to systematically review the existing literature that addresses the conservative treatment of muscle injuries in adult (skeletally mature) athletes.

3.2. Methods

Electronic databases searched for the purpose of this systematic review included: Medline and PubMed.

The research question (PICO) was defined with the following criteria:

P: Adult (skeletally mature) athletes; I: conservative treatment; C: other treatment or no treatment; O: recovery of pre-injury muscle parameters and functional activities.

P I C O	Populations/Patient	Adult (skeletally mature) athletes
	Intervention	Conservative treatment
	Comparison intervention	Other treatment or no treatment
	Outcome	Recovery of pre-injury muscle parameters and functional activities

The following search method was used:

("Athletic injuries"(Mesh) OR "Muscle, Skeletal/injuries"(Mesh) OR "Sprains and strains"(Mesh) OR Muscle injur*(Tw)) AND ("Rehabilitation"(Mesh) OR "Rehabilitation programs"(TW) OR Treatment(Tw) OR "Physical therapy modalities"(Mesh) OR "Therapeu-tics"(Mesh)) AND ("Treatment outcome"(Mesh) OR "Muscle strength"(Mesh) OR "Recovery of function"(Mesh) OR "Evidence based medicine"(Mesh))

Filters: Randomized Controlled Trial; Systematic Reviews; Guideline; published in the last 10 years

For more details on the search strategy see Appendix 1.

3.3. Results

Initially, 488 papers were identified for potential inclusion. After an analysis about the internal requirements of the studies, only five reports met the inclusion searching criteria. "The Physiotherapy Evidence Database (PEDro) Scale was used by two independent reviewers to assess the methodological quality of each included full text article" (Centre for Evidence-Based Physiotherapy. Physiotherapy Evidence Database (PEDro) Scale. Available at: http://www.pedro.fhs.usyd.edu.au/scale_item.html.)

To view the studies included and excluded from this review of the literature see appendix 2.

From the analysis of the few items found arises that there is no research on therapeutic interventions of muscle injuries. There are only a few studies on hamstring muscle injuries, which may not provide strong scientific evidence.

A recent Cochrane review (Mason et al., 2012) highlights the lack of studies about the thera-peutic interventions of muscle injuries, especially that there are not right drawings studies, precisely Randomized Controlled Trials. The authors contend that at the moment there is limited evidence to suggest an increased frequency of daily stretching to reduce recovery time and the percentage of recurrence.

Some preliminary scientific evidence available, suggests exercises to improve movement dysfunction. Another recent systematic review (Reurink et al., 2012) demonstrates that the therapeutic interventions for acute hamstring injuries such as stretching, agility and trunk stabilization exercises have limited evidence.

Sherry and Best (2004) performed a prospective randomized study to compare two rehabili-tation programs for the treatment of acute hamstring muscle injury. The study concludes that a rehabilitation program which consisted of exercises of agility and trunk stabilization was more effective than a program emphasizing isolated stretching and selective strengthening exercises of the hamstring muscles.

3.4. Discussion

Following a comprehensive appraisal of the available literature five studies were included in this systematic review. Our findings suggest a lack of research studies that addresses the conservative management of muscle injuries. All five studies included in this review concern the hamstring muscle injuries. As a consequence this limits the possibility to effectively generalize these findings to the clinical settings. The limited number of relevant articles as well as their focus only on the hamstring muscle injuries, highlights the need for future well-designed randomized controlled trials to conclusively evaluate the effectiveness of conservative treatment in the management of muscle injuries, particularly for muscles other than the hamstrings.

IMPLICATION FOR RESEARCH

In order to standardize the therapeutic approach and intervention strategies for muscular injuries should produce scientific literature characterized by an appropriate design of studies (RCT) as well as a high methodological quality.
In addition, researchers should also produce studies on alternatives muscle groups and not only hamstring muscles.

3.5. Author's conclusions

There is no consensus regarding treatment for muscle injuries. Most proposed conservative rehabilitation treatment of muscle injuries have not been assessed using randomized controlled trials. Even when randomized controlled trials have been conducted, most have low total numbers of injured athletes, which potentially explains the variability among study results. Most other studies do not provide a level of evidence greater than expert opinion. Although the initial treatment of rest, ice, compression, and elevation is accepted for muscle injuries, no consensus exists for their rehabilitation. Until further evidence is available, current practice and widely published rehabilitation protocols cannot either be supported or refuted. As medical science does not help us we have to turn our attention to the basic sciences to have an approach based on biomedical fundamentals. Thus, factors that impact skeletal muscle structure, function and regeneration are of great importance and interest not only scientifically but also clinically.

TAKE HOME MESSAGE

There is no consensus regarding the rehabilitation treatment for muscle injuries.
There is a very low production of research studies about therapeutic interventions.
The basic sciences are a benchmark for developing a rehabilitation program to manage the muscle injuries.

Despite the inconclusive results of our review, we will try to provide the reader with the tools to build a reasoned approach to manage the muscle injuries, having as a benchmark the basic sciences and the few available evidences from clinical studies.

4. Conservative treatment: from scientific evidence to clinical practice

---

Keys points

- Describe the stages of tissue healing and the importance of application of this knowledge in rehabilitation.
- Identify characteristics of the different grades of strains and application of this to rehabilitation.
- State aspects of the clinical evaluation.
- Design appropriate interventions for describe the conservative treatment from scientific evidence to clinical practice.

4.1. End points of therapy

Although a variety of conservative treatment strategies exist for the management of muscle injuries, and the "RICE (Rest, Ice, Compression, Elevation) approach" is widely accepted, there is still no consensus regarding the best conservative treatment to offer to patients with muscle injuries.

Knowledge of basic principles of skeletal muscles regeneration and repair mechanisms may help to define a rational rehabilitation program. Many authors highlighted that the healing process of an injured skeletal muscle is characterized by three phases. The first phase or *destruction phase*, is characterized by disruption and subsequent necrosis of muscle myofibrils, by the formation of a hematoma between the stumps muscle and by the inflammatory reaction. The second phase or *repair phase* consists in the phagocytosis of necrotized tissue with the regeneration of myofibers and the concomitant production of connective tissue scar and revascularization into the injured area. The third phase or *remodeling phase*, characterized by the maturation of the regenerated myofibers, contraction and reorganization of the scar tissue and recovery of the functional capacity of the muscle. Relying on the basic knowledge on connective tissue healing, an ideal treatment and rehabilitation program of an acute soft-tissue injury has been formulated to fulfill some requirements.

Firstly, immediately after the injury, the ideal treatment should follow RICE (rest, ice, compression, elevation) principles; allowing to minimized pain, swelling, inflammation, and hemorrhage, to offering the best possible condition for the healing process.

The second requirement is protection and immobilization of the damaged muscle area. To prevent additional bleeding to injury site, muscle secondary strains, and early lengthening of injured structures. A short period of immobilization following muscle injury is beneficial for the healing process. However, it was suggested that restricting the length of immobilization to a period of less than a week, the adverse effects of immobility per se can be minimized.

Thirdly, 2-3 weeks after injury, during the maturation and remodeling phase, scar tissue forms initially in a random pattern. However, perform gentle and controlled movements along the main axis of injured muscle that does not produce or increase pain at the injury site leads to a better healing process allowing to the scar tissue to align parallel to muscle fascicles ("mobile scar"). Gentle and controlled movements along the main axis of injured muscle that do not produce or increases pain at the injury site stimulates the healing process allowing to the scar tissue to assume a structural architecture with an alignment parallel to the muscle fascicles.

Finally, 6-8 weeks after injury, there are no reasons to continue to protect the affected area.

And so the rehabilitation is directed towards quick and complete return to exercise and sport activities.

From these principles we must try to build our treatment plan; will develop methods of approach to the pathological condition and therapeutic intervention strategies to be used.

It's important to understanding tissue-healing phases before discussing pathology and ultimately deciding appropriate treatment, because knowledge of tissue-healing phases will help guide the decision-making process during patient rehabilitation treatment.

Most muscle injuries will respond to rehabilitation treatment without complications. However, in cases of excessive fibroblast proliferation or of abnormal response of myoblasts to bone morphogenetic protein, exuberant scar tissue or myositis ossificans can form, respectively.

4.2. Purposes of therapy

As with other athletic injuries, the primary objective of a rehabilitation treatment for muscle injuries management is to return the athlete to sporting activities at the pre-injury level of performance with a minimal risk of injury recurrence. There are some factors that can increase the recurrence in a muscle injury such as the formation of non-functional scar tissue that is associated with an alteration in muscle tissue lengthening mechanics, reduced flexibility, muscle weakness, alteration in lower limb biomechanics (Malliaropoulos et al., 2010). It should keep in mind these factors when a rehabilitation program is prepared.

4.3. Clinical and diagnostic evaluation

As previously suggested (Askling et al. 2006), the diagnosis of muscle injuries is mainly clinical, based on detailed history of trauma and physical examination with inspection, palpation, ROM tests, manual muscle testing, and special tests.

Although clinical evaluation remain very important, imaging examinations such as ultrasound (US) and magnetic resonance (MR) provide useful information for defining the injury more precisely. It has been shown that appropriate management decisions, return to training and competitions, and prediction of injury recurrence may all be enhanced with appropriate imaging examination (Verrall et al., 2003; Gibbs et al., 2004; Cross et al., 2004; Hasselman et al., 1995). Usually, US is the imaging modality of choice in visualizing sport-related muscle injuries, since it is widely available, safe, and inexpensive tool and allows dynamic evaluation which often can be helpful in distinguishing between a partial or complete tear of injured muscle. It has the disadvantage of being examiner-dependent. In athletes in whom an US examination does not provide an adequate assessment of a suspected muscle injury, MRI should be the next imaging modality to be used. MR imaging is more sensitivity in depicting edema and extent of injury, as well as in evaluating muscle-tendon injuries.

The initial assessment is often carried out within 12h to 2 days post-injury (Askling et al., 2007).

Possible signs of swelling and ecchymosis may arise a few days later the injury and consequently may not be noticed at the initial examination (Wood et al., 2008; Askling et al., 2006).

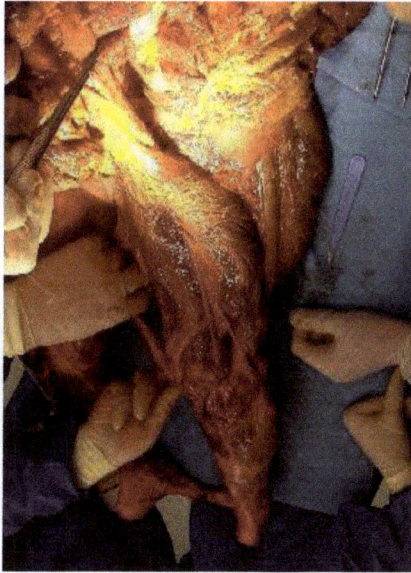

Figure 1. The cadaver anatomy hamstring

A rapid phase change of muscle contraction from eccentric to concentric has been suggested as the underlying mechanism for hamstring injuries. During running, especially fast running, the bi-articular arrangement of the hamstring muscles across the hip and knee allow the hamstrings to work eccentrically during late swing phase to decelerate the lower leg and control knee extension. A concentric contraction follows to initiate hip extension prior to heel strike. So that hamstrings are maximally loaded and lengthened during this rapid change from eccentric to concentric contraction (Proske et al., 2004). In case of an acute hamstring injury, the hip and knee ROM of the injured leg is significantly decreased compared to the uninjured leg. However, the flexibility of the hip in the acute situation is often influenced by pain as a consequence of which the test may be poor accurate.

Active ROM is decreased in the acute phase of the injury and it is advised to be measured at the end of the second day. Knee active ROM deficit 48 h after a unilateral posterior thigh muscle injury is an objective and accurate measurement.

No difference was found between active and passive ROM tests. Knee flexion and extension ROM can be estimated with a goniometer.

Strength of the hamstring muscles can be tested with the patient lying in a prone position by applying a manual resistance at the heel. The prone-resisted knee flexion should be done with different angles of knee flexion (e.g. 90°, 30°, and 15°), and with internal or external tibial rotation to target the medial (semimembranosus and semitendinosus) and lateral (biceps femoris) hamstring muscles, respectively. Due to their biarticular nature, the hamstring muscles also extend the hip, so it is recommend that hip extension strength is assessed with the knee positioned at 90° and 0° of flexion while resistance is applied to the distal posterior thigh and heel, respectively.

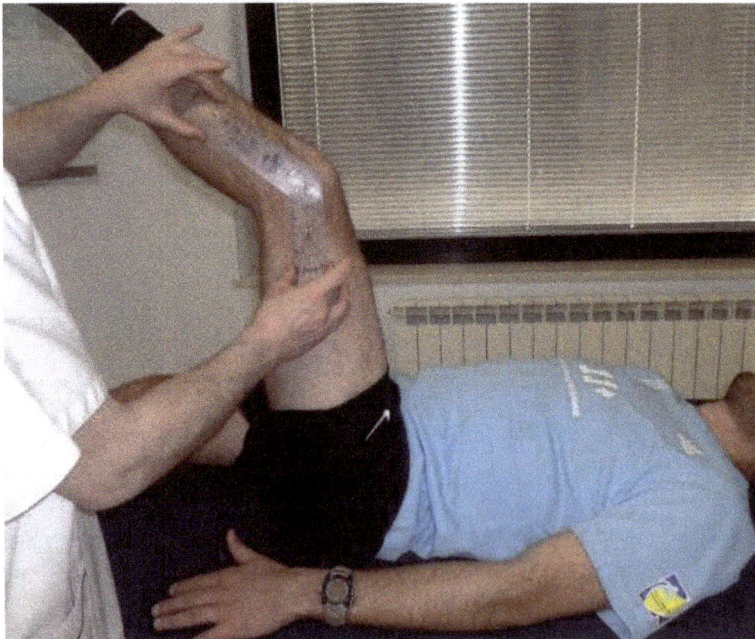

Figure 2. Test ROM knee with goniometer

Although is important evaluate also the eccentric component of strength, this should not be evaluated after an acute muscle injury due to the high load that eccentric contraction causes on the muscle structures.

Differential diagnosis of posterior thigh pain should include sciatic pain caused by nerve roots compression by herniated disc at L4-L5 or L5-S1 levels, sacro-iliac joint referred pain, gluteal trigger point referred pain, as well as other neural syndromes such as piriformis syndrome and hamstring syndrome.

Keeping in mind that "back related" hamstring injuries are characterized by a gradual buildup of pain, if these conditions are suspected, the active slump test can be used to confirm whether a patient has a neural component to their hamstring pain (Orchard et al., 2004). To completing patient evaluation also an MRI could be used to rule out these conditions.

Although imaging evaluation may not be necessary in all cases of muscle injuries, its use not only confirms the diagnosis of muscle injury but also supplies information that helps to determine the degree and location of a muscle injury, and to predict the time to sport resumption in professional and recreational athletes.

Several groups (Koulouris and Connell, 2006; De Smet and Best 2000) compared the performance of US and MRI. Among them, a prospective study (Connell et al., 2004) found US to be as useful as MRI in detecting the presence of an acute muscle (hamstrings, in this case) injury. However, the same authors affirm that more detailed analysis of the injury profile was achieved using MRI during the healing phase.

Gibbs et al. (2004) and Verrall et al. (2003) found that MRI negative hamstring strains had a significantly faster rehabilitation interval (6.6 and 16 days, respectively) compared with MRI positive strains (20.2 and 27 days, respectively) in their studies of elite Australian footballers. However, it should be keeping in mind that repeat MR imaging of athletes who have been cleared to return to sport, often show persistent high signal changes and muscle edema (Slavotinek et al., 2002; Connellet al., 2004).

In the only study to relate radiological parameters of hamstring injury to injury recurrence on return to competition Verrall et al. (2006) showed that a larger size of hamstring injury was indicative of higher risk for recurrent injury but only after the subsequent playing season was considered along with the same playing season.

4.4. Treatment strategies: How—to—treat

Determining the appropriate grade of strain will help guide the clinician through the rehabilitation process. A grade 1 strain may leave the athlete with slight discomfort and minimal swelling but full ROM and little functional deficit. A grade 2 strain is characterized by a small to moderate palpable area of involvement along with increased pain and swelling. A grade 2 muscle strain will often demonstrate restricted ROM and impaired gait. A grade 3 muscle strain is typified by a moderate to severe palpable area of involvement and sometimes a defect at the site of injury. The patient demonstrates significant deficits in ROM, and functional mobility will be severely impaired (Järvinen et al., 1978).

Today, we have a considerable amount of scientific, mostly experimental, evidence to support the early mobilization treatment approach of muscle injuries. It has been shown that early mobilization induces more rapid and intensive capillary ingrowth into the injured area, better regeneration of muscle fibers and more parallel orientation of the regenerating myofibers in comparison to immobilization, the previously preferred treatment for injured muscle (Järvinen, 1976; Järvinen and Sorvari, 1975; Järvinen, 1975; Järvinen, 1978).

The positive effects of early mobilization on the regeneration of the injured skeletal muscle are not only limited to morphostructural changes, since it has been shown that the biomechanical strength of the injured muscle achieved the level of uninjured muscle more rapidly using active mobilization rather than immobilization after a muscle injury. (Järvinen, 1976)

A short period of rest relative after muscle injury is beneficial, but it should be limited only to the first few days after the injury. This rest period allows the scar tissue connecting the injured muscle stumps to gain the required strength to withstand the contraction-induced forces applied on it without a re-injury, but being restricted to the first few days only, the adverse effects of immobility can be limited to a minimum. The experimental data showing that beginning active mobilization after the short period of immobilization enhances the penetration of muscle fibers through the connective tissue scar, limits the size of the permanent scar, facilitates the proper alignment of the regenerating muscle fibers, and helps in regaining the tensile strength of the injured muscle.

The immediate treatment of the injured skeletal muscle is known as RICE principle - Rest, Ice, Compression and Elevation. The overall justification for the use of the RICE principle is very practical, as all 5 means aim to minimize bleeding into the injury site. It needs to be stressed that there is not a single, randomized clinical trial to prove the effectiveness of the RICE principle in the treatment of soft tissue injury. However, there is scientific proof for the appropriateness of the distinct components of the concept, the evidence being derived from experimental studies. The most persuasive proof for the use of rest has been obtained from studies on the effects of immobilization on muscle healing. By placing the injured extremity to rest immediately after the trauma, one can prevent further retraction of the ruptured muscle stumps (the formation of a large gap within the muscle) as well as reduce the size of the hematoma and, subsequently, the size of the connective tissue scar. Regarding the use of ice, it has been shown that the early use of cryotherapy is associated with a significantly smaller hematoma between the ruptured myofiber stumps, less inflammation, and somewhat accelerated early regeneration (Deal et al., 2002; Hurme et al., 1993).

Although compression reduces the intramuscular blood flow to the injured area, (Kalimo et al., 1997) it is debatable whether compression applied immediately after the injury actually accelerates the healing of the injured skeletal muscle (Thorsson et al., 1997).

However, according to the prevailing belief, it is recommended that the combination of ice (cryotherapy) and compression be applied in shifts of 15 to 20 minutes in duration, repeated at intervals of 30 to 60 minutes, as this kind of protocol has been shown to result in a 3° to 7° C decrease in the intramuscular temperature and a 50% reduction in the intramuscular blood flow (Thorsson et al., 1987; Thorsson et al., 1985).

Finally, concerning the last component of the RICE principle, elevation, the rationale for its use is based on the basic principles of physiology which suggests as the elevation of an injured extremity above the level of the heart results in a decrease in hydrostatic pressure and, subsequently, reduces the accumulation of interstitial fluid.

The patient to move very carefully for the first 3 to 7 days after the injury to prevent the injured muscle from stretching.(Järvinen and Lehto, 1993).

After this period of relative rest, more active use of the injured muscle can be started gradually within the limits of pain.

The use, in this phase, of some neuromuscular control exercises of the lumbo-pelvic region are essential for optimal functional recovery. Furthermore, the normal gait should be implemented as soon as the pain allows.

Both passive and active exercises that apply a longitudinal strain to the injured structure will help the tissue accommodate to the new stress.

The treatment practiced in most of the muscle injury is the "deep transverse friction" massage. This procedure is widely used, and based on a biological hypothesis feasible with regard to the proposed mechanism of action, but the scientific evidence regarding the clinical effectiveness of "deep transverse friction" has been negative.

The request for sports massage among competitive athletes is high, but the scientific support for the effect of sport massage is very limited.

In the DOMS, massage administered 2 hours after muscle insult did not improve the function of the hamstring, but reduced the intensity of pain 48 hours after the muscle insult (Hilbert et al., 2003).

Pain-free stretching and strengthening exercises are essential to regain flexibility and strength and prevent further injury and should be initiated quickly at the end of inflammatory response phase.

Stretching exercises should be included to determine the stress lines along which collagen will be oriented. The type, duration, and frequency of stretches are three factors, which may influence or even determine its effectiveness.

Strengthening exercises program is a composite of different variables that include: muscle actions used, resistance used, volume (total number of sets and repetitions), exercises selected and workout structure (e.g., the number of muscle groups trained), the sequence of exercise performance, rest intervals between sets, repetition velocity, and training frequency. Manipulation of the program variables should be performed to be beneficial to recovery progression. Progression may be maximized by the incorporation of progressive overload, specificity, and training variation in the program.

During a rehabilitation program, strengthening exercises should begin with isometric type, and progress with isotonic type, initially without and then with the application of an external resistance such as elastic devices, dumbbells, barbells, weight-machines, etc.

In the isometric training (ie, muscle contractions in which the length of the muscle remains constant and the tension improves) all the contractions must be done without pain. Isometric training can begin with short-duration and progress to long-duration muscle contractions. Strength training with isometric contractions produces large but highly angle-specific adaptations, thus it is important to exert the muscle at different joint angles as well as in sport specific positions.

Isotonic training (i.e., the muscle length changes and the tension remains constant during muscle contraction) can be started when long-duration muscle contraction of isometric training can be performed pain free. Isotonic exercises should be firstly performed without an external resistance, which should then be introduced and progressively increased. The strength training includes single-joint exercises, multiple-joint exercises, but above all functional exercises that mimic the actual sport actions. Weakness after painful musculoskeletal injury is typically mediated by both muscular and neural adaptations. After a knee injury with anterior cruciate ligament rupture, maximal voluntary activation of the quadriceps is reduced despite restoration of knee stability over the years. In the muscle injuries little attention has been paid to the possibility that prolonged deficits in muscular activation due to a reduction of the nervous system constitutes a strategy to unload damaged tissues. The athlete often expressed fear in carrying out the action that caused the injury. The execution of this action must be re-programmed, performed, and correct if necessary. The training in specific position may prepare in an optimal manner the structure to stress that then can expect during sport activities. The progression of exercises should consider also the ROM andThe training in specific position may prepare in an optimal manner the structure to stress that then can expect during sport in to injuryangular velocity of joint. The eccentric exercises are also important. It consists in a "negative" muscular activity (muscle-tendon system absorbs energy) in which there is an overall lengthening of the muscle while under tension, in response to an external load (such as a weight) that is greater than the force generated by the muscle.

Scar tissue increasing passive stiffness of the muscle-tendon unit and making it more susceptible to injury during large eccentric contractions. Optimum tension-length curve of healthy or injured muscle can be optimized (such that peak tension is generated at longer muscle lengths) by eccentric training. Given the length-dependent nature of muscle damage in hamstring strains near end range, this structural adaptation optimizes the angle of peak torque to reduce the risk for potential injury. Despite the inherent limitations and lack of supporting evidence, Croisier et al. (2002) recommended that eccentric exercise should be included in the rehabilitation of hamstring injuries to help prevent recurrent injuries.

It has been suggested that all rehabilitation treatments should always start with an adequate warm-up of the injured muscle (Magnusson et al., 1995; Safran et al., 1988; Safran et al., 1989).

When warm-up is combined with stretching, the flexibility of muscle is improved. Painless elongation of the scar tissue can be achieved by stretching the duration of which should be gradually increased from 15 seconds to 1 minute.

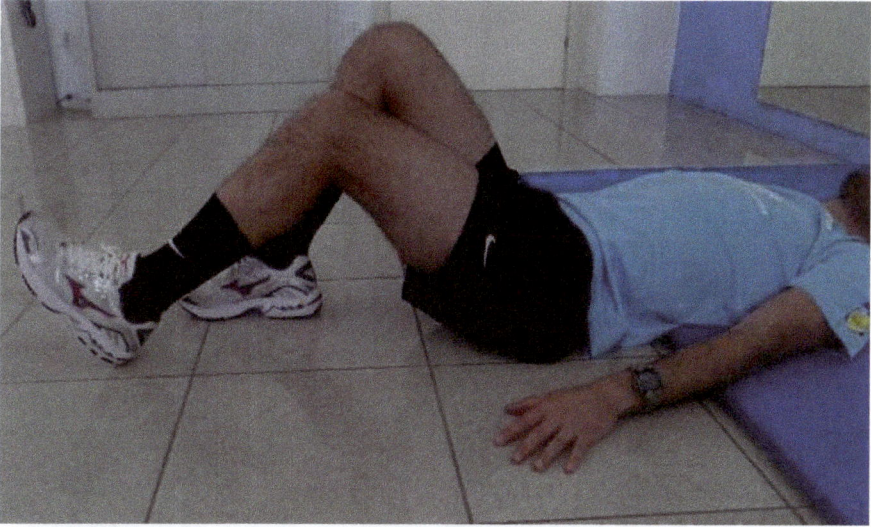

Figure 3. The patient is lying on the ground: submaximal to maximal isometric contractions at different knee angles. 5 sec of contraction 5 sec of rest for 6 times. 4 – 5 times / day.

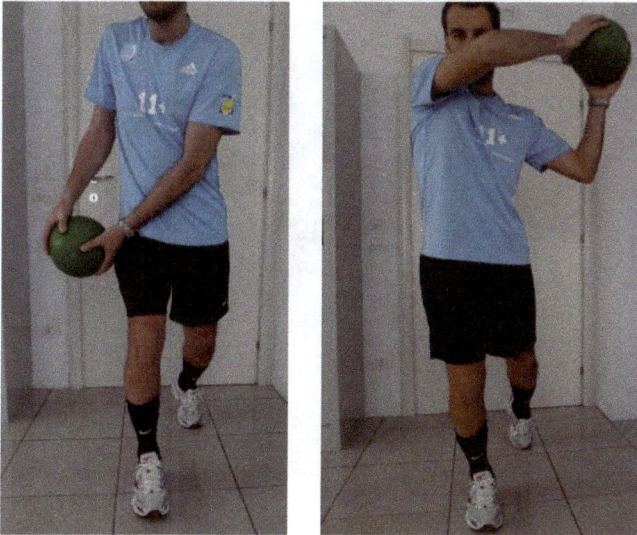

Figure 4. The patient should rotate the trunk as for kicking with the aim to train the core muscolature.

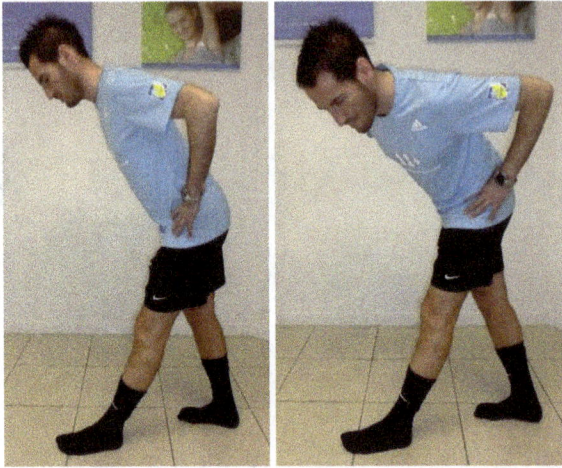

Figure 5. Walking hamstring stretch: the patient is in standing position. The injured limb is extended. Trunk flexion to stretch the hamstring muscles.

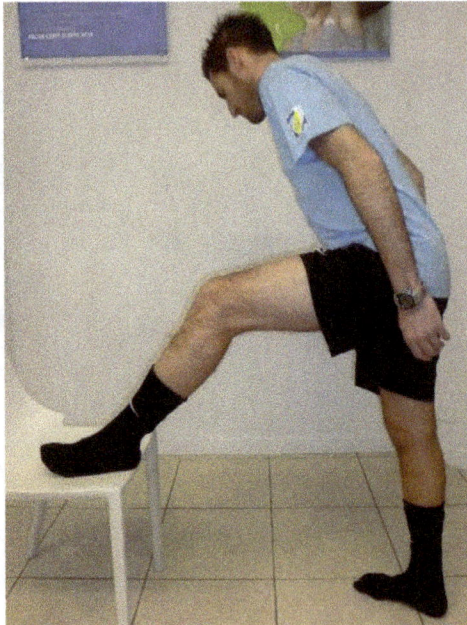

Figure 6. Hamstring stretch: swing phase position with slow side to side rotation and flexion extension of the knee.

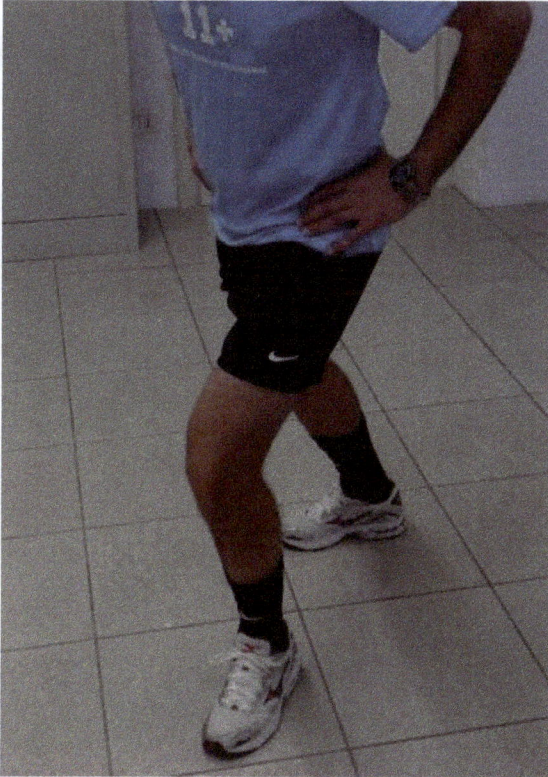

Figure 7. Lunges in all planes of motion. The patient is in standing position: must make small steps in all directions as to a change of direction.

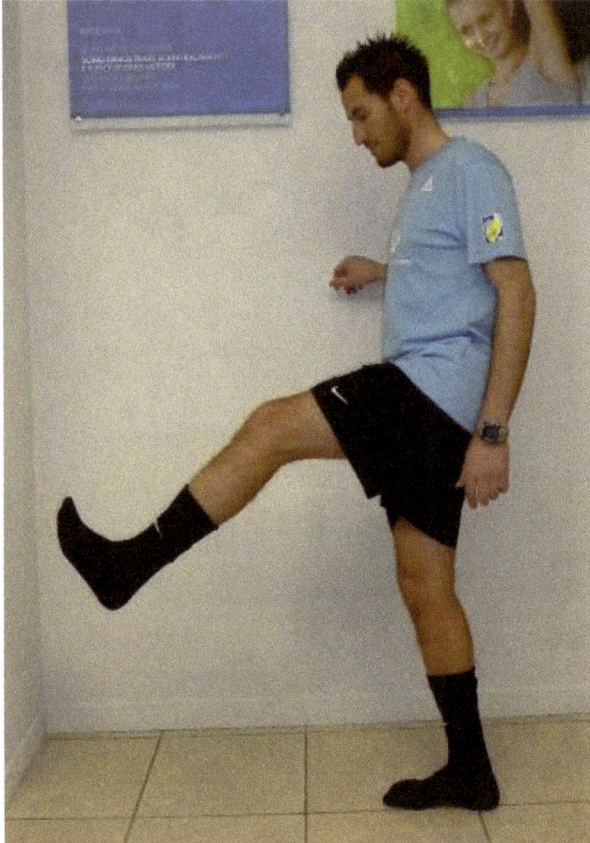

Figure 8. Foot catch exercise. The athlete stands parallel to a wall, and simulates the swing phase of walking at the first phase and after of the running. During the swing phase, the athlete performs a quick quadriceps contraction and then attempts to catch or stop the lower leg before reaching full knee extension by a hamstring contraction. In first phase with a little hip and knee extension. In a second phase increase hip and knee extension and the velocity.

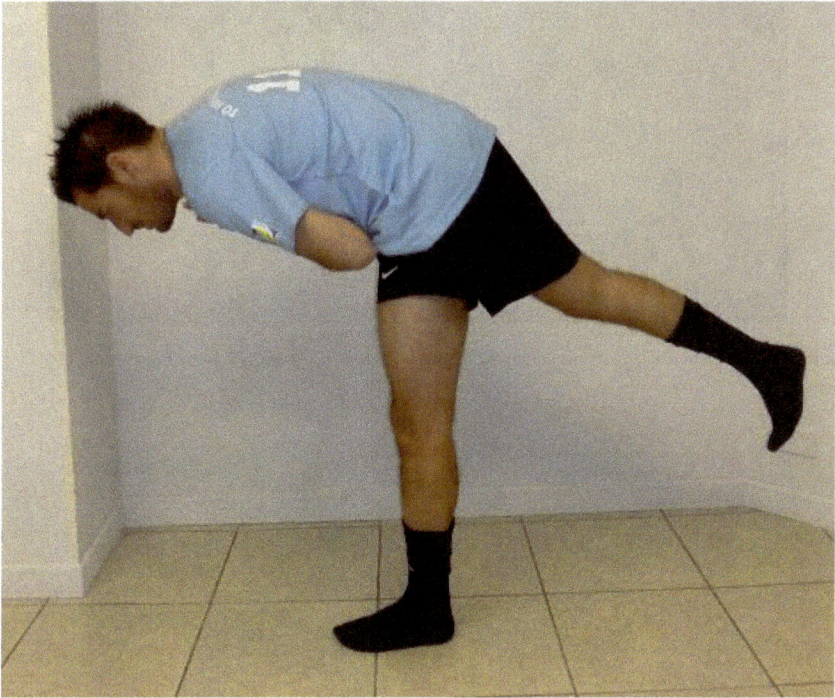

Figure 9. The patient is in an upright position on a single leg. Flexion of the trunk in all directions.

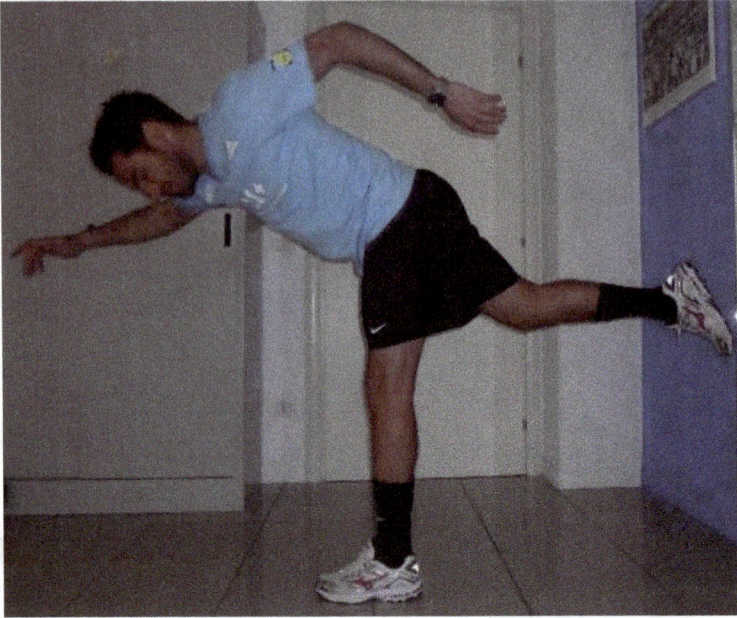

Figure 10. The patient is in an upright position on a single leg: flexion of the trunk with arms that push forward to increase the difficulty.

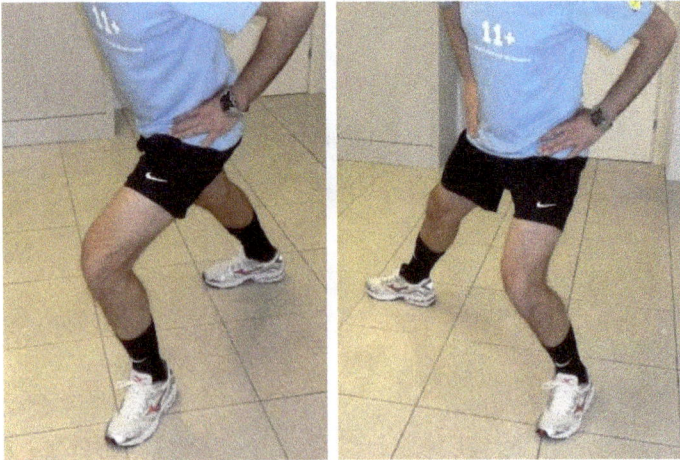

Figure 11. Lunges in all planes with return to start position. Increasing the length of the step and / or the execution speed of each sitting to vary the training stimulus.

4.5. How to monitor treatment and clinical outcomes

Although many athletes will return to activity before the MR imaging findings are resolved, follow-up imaging is useful in the case of complications and in order to provide additional information of clinical progress through a rehabilitation program and consequently to support the decision-making for return to sports.US and MRI are both useful imaging modalities in defining the location, extent and severity of muscle injury.

These modalities can assess healing or scar formation, detect associated complications, predict prognosis and monitor treatment response in muscle injuries. Greater availability, low cost, short imaging time, no contraindications (e.g., pacemakers), and dynamic capability of US favors its use in the initial assessment and subsequent follow-up of the majority of muscle injuries. However, overall its limitations, including user dependence and lower sensitivity, tend to outweigh its advantages as far as accurate pathology delineation in elite athletes is concerned. Moreover, MRI due to its higher contrast resolution appears to be the technique of choice for follow-up imaging evaluations.

The optimum time to carry out assessments of imaging follow-up is different for each case, and so it is difficult to generalize. However, it should to keep in mind that abnormalities appear to resolve sooner on US than on MRI, and US detected fewer abnormalities than MRI at 2 and 6 weeks.

The choice of imaging modality selected for the evaluation of muscle injuries will also depend on availability, cost, and operators expertise.

Since the re-injury rate can be as high as 34% after 1 year, it's very important monitor rehabilitation treatment progress by imaging evaluations. (Orchard and Best, 2002)

5. Conclusions

While efforts have been made to minimize their effect, several limitations are present in this review and it is possible that some relevant articles may have been overlooked. However, we can conclude that due to a real lack of published scientific studies until now there is no consensus about the rehabilitation treatment of muscle injuries.

A consensus classification system for muscle injuries currently does not exist, but classify muscle injuries according to their severity it may be useful for a prognosis and for establish an adequate rehabilitation treatment program.

Diagnosis of a muscle injury is mainly clinical, but enhanced by imaging findings which allow to determine its degree and location, and to predict return to sport in professional and recreational athletes.

Although commonly recommended, there is little evidence to support the RICE principles. Early mobilization for lower grade injuries and brief (1-3 days) immobilization of the extremity for higher grade injuries appear to be beneficial.

Most muscle injuries will respond to rehabilitation treatment without complications. Grade I strains have a low risk of tear extension and heal within 2 weeks with conservative management. Grade II strains require at least 4 weeks of conservative management, with a significant risk of tear extension if the patient returns to full exercise too early. It has been shown that if more than 50% of the cross-sectional area of the hamstring is torn, this correlates well with a convalescence period of greater than six weeks. Increasing length of a strain has also been correlated with an increased period of convalescence.

Prevention strategies, although promising, have not yet proven their effectiveness. Currently, there are very few scientific evidences that a determined preventative protocol has been effective, leading to a statistically significant decrease in muscular injuries. Therefore further research is needed to define its role.

Due to the lack of experimental studies on treatment of muscle injuries, basic sciences are fundamentals to build up a rationale rehabilitation treatment program.

From scientific evidence to clinical practice

\# Muscle injuries are one of the most common injuries in sports.

\# Muscle injuries heal with a scar that impedes complete regeneration.

\# Muscle injuries are classified according to the clinical impairment they cause.

\# Diagnosis of a muscle injury is instrumental

\# Ultrasonography and magnetic resonance imaging (MRI) can be used to assist diagnosis in the elite sportive

\#Ultrasonography is equally useful at identifying hamstring muscle injuries and may be preferable because of lower costs.

\# Injured skeletal muscle should be placed to relative rest after the injury for 3–7 days.

\# Immediate first aid aims at reducing the bleeding to the injured area.

\# Diagnosis can wait for the immediate treatment, icing should last for 48 hours after the injury.

\# Immediate treatment follows the 'RICE'-principle; Rest, Ice, Compression and Elevation.

\# Mobilization with manual therapy and active exercise of the injured muscle should be carried within limits of pain.

\# Mobilization program include exercises for the injured muscle,

with exercises improving agility and trunk stabilization.

\# Stretching is an important part of the mobilization programme.

\# For the most part muscle injuries to heal conservatively.

\# Non-steroidal anti-inflammatory drugs (NSAIDs) are recommended after skeletal muscle injury.

\# Corticosteroids should not be injected nor given orally to the patient with a skeletal muscle injury.

\# Therapeutic ultrasound does not have proven therapeutic effect on the regeneration of injured skeletal muscle.

\# Muscle strengthening consisting of eccentric exercise are very effective in preventing muscle injuries.

\# Massage in reducing pain instead seems to be unique on the psychological effects.

Among different therapeutic interventions, exercise plays a very important role in the prevention and treatment of muscle injuries.

Appendix

Therapeutic exercise

PHASE 1
Goals:
Correct gait
Start Isometric training
Gentle stretch pain free

---

1. 5' of low stationary biking with no resistance or 5' walking if it possibile
2. Supine hip flexion with knee exstension stretch 3 x 30 sec
• Submaximal isometric hamstrings sets 5 sec x 6 times 4 – 5 times/days
• Neuromuscolar exercise for the lumbopelvic region. 20 – 30 repetitions (foto 6 – 7)
• Ice in long sitting position for 20min.

---

1. Progression from phase 1 to phase 2 is allowed when the athlete showed a normal gait pattern, and can perform a pain-free isometric contraction against submaximal (60%-80%) resistance during prone knee flexion (90°) manual strength test.

PHASE 2
Goals:
Start isotonic training
Stretching training
Cardiovascular training

• 10' of low stationary biking with little resistance or 10' walking
• Standing hip flexion with knee extension stretch with slow side to side rotation. Standing
• hamstring stretch sport position. 3 x 30 sec
• Prone or standing position knee flexion . 3 – 4 x 12 – 15
• Light lunges in all planes (foto 10) 5 x 15 sec

2.   progression from phase2 to phase 3 is allowed when the athlete can perform all activities
     without pain.

PHASE 3
Goals:
Stretch training
Isotonic training
•10′ of low stationary biking with little resistance or 10′ walking •Non–weight-bearing "foot catches" 6 – 8 rep •Single leg deadlifts 5 x 8 – 10 rep •Single leg standing 2 x 6 – 8 rep •Nordic hamstring exercise 2 x 6 rep lunges in all planes with return to start position with different velocity 5 x 30 sec

Key: All the exercises must be performed without pain. In a first phase low intensity, a velocity
of movement that is less than or near that of normal walking; in a second phase moderate
intensity, a velocity of movement greater than normal walking but not as great as sport; in a
third phase high intensity, a velocity of movement similar to sport activity.

Appendix 1: Search strategies

Pubmed/Medline

1.   "Athletic injuries"(Mesh)

2.   "Muscle, Skeletal/injuries"(Mesh)

3.   "Sprains and strains"(Mesh)

4.   Muscle injur*(Tw)

5.   "Athletic injuries"(Mesh) OR "Muscle, Skeletal/injuries"(Mesh) OR "Sprains and
     strains"(Mesh) OR Muscle injur*(Tw)

6.   "Rehabilitation"(Mesh)

7.   "Rehabilitation programs"(TW)

8.   Treatment(Tw)

9.   "Physical therapy modalities"(Mesh)

10. "Therapeutics"(Mesh)

11. "Rehabilitation"(Mesh) OR "Rehabilitation programs"(TW) OR Treatment(Tw) OR "Physical therapy modalities"(Mesh) OR "Therapeutics"(Mesh)

12. "Treatment outcome"(Mesh)

13. "Muscle strength"(Mesh)

14. "Recovery of function"(Mesh)

15. "Evidence based medicine"(Mesh))

16. "Treatment outcome"(Mesh) OR "Muscle strength"(Mesh) OR "Recovery of function"(Mesh) OR "Evidence based medicine"(Mesh))

17. "Athletic injuries"(Mesh) OR "Muscle, Skeletal/injuries"(Mesh) OR "Sprains and strains"(Mesh) OR Muscle injur*(Tw) AND "Rehabilitation"(Mesh) OR "Rehabilitation programs"(TW) OR Treatment(Tw) OR "Physical therapy modalities"(Mesh) OR "Therapeutics"(Mesh) AND "Treatment outcome"(Mesh) OR "Muscle strength"(Mesh) OR "Recovery of function"(Mesh) OR "Evidence based medicine"(Mesh))

18. "Athletic injuries"(Mesh) OR "Muscle, Skeletal/injuries"(Mesh) OR "Sprains and strains"(Mesh) OR Muscle injur*(Tw) AND "Rehabilitation"(Mesh) OR "Rehabilitation programs"(TW) OR Treatment(Tw) OR "Physical therapy modalities"(Mesh) OR "Therapeutics"(Mesh) AND "Treatment outcome"(Mesh) OR "Muscle strength"(Mesh) OR "Recovery of function"(Mesh) OR "Evidence based medicine"(Mesh))Filters: Randomized Controlled Trial; Systematic Reviews; Guideline; published in the last 10 years

Appendix 2

Included studies

- Mason DL, Dickens VA, Vail A. Rehabilitation for hamstring injuries. Cochrane Database Syst Rev. 2012 Dec 12;12:CD004575.

- Reurink G, Goudswaard GJ, Tol JL, Verhaar JA, Weir A, Moen MH. Therapeutic interventions for acute hamstring injuries: a systematic review. Br J Sports Med. 2012 Feb;46(2):103-9.

- Copland ST, Tipton JS, Fields KB. Evidence-based treatment of hamstring tears. Curr Sports Med Rep. 2009 Nov-Dec;8(6):308-14.

- Petersen J, Hölmich P. Evidence based prevention of hamstring injuries in sport. Br J Sports Med. 2005 Jun;39(6):319-23.

- Sherry MA, Best TM. A comparison of 2 rehabilitation programs in the treatment of acute hamstring strains. J Orthop Sports PhysTher. 2004 Mar;34(3):116-25.

Excluded studies

Study	Reason for exclusion
ElMaraghy AW, Devereaux MW. A systematic review and comprehensive classification of pectoralis major tears. J Shoulder Elbow Surg. 2012 Mar;21(3):412-22.	This systematic review examines scientific literature of pectoralis major tears to identify incidence and injury patterns, while doesn't investigate interventions to treat muscle injuries.
Andia I, Sánchez M, Maffulli N. Platelet rich plasma therapies for sports muscle injuries: any evidence behind clinical practice? Expert OpinBiolTher. 2011 Apr;11(4):509-18.	Platelet-rich plasma (PRP) therapies don't represent a physical therapy treatment.
Hamilton BH, Best TM. Platelet-enriched plasma and muscle strain injuries: challenges imposed by the burden of proof. Clin J Sport Med. 2011 Jan;21(1):31-6.	Platelet-enrich plasma (PRP) therapies don't represent a physical therapy treatment.
Prins JC, Stubbe JH, van Meeteren NL, Scheffers FA, van Dongen MC. Feasibility and preliminary effectiveness of ice therapy in patients with an acute tear in the gastrocnemius muscle: a pilot randomized controlled trial. ClinRehabil. 2011 May;25(5):433-41.	This report don't study a specific sports athletes population.
Harris JD, Griesser MJ, Best TM, Ellis TJ. Treatment of proximal hamstring ruptures - a systematic review. Int J Sports Med. 2011 Jul; 32(7):490-5.	This systematic review analyzes surgical repair treatments of tendinous or bony tuberosity avulsion in the proximal hamstring. This is not a systematic review of muscle injuries.
O'Sullivan K, Murray E, Sainsbury D. The effect of warm-up, static stretching and dynamic stretching on hamstring flexibility in previously injured subjects. BMC MusculoskeletDisord. 2009 Apr 16;10:37.	This study examined the short-term effects of warm-up, static stretching and dynamic stretching on hamstring flexibility in individuals with previous hamstring injury. It didn't analyze actual muscle injuries and so treatment techniques for the rehabilitation.

Author details

Andrea Foglia[1], Massimo Bitocchi[1], Manuela Gervasi[1], Gianni Secchiari[1] and
Angelo Cacchio[2]

1 Department of Physiotherapy, "Riabilita" Centre, Civitanova Marche (MC), Italy

2 Department of Life, Health & Environmental Sciences, School of Medicine, University of
L'Aquila, L'Aquila, Italy

References

[1] Garrett W.E. (1996). Muscle strain injuries. Am. J. Sports Med. 24, S2-S8.

[2] Croisier J.L., Forthomme B., Namurois M.H., Vanderthommen M. and Crielaard J.M. (2002). Hamstring muscle strain recurrence and strength performance disorders. Am. J. Sports Med. 30, 199-203.

[3] Jarvinen TA, Jarvinen TL, KaariainenM, et al. Muscle injuries: biology and treatment. Am J Sports Med 2005;33:745–64.

[4] Verrall G.M., Slavotinek J.P., Barnes P.G., Fon G.T. and Spriggins A.J. (2001). Clinical risk factors for hamstring muscle strain injury: a prospective study with correlation of injury by magnetic resonance imaging. Br. J. Sports Med. 35, 435-439; discussion 440.

[5] Orchard J. and Best T. (2002). The management of muscle strain injuries: an early return versus the risk of recurrence. Clin. J. Sport Med. 12, 3-5.

[6] Volpi P, Melegati G, Tornese D, et al. Muscle strains in soccer: a five-year survey of an Italian major league team. Knee Surg Sports TraumatolArthrosc 2004;12:482–5.

[7] Huard J, Li Y, Fu FH. Muscle injuries and repair: current trends in research. J Bone Joint Surg Am. 2002 May;84-A(5):822-32.

[8] Ekstrand J, Gillquist J. Soccer injuries and their mechanisms: a prospective study. Med Sci Sports Exerc 1983;15:267-270.

[9] Verrall G, Slavotinek J, Barnes P, et al. Diagnostic and prognostic value of clinical findings in 83 athletes with posterior thigh injury: comparison of clinical findings with magnetic resonance imaging documentation of hamstring muscle strain. Am J Sports Med. 2003;31:969-973.

[10] Brockett C, Morgan D, Proske U. Predicting hamstring strain injury in elite athletes. Med Sci Sports Exerc. 2004;36:379-387.

[11] Gibbs N, Cross T, Cameron M, et al. The accuracy of MRI in predicting recovery and recurrence of acute grade one hamstring muscle strains within the same season in Australian Rules football players. J Sci Med Sport. 2004;7:248-258.

[12] Cross T, Gibbs N, Cameron M, et al. Acute quadriceps muscle strains: magnetic resonance imaging features and prognosis. Am J Sports Med. 2004;32:710-719.

[13] Orchard J, Best T. The management of muscle strain injuries: an early return versus the risk of recurrence. Clin J Sport Med. 2002;12:3-5.

[14] Sherry M, Best T. A comparison of 2 rehabilitation programs in the treatment of acute hamstring strains. J Orthop Sports PhysTher. 2004;34:116-125.

[15] Cacchio A, Melegati G, Volpi P. Return to Play. In: Volpi P (Ed), Football Traumatology - Current Concepts: from prevention to Treatment. Springer - Verlag, Milan, Italy, 2006; pp. 389-399.

[16] Gleim GW, McHugh MP. Flexibility and its effects on sports football medical research program: an audit of injuries in injury and performance. Sports Med 1997;24:189-99.

[17] Garrett WEJr, Nikolaou PK, Ribbeck BM, et al. The effect of muscle architecture on the biomechanical failure properties of skeletal muscle under passive extension. Am J Sports Med 1988;16:7–12.

[18] Hasselman CT, Best TM, Hughes C, et al. An explanation for various rectus femoris strain injuries using previously undescribed muscle architecture. Am J Sports Med 1995;23:493-499.

[19] Hughes C. 4th, Hasselman C.T., Best T.M., Martinez S. and Garrett W.E. Incomplete, intrasubstance strain injuries of the rectus femoris muscle. Am. J. Sports Med. 1995; 23, 500-506.

[20] Kasemkijwattana C., Menetrey J., Somogyi G., Moreland M.S., Fu F., Buranapanitkit B., Watkins S.C. and Huard J. Development of approaches to improve the healing following muscle contusion. 1998. Cell Transplant. 7, 585-598.

[21] Järvinen M, Lehto MUK. The effect of early mobilization and immobilization on the healing process following muscle injuries. Sports Med. 1993;15:78-89.

[22] Crisco JJ, Jokl P, Heinen GT, Connell MD, Panjabi MM. A muscle contusion injury model: biomechanics, physiology, and histology. Am J Sports Med. 1994;22:702-710.

[23] Warren G.L., Ingalls C.P., Lowe D.A. and Armstrong R.B. What mechanisms contribute to the strength loss that occurs during and in the recovery from skeletal muscle injury? J. Orthop. Sports Phys. Ther.2002; 32, 58-64.

[24] Barash I.A., Peters D., Friden J., Lutz G.J. and Lieber R.L. Desmin cytoskeletal modifications after a bout of eccentric exercise in the rat. Am. J. Physiol. Regul. Integr. Comp. Physiol. 2002;283, R958- R963.

[25]   Lieber R.L., Shah S. and Friden J. Cytoskeletal disruption after eccentric contraction-induced muscle injury. Clin. Orthop. 2002;403, S90-S99.

[26]   MacIntyre D.L., Reid W.D., Lyster D.M., Szasz I.J. and McKenzie D.C. Presence of WBC, decreased strength, and delayed soreness in muscle after eccentric exercise. J. Appl. Physiol. 1996;80,1006-1013.

[27]   Kujala UM, Orava S, Järvinen MJ. Hamstring injuries: current trends in treatment and prevention. Sports Med 1997;23:397-404.

[28]   Mason DL, Dickens V, Vail A. Rehabilitation for hamstring injuries. Cochrane Database Syst Rev. 2007;CD004575.

[29]   Mueller-Wohlfahrt HW, Haensel L, et al. Terminology and classification of muscle injuries in sport: The Munich consensus statement. Br J Sports Med. 2013;47:342-50.

[30]   Chan O, Del Buono A, Best TM, Maffulli N. Acute muscle strain injuries: a proposed new classification system. Knee Surg Sports TraumatolArthrosc. 2012;20:2356-62.

[31]   Inklaar H. Soccer injuries II: aetiology and prevention. Sports Medicine 1994;18:81-93.

[32]   Taimela S, Kujala UM, Osterman K. Intrinsic risk factors and athletic injuries. Sports Med 1990;9:205-215.

[33]   Gabbe BJ, Branson R, Bennell, KL. A pilot randomised controlled trial of eccentric exercise to prevent hamstring injuries in community-level Australian Football. J Sci Med Sport 2006;9:103-109.

[34]   Greig M, Siegler JC. Soccer-specific fatigue and eccentric hamstrings muscle strength. J Athl Train. 2009;44:180-184.

[35]   Hagglund M, Walden M, Ekstrand J. Previous injury as a risk factor for injury in elite football: a prospective study over two consecutive seasons. Br J Sports Med. 2006;40:767-772.

[36]   Gabbe BJ, Schneider-Kolsky M, Bennell KL. Clinical predictors of time to return to competition and of recurrence following hamstring strain in elite Australian footballers. Br J Sports Med. 2010;44:415-419.

[37]   Agre JC. Hamstring injuries. Proposed aetiological factors, prevention, and treatment. Sports Med 1985;2:21-33.

[38]   Askling C, Karlsson J, Thorstensson A. Hamstring injury occurrence in elite soccer players after preseason strength training with eccentric overload. Scand J Med Sci Sports. 2003;13:244-250.

[39]   Croisier JL, Ganteaume S, Binet J, et al. Strength imbalances and prevention of hamstring injury in professional soccer players: a prospective study. Am J Sports Med. 2008;36:1469-1475.

[40] Hawkins RD, Fuller CW. A prospective epidemiological study of injuries in four English professional football clubs. Br J Sports Med 1999;33:196-203.

[41] Foreman TK, Addy T, Baker S, et al.. Prospective studies into the causation of hamstring injuries in sport: a systematic review. PhysTher in Sport 2006;7:101-109.

[42] Goldman EF, Jones DE. Interventions for preventing hamstring injuries: a systematic review. Physiotherapy. 2011 Jun;97(2):91-9.

[43] Van Mechelen W, Hlobil H, Kemper HC. Incidence, severity, aetiology and prevention of sports injuries. A review of concepts. Sports Med 1992;14:82-99.

[44] van Mechelen W, Hlobil H, Kemper HC, et al. Prevention of running injuries by warm-up, cool-down, and stretching exercises. Am J Sports Med 1993;21:711-719.

[45] Emery CA, Rose MS, McAllister JR, et al. A prevention strategy to reduce the incidence of injury in high school basketball: a cluster randomized controlled trial. Clin J Sports Med 2007;17:17–24.

[46] Verrall GM, Slavotinek JP, Barnes PG. The effect of sports specific training on reducing the incidence of hamstring injuries in professional Australian Rules football players. Br J Sports Med 2005;39:363-368.

[47] Opar DA, Williams MD, Shield AJ. Hamstring strain injuries: factors that lead to injury and re-injury. Sports Med 2012;42:209–26.

[48] Boening D. Delayed-onset muscle soreness (DOMS). DtschArztebl 2002;99:372–77.

[49] Ong A, Anderson J, Roche J. A pilot study of the prevalence of lumbar disc degeneration in elite athletes with lower back pain at the Sydney 2000 Olympic Games. Br J Sports Med 2003;37:263–6.

[50] Orchard JW, Farhart P, Leopold C. Lumbar spine region pathology and hamstring and calf injuries in athletes: is there a connection? Br J Sports Med 2004; 38:502–4.

[51] Orchard JW. Intrinsic and extrinsic risk factors for muscle strains in Australian football. Am J Sports Med 2001;29:300–3.

[52] Woods C, Hawkins RD, Maltby S, et al. The Football Association Medical Research Programme: an audit of injuries in professional football—analysis of hamstring injuries. Br J Sports Med 2004;38:36–41.

[53] Malliaropoulos N Papacostas E, Kiritsi O, Papalada A, Gougoulias N, Maffulli N (2010) Posterior thigh muscle injuries in elite track and field athletes. Am J Sports Med 38:1813–1819.

[54] Askling CM, Tengvar M, Saartok T, et al. Acute first-time hamstring strains during high-speed running: a longitudinal study including clinical and magnetic resonance imaging findings. Am J Sports Med 2007;35:197–206.

[55] Wood DG, Packham I, Trikha SP, Linklater J (2008) Avulsion of the proximal ham-string origin. J Bone JtSurg Am 90:2365–2374.

[56] Askling C, Saartok T, Thorstensson A 2006 Type of acute hamstring strain affects flexibility, strength, and time to return to pre-injury level. Br J Sports Med 40:40–44.

[57] Connell DA, Schneider-Kolsky ME, Hoving JL, Malara F, Buchbinder R, Koulouris G, Burke F, Bass C (2004) Longitudinal study comparing sonographic and MRI assess-ments of acute and healing hamstring injuries. AJR Am J Roentgenol 183:975–984.

[58] Proske U, Morgan DL, Brockett CL, et al. Identifying athletes at risk of hamstring strains and how to protect them. ClinExpPharmacol Physiol. 2004; 31:546-550.

[59] Koulouris G, Connell D. Imaging of hamstring injuries: therapeutic implications. EurRadiol. 2006;16(7):1478–1487.

[60] De Smet AA, Best TM. MR imaging of the distribution and location of acute ham-string injuries in athletes. AJR Am J Roentgenol. 2000;174(2):393–399.

[61] Koulouris G. and Connell D. Imaging of hamstring injuries: therapeutic implications. Eur Radiol. 2006 Jul; 16(7):1478-87.

[62] De Smet AA. and Best TM. MR imaging of the distribution and location of acute hamstring injuries in athletes. AJR Am J Roentgenol. 2000 Feb;174(2):393-9.

[63] Connell DA, Schneider-Kolsky ME, Hoving JL, et al. Longitudinal study comparing sonographic and MRI assessments of acute and healing hamstring injuries. AJR Am J Roentgenol. 2004;183(4):975–984.

[64] Gibbs, N., T. Cross, et al. (2004). "The accuracy of MRI in predicting recovery and re-currence of acute grade one hamstring muscle trains within the same season in Aus-tralian Rules football players." Journal of Science and Medicine in Sport 7(2): 248-58.

[65] Verrall, G. M., J. P. Slavotinek, et al. (2003). "Diagnostic and prognostic value of clini-cal findings in 83 athletes with posterior thigh injury: comparison of clinical findings with magnetic resonance imaging documentation of hamstring muscle strain." Am J Sports Med 31(6): 969-73

[66] Slavotinek, J. P., G. M. Verrall, et al. (2002). "Hamstring Injury in Athletes: Using MR Imaging Measurements to compare extent of muscle injury with amount of time lost from competition." Am J of Roentgenol 179: 1621-1628.

[67] Connell DA, Schneider-Kolsky ME, Hoving JL, et al. Longitudinal study comparing sonographic and MRI assessments of acute and healing hamstring injuries. AJR Am J Roentgenol. 2004;183(4):975–984.

[68] Verrall, G. M., J. P. Slavotinek, et al. (2006). " Assessment of physical examination and magnetic resonance imaging findings of hamstring injury as predictors for recurrent injury." J Orthop Sports PhysTher. 36 (4): 215-24.

[69] Järvinen M, Sorvari T. A histochemical study of the effect of mobilization and immobilization on the metabolism of healing muscle injury. In: Landry F, ed. Sports Medicine. Miami, Fla:Symposia Specialists, Orban WAR; 1978:177-181.

[70] Järvinen M. Healing of a crush injury in rat striated muscle, 3: a microangiographical study of the effect of early mobilization and immobilization on capillary ingrowth. ActaPatholMicrobiol Scand. 1976;84A:85-94.

[71] Järvinen M, Sorvari T. Healing of a crush injury in rat striated muscle, description and testing of a new method of inducing a standard injury to the calf muscles. ActaPatholMicrobiol Scand.1975;83A:259-265.

[72] Järvinen M. Healing of a crush injury in rat striated muscle, 2: a histological study of the effect of early mobilization and immobilization on the repair processes. ActaPatholMicrobiol Scand. 1975;83A:269-282.

[73] Deal DN, Tipton J, Rosencrance E, Curl WW, Smith TL. Ice reduces edema: a study of microvascular permeability in rats. J Bone Joint Surg Am. 2002;84:1573-1578.

[74] Hurme T, Rantanen J, Kalimo H. Effects of early cryotherapy in experimental skeletal muscle injury. Scand J Med Sci Sports. 1993;3:46-51.

[75] Kalimo H, Rantanen J, Järvinen M. Muscle injuries in sports. BaillieresClinOrthop. 1997;2:1-24.

[76] Thorsson O, Lilja B, Nilsson P, Westlin N. Immediate external compression in the management of an acute muscle injury. Scand J Med Sci Sports. 1997;7:182-190.

[77] Thorsson O, Hemdal B, Lilja B, Westlin N. The effect of external pressure on intramuscular blood flow at rest and after running. Med Sci Sports Exerc. 1987;19:469-473.

[78] Thorsson O, Lilja B, Ahlgren L, Hemdal B, Westlin N. The effect of local cold application on intramuscular blood flow at rest and after running. Med Sci Sports Exerc. 1985;17:710-713.

[79] Stratford P. Reliability: consistency or differentiating among subjects? Phys Ther. 1989 Apr;69(4):299-300.

[80] Hilbert J.E., Sforzo G.A., Swensen T. The effects of massage on delayed onset muscle soreness. Br J Sports Med. 2003 Feb;37(1):72-5.

[81] Magnusson SP, Simonsen EB, Aagaard P, GleimGW, McHugh MP, Kjaer M. Viscoelastic response to repeated static stretching in the human hamstring muscle. Scand J Med Sci Sports. 1995;5:342- 347.

[82] Safran MR, Garrett WE Jr, Seaber AV, Glisson RR, Ribbeck BM. The role of warm-up in muscular injury prevention. Am J Sports Med.1988;16:123-129.

[83] Safran MR, Seaber AV, Garrett WE Jr. Warm-up and muscular injury prevention. An update. Sports Med. 1989;8:239-249.

[84] Takala TE, Virtanen P. Biochemical composition of muscle extracellular matrix: the effect of loading. Scand J Med Sci Sports. 2000;10:321-325.

[85] Schneider-Kolsky ME, Hoving JL, Warren P, Connell DA. A comparison between clinical assessment and magnetic resonance imaging of acute hamstring injuries. Am J Sports Med. 2006;34(6):1008-1015.

[86] Kornberg C, Lew P. The effect of stretching neural structures on grade one hamstring injuries. J Orthop Sports PhysTher. 1989; 10(12):481-487.

[87] Turl SE, George KP. Adverse neural tension: a factor in repetitive hamstring strain? J Orthop Sports PhysTher. 1998;27(1):16-21.

Chapter 6

The Treatment of Muscle Hematomas

Maria Conforti

Additional information is available at the end of the chapter

1. Introduction

Muscle injuries with hematomas are one of the most common events occurring in sport traumatology and require careful clinical and instrumental evaluation and timely treatment in order to restore a good functional outcome. The consequences of a failed treatment can be very serious, postponing an athlete's return to sports for weeks or months because of possible recurrences and complications (Gabbett, 2000).

2. Epidemiology

Muscle contusion is one the most common cause of morbidity from sports-related injuries, together with sprains and strains. Muscle trauma mainly results from sporting activities and accounts for 15 to 50% of sports injuries. Muscle injuries are the most common injuries in sports, with hamstring injuries accounting for 29% of all injuries in athletes. The playing style, refereeing, extent and intensity of match play might influence changes in the incidence of injuries in top-level tournaments. Strict application of the Laws of the Games is an important means of injury prevention (Junge and Dvorak, 2013). A good training and a good warming-up are suggested to reduce muscle injuries.

3. Etiology

The muscle hematoma can be the consequence of an impact against an external blunt or against a bone (direct trauma) or of a excessive or uncoordinated contraction (indirect trauma) (Fig 1). In a direct trauma, when the muscle is contracted, the contusion will impact more superficial tissues while, in a relaxed muscle, the structural damage and the consequent hematoma, generally occur in depth, nearest the bone. The severity of the lesion depends on the site of impact, the activation status of the muscles involved, the age of the patient, and the presence of fatigue.

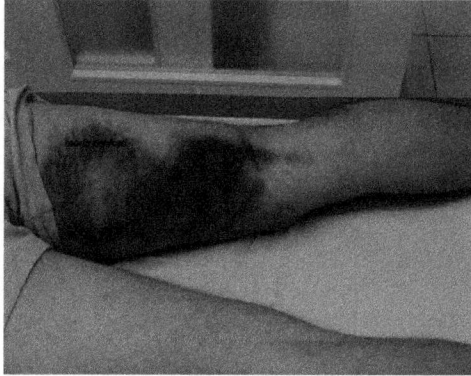

Figure 1. Hamstring subcutaneous hematoma occurred in consequence to a muscle rupture after a sudden eccentric contraction

The size of the effusion can be more or less conspicuous depending on the athlete's muscle status of contraction and on the athlete's characteristics of vascularization and coagulation. Very influent in the severity of hematoma are inherited abnormalities of coagulation like Antitrombine III or C protein or S protein deficit, or quantitative abnormalities in Leiden V or VIII or IX factors or anti-coagulants therapies or massive anti-inflammatory drugs use. External condition like a delayed or insufficient compression is important as well.

4. Classification

Many classifications of muscle injuries have been performed in according with anatomical location, pathophysiological characteristics, clinical and radiological features (Tol et al., 2013) (Chan, N. Maffulli et al classification 2012) (The Munich Consensus Statement). Depending on the muscular structures involved, muscle injuries are distinguished in intramuscular, myofascial, myofascial/perifascial and musculo-tendinous.

The **intramuscular** hematoma is characterized by the integrity of epimysium and by blood extravasation into the body of the muscle affected by the trauma. This causes an increasing of the intramuscular pressure with consequent compression of the capillary bed, which contrasts the bleeding; therefore clinical signs and symptoms remain localized. Since the presence of blood flow may cause an increase in the osmotic gradient, the swelling may increase more than 48 hours after the traumatic event. This change of the osmotic gradient causes a passage of the

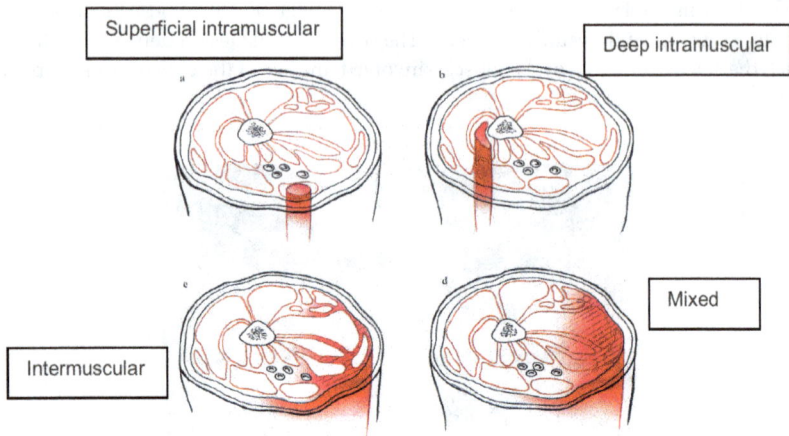

Figure 2. From Orthopaedic Sports Medicine: Principles and Practice Delee, Jesse C. M.D.; Drez, David Jr. Saunders Company, 1994

interstitial fluid through the muscle fascia, in order to balance the same osmotic gradient. This fact causes a further increase in the swelling of the injured muscle up to the limits of extensibility of the muscle fascia or the muscle itself. The main symptoms related to the onset of an intramuscular hematoma consists of pain, especially during the first 72 hours after the trauma and, after a few days, involve a decreased contractility and muscle functionality and extensibility. The prognosis for intramuscular hematomas is worse than for intermuscular hematomas, and experts' opinions suggest treating these with drainage in order to avoid potential post-traumatic myositis ossificans or fibrosis.

Although **intermuscular** hematomas appear initially more dramatic due to the resultant bruising and swelling, intramuscular hematomas are considered a more serious condition because the intact fascia creates an increasing of muscle pressure.

In intermuscular hematoma the muscle fascia looks damaged thereby allowing the extravasation of blood flow between muscles and fascia. This causes the formation of a more or less wide livid and swelling area. Contrary to the intramuscular hematoma, the intermuscular hematoma causes a painful symptoms limited to the first 24 hours post-trauma.

Finally in case of a **mixed** hematoma, after a first stage characterized by a temporary pressure increasing due to an extravasation, a rapid decrease in blood pressure can be observed. The swelling due to a blood extravasation appears usually after 24-48 hours, but after a sudden increase in pressure and swelling, the symptoms decrease and functional recovery is fairly rapid with an usually complete healing.

The knowledge of skeletal muscle regeneration principles and healing processes can help in respecting the timing for return to competitions (Klein, 1990).

Muscle repair is a multistep process which includes myofibers degeneration, regeneration and remodeling by acute inflammatory response (Clever JL, Sakai Y, Wang RA, Schneider DB 2010).

The phases of **inflammation** are, in order: organization of the hematoma, necrosis and finally, degeneration of muscle fibers with diapedesis[1] of macrophages and phagocytosis of necrotic material Anti-inflammatory drugs which target cyclooxygenase-2 are found able of hindering the skeletal muscle repair process. Muscle regeneration phase can be aided by growth factors, including insulin-like growth factor-1 and nerve growth factor, but these factors are typically short-lived, and thus more effective methods of healing are needed. Skeletal muscle injuries are repaired by muscle cells, myoblasts in condition of oxygenation. The stem cells repair the tissue with paracrine effects, leading to neovascularization of injured site. The *Gharaibeh B'*Group of University of Pittsburgh has found that factor invoked in paracrine action is Angiotensin II, the hormone of blood pressure control.The "LOSARTAN", a drug receptor blocker, in fact reduces fibrotic tissue formation and improves repair of murine injured muscle(Gharaibeh et al. 2012)Other authors hypothesized that a combination of platelet-rich plasma (PRP) injection and oral administration of LOSARTAN, as antifibrotic agent, could enhance muscle healing by stimulating muscle regeneration and angiogenesis and by preventing fibrosis in contusion-injured skeletal muscle Terada et al., 2013.

The stage of **regeneration** includes all final phases of the healing process: the production of connective tissue scar and neoangiogenesis, phases very important for the restoration of the muscle visco-elastic properties. The low neovascularization would cause fibrosis, due to local ischemia and low O2 tension. So, in this phase, it's important the utilization of physical therapies which cause vasodilatation and neovascularization.

The regeneration process requires the activation of a myogenic stem cells population,, which give rise to proliferating myoblasts. Today we know that repair of muscle takes place with the increase of protein synthesis and activation of satellite cells (stem cells) The satellite cells are quiescent myogenic precursor cells located between the basal membrane and the sarcolemma of myofiber. The adaptation of skeletal muscles to altered use is governed by three major processes: satellite (stem) cell activity, gene transcription, and protein translation. A defect in any of these processes could interfere with muscle maintenance and regeneration. (Shefer G 2012).

In the **remodeling** phase we can observe the "restitutio funtio lesa".

Myoblasts differentiate and unite together into regenerated myofibers. During the final stages of muscle repair, myofibers remodel to produce mature muscle fibers and recover the contractile capacity of the injured muscle (Mayssa et al 2012)

In response to stimuli such as injury or exercise, satellite cells become activated and express myogenic regulatory factors (MRFs, transcription factors of the myogenic lineage including Myf5, MyoD, myogenin, and Mrf4) that proliferate and differentiate into myofibers. The MRF

---

1 Passage of corpuscular elements of the blood through the capillary walls, typical of inflammatory states.

family of proteins controls the transcription of important muscle-specific proteins such as myosin heavy chain and muscle creatine kinase.

The MGF mechano-growth factor isoform appears to work by activating satellite cells MGF expresses the level of mechanical stress in muscles and other tissues and could have a important role in muscle growth and repair.

5. Clinical examination and prognosis

We extend these new findings to clinical practice to propose an evidence-based approach for the diagnosis and optimal treatment of skeletal muscle hematomas. Optimal treatment of skeletal muscle injuries start with the right diagnosis (Jarvinen et al., 2005). The clinical diagnosis of a surface hematoma is rather easy thanks to the detection of a bruised area of variable extension depending on the extent of the trauma, contextual to swelling and loss of muscle function. On the other hand, the clinical diagnosis of a deep hematoma may be much more complicated. In this case, the clinical diagnosis must necessarily be supported by the imaging consisting of ultrasonography and / or MR. However, the formulation of a precise and definitive diagnosis in case of an intramuscular hematoma, becomes possible only after 12-72 hours from the detrimental event, since the formation of the hematoma may also appear over three days after the trauma, thereby preventing a possible early diagnosis. A more detailed characterization of the injury can be made using imaging (ultrasound or MRI) repeated at second, seventh and fifteenth day, and certainly at the time of going back to aerobic and anaerobic work (Nanni and Roi, 2013).

A decrease in swelling, a reduction in pain, in the appearance of an area in the first 24 hours post-traumatic and a recovery of muscle function, are indicators of a favorable prognosis. On the contrary, an increase or a persistent swelling after 48-72 hours, an increase in pain, a decrease of peripheral pulses, a prolonged or progressive limitation of joint caused by pain or muscle weakness, a numbness and a sense of / or paresthesia below the area of injury, are all negative prognostic factors.

In any case, there is a better prognosis in the case of intermuscular compared intramuscular hematoma In case of intermuscular hematoma is possible an early mobilization and the patient returns to the sport activity between 1 and 10 weeks. On the contrary, the intramuscular hematoma, especially if is extended, requires greater caution in order to avoid the worrying complications, the myositis ossificans or the fibrosis. For this reason, in the case of intramuscular hematoma, return to sport activity is generally not possible before a period of 10-20 weeks (Ryan, 1999).

6. Imaging

The evaluation of the longitudinal size (measured in mm) is a more important severity predictor than the cross section of the lesion and the entity of the hematoma. Ultrasonography, with panoramic vision, performed after 24-48 hour is useful in localizing the hematoma and in characterizing its different types. Findings can include the following: circumscribed lesion, anechoic lesion compatible with a liquefied hematoma, circumscribed lesion of mixed echogenicity compatible with areas of liquefied hematoma, coagulated blood, and edema. Considerations could also be made on investigation methods: Ultrasound (Fig. 3 and Fig. 4) is considered an operator-dependent method while MRI (Fig. 5 and Fig. 6) appears to be more sensitive to follow the evolution and to well evaluate extensive lesions.

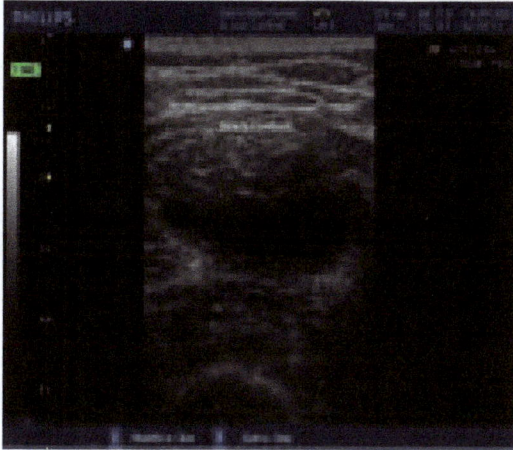

Figure 3. Transversal section: 4,6 x 2 cm lesion in Rectus femoris at day 6, before drainage

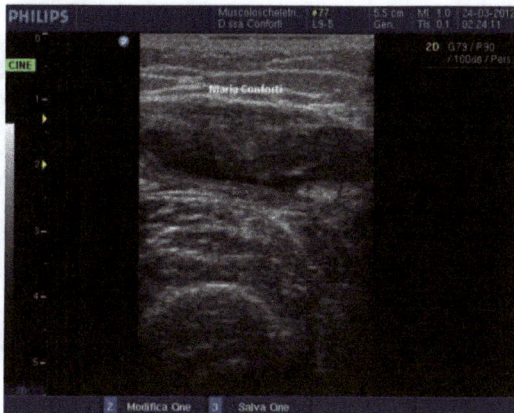

Figure 4. After drainage at day 6

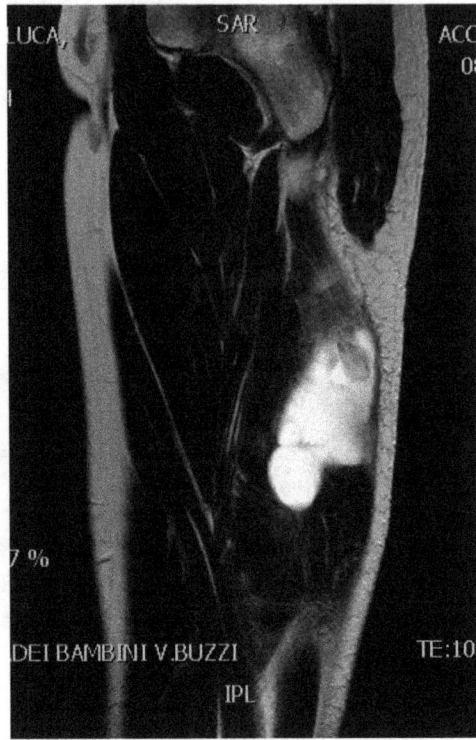

Figure 5. Axial and Coronal MR of hematoma in the hamstring muscle group at day 10.

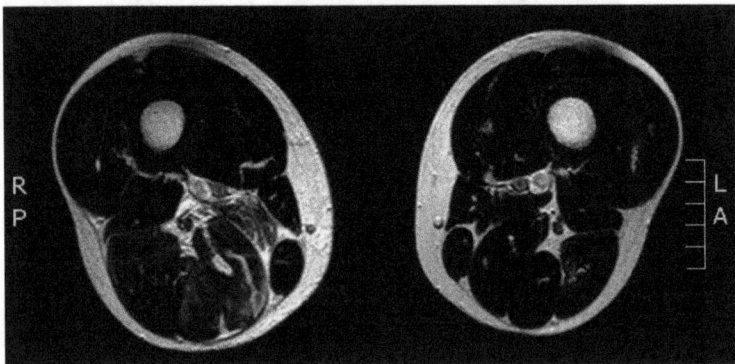

Figure 6. Axial and Coronal MR of hematoma in the hamstring muscle group at day 10.

Aside from the different degrees of seriousness in muscle damages, it is necessary to consider the anatomical location where the damage occurred in order to plan the most proper rehabilitation treatment.

7. Treatment

The first aid for any kind of muscle injury is the **RICE** (Rest, Ice, Compression and Elevation) principle or **PRICE** (Protection, Rest, Ice, Compression and Elevation) principle. The aim of RICE is to stop the injury-induced bleeding into the muscle tissue and thereby to reduce the extent of the injury (Thorsson et al., 1997).

7.1. Rest

Rest is recommended during the first 24-72 hours following the traumatic event (Reström and Peterson, 2001), in order to prevent further bleeding and exacerbation of fibrillar necrosis at the site of the lesion, thus allowing a better scar (Reström, 2003). Some authors recommend, in case of important hematoma in the lower limb, the total abstention from the load for 48 hours (Lachmann and Jenner, 1994; Reström, 2003). The duration of the rest period depends on the extent of the trauma and the pain symptoms of the patient.

7.2. Elevation

The elevation of the injured limb may contribute to the resolution of the hematoma reducing blood pressure and increasing venous return (Gray, 1977; Williams, 1980; Peterson and Reström, 2001; Reström, 2003;).

7.3. Compression

The aim for applying a compression bandage on the injured area is to limit a further haemorrhage (O'Donoghe, 1984; Klein, 1990; Peterson and Reström, 2001). The compression bandage should be maintained for a period of 2 -7 days, but not neglected until a substantial decrease in the swelling and a fluctuation reduction of the palpable mass is obtained (Thorsson et al., 1987; Thorsson et al., 1997). The amount of compression due to the different types of bandage causes different responses at the site of the lesion: high compression, approximately 85 mmHg, obtain an immediate stop of intramuscular blood flow, while a low compression, in the order of 40-45 mmHg, reduces blood flow about 50%. In the bibliography there are not studies on the optimal compression intensity in the case of intra-or intermuscular hematoma. Certainly the patient should not feel pain or have ischemia symptoms.

7.4. Ice

The cooling of a body area involves a complex of physiological responses that Fu et al. (2007) summarized in: Vasoconstriction-Analgesia-Reduction of edema - Muscle contracture. This initial response induces respectively:

- A decrease in capillary blood flow

- An improvement of lymphatic drainage.

- A reduction in the local metabolism

- A reduction in the enzymatic liberation

- A decrease in histamine liberation

- A decrease in nerve conduction velocity and a change in sympathetic activity

The lowering of the temperature causes an increase in blood viscosity with a reduction of blood flow and a reduction of vascular permeability in the cooling area. This physiological effect induced by cold is the key mechanisms in the reduction of edema due to the increasing of venous diameter and of the inflammatory reaction (Smith et al., 1993; Low and Reed, 2000).

A crucial point in cryotherapy application is the duration of cooling. The cooling of a healthy body area initially causes a reflex vasoconstriction, for a period between 9 to16 minutes, followed by a vasodilatation phase between 4 and 6 minutes, after which vasoconstriction reappears. For this reason the application of cold pack on a hematoma should have a duration between 12 and 15 minutes, with interruption of about 10 minutes. The total duration of treatment cryotherapy, however, must be appropriate to the level of the lesion (Lindsey, 1990), because unfortunately is based on empiricism (Bleakeley et al., 2004). We recommend ice bag for 20 minutes (Meaney et al., 1979) or airjet cryotherapy at -3°C for 5 minutes applied several times in a day. The muscle becomes tenser, stiffer, and less elastic as a result of cooling, and the mechanical properties are not fully recovered even after 15 min. So, in results of muscle injuries, warming-up is suggested after cooling to enable normalization of mechanical properties of the muscle.In any case cryotherapy appears particularly indicated in the first 24 hours post-trauma (Gray, 1977; Williams, 1980; Klein, 1990; Lachmann and Jenner, 1994; Renström and Peterson, 2001; Prentice, 2004).

Cryotherapy is used to prevent muscle damage, (Bailey et al 2007) either separate or associated to stretching in the stretching -spray technique (Taylor et al., 1995). Cryoultrasound (cryotherapy with ultrasound) therapy has more scientific evidence in treatment of tendonitis thank in muscle injury (Costantino et al., 2005).

7.5. Mobilisation

In the treatment of injured skeletal muscle, an immobilization should immediately be carried out or, at least, an avoidance of muscle contractions should be encouraged. The key to a right therapy consists in the appropriate timing between immobilization and mobilization. However, the duration of immobilization should be limited to a short period, sufficient to produce a scar able to bear the forces induced by re-mobilization, thus avoiding to mobilize a lesion healed with type I collagen fibers that would facilitate re-injury. The muscle activity (mobilization) should be started gradually respecting the physiological phases of wound healing and with the limits of not pain. On the other hand, early return to activity is desirable to optimize the regeneration of healing muscle and recovery of the flexibility, elasticity and strength of the injured skeletal muscle to pre-injury levels.

The interval to muscle repair might be shortened by certain adjuvant therapies which induce higher metabolic turnover.

In case of a not yet organized blood mass, it may be appropriate, from the seventh to twelfth day, to drain the hematoma, under ultrasound guidance. This is possible when blood is melted (Sofka et al., 2001; Del Cura et al., 2010; Zabale and Corta 2010).

Ultrasound is the most appropriate tool for interventional procedures on the hematoma when the lesion is visible with this methodology. The target area is easily identified with ultrasound and needle or catheter position is easily and efficacy documented (fig 7). Advantages of US-guided procedures include the absence of ionizing radiation, real-time monitoring during needle placement, decreased risk of injury to vessels and nerves, real time confirmation of procedure success of complete fluid aspiration. Complications are rare and can be avoided by using proper sterile technique and evaluate for potential contra-indications to the procedure.

8. Kinesiotaping

Kinesiotaping (KTT) is no more clinically effective than the usual care tape/elastic bandage. There was limited evidence that KTT in conjunction with physiotherapy was clinically beneficial for plantar fasciitis related pain in the short term; however, there are serious questions around the internal validity of this treatment. (Fig. 8 and 9) It currently exists insufficient evidence to support the use of KTT over other modalities in clinical practice but, in reality, it is largely used in practice by physiotherapists and masseurs (Morris et al., 2012).

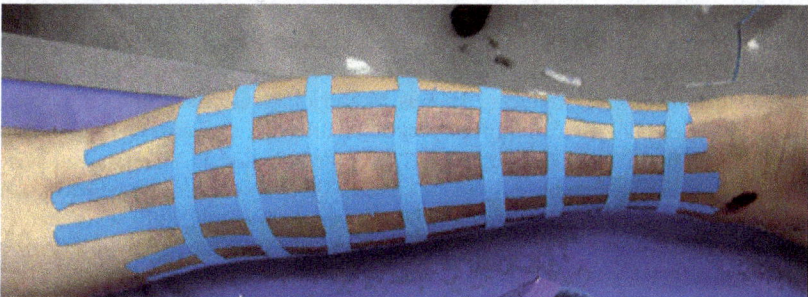

Figure 7. Kinesiotaping in medialis gastrocnemius in "tennis leg" injury

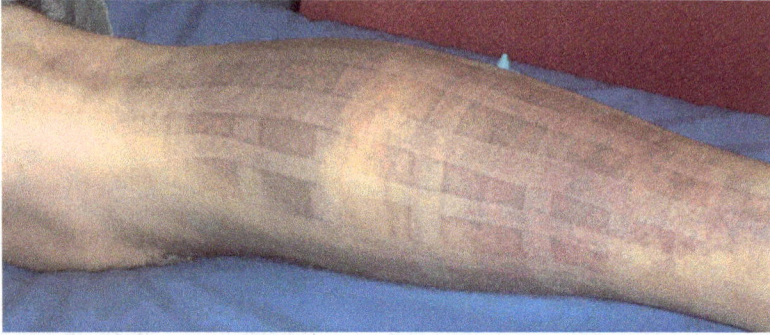

Figure 8. Evolution of the lesion after 3days

9. T.E.CA.R. THERAPY (Transfer Energetic Capacitive and Resistive)

The diathermy is based on application of electromagnetic waves; those oscillations induce a transfer of kinetic energy which is readily converted into heat. This effect of heat production in the tissues is called "Joule effect". The diathermy and every other exogenous form of application of heat is indicated only in the resolution phase of the hematoma and never in the immediate post-traumatic period. The rational application of various forms of diathermy is based on accelerating the rate of absorption of the residual hematoma, due to increased blood circulation induced by the temperature (Costantino et al., 2005).

9.1. Hyperthermia

Notoriously, heat in depth may be very helpful instrumental in hematomas re-absorption.

Also microwave diathermy (the old Marconi therapy) induced hyperthermia into the tissues and can stimulate the repair processes, allowing more efficient relief from pain, helping in the removal of toxic metabolites, reducing the muscles and joints stiffness. Moreover, hyperthermia induces hyperemia, which improves local tissue drainage, increases metabolic rate and induces alterations in the cell membrane. The biological mechanism that regulates the relationship between the thermal dose and the healing process of soft tissues with low or high water content or with low or high blood perfusion is still under study. Microwave diathermy treatment at 434 and 915 MHz can be effective in the short-term management of musculoskeletal injuries (Lehmann et al., 1993) also combined with massage therapy.

9.2. Massage therapy

Massage therapy and intense eccentric exercise, practical and non-invasive forms of therapy, also seem to have certain usefulness in preventing fibrosis.

Several studies have also shown that vascular endothelial growth factor (VEGF) can increase the efficiency of skeletal muscle repair by increasing angiogenesis and, at the same time, reducing the accumulation of fibrosis. The biological mechanism(s) behind the beneficial effect of massage are still unclear and require further more investigations and randomized human clinical studies (Best et al., 2012).

9.3. Lasertherapy

For a correct use of high power laser therapies, a practical classification is based on the precise localization in depth and on presence-absence of hematoma in muscular injuries.

On the basis of this, the following classification can be purposed:

A) Injury to a depth of 0.5 to 2.5 cm, without hematoma

B) Lesion to a depth of 0.5 to 2.5 cm, with hematoma

C) Injury to a depth of more than 2.5 cm, without hematoma

D) Injury to a depth of more than 2.5 cm, with hematoma (Conforti et.al. 2004)

High energy **laser therapy** had developed in the last twenty years and offers today an effective help by acting in all phases of inflammation and regeneration. At the basis of biological reparative processes is a photochemical reaction able to speed up the reabsorption of intra-muscular or intermuscular hematoma and repair processes like capillarization and neoangio-genesis (Algeri et al., 2011).

It was demonstrated that laser promotes an increase in collagen IV immunolabeling in skeletal muscle in the first 7 days after acute trauma caused by cryoinjury, but does not modify the duration of the tissue-repair process. Even with LLLT (low-level laser therapy), the injured muscle tissue needs ~21 days to achieve the same state of organization as that in the non-injured muscle (Baptista et al., 2011).

The laser therapy, in the first 48 h, reduces the intensity of inflammation, in a second phase, about two weeks, it accelerates the healing process and in the third stage, about third and fourth week, of proliferative and restorative healing, it helps to avoid fibrosis, scarring or inelastic metaplasia. Distinction in soft, mid and laser power is no longer accepted, it is preferable to classify laser depending on the wavelength, the power density and the density of energy transferred for unity of surface. The choice of treatment is not empirical but based on the study of Laser radiation interaction -tissue.

The Nd-YAG laser, with 1064 nm, continuous emission is, since fifteen years, the most accredited and used method for treatment of muscle injuries due to its penetration ability, not absorption in Hb and low coefficient of water and melanin absorption (Castellacci et al., 2003)

It is known for effective possibility of transferring the right amount of energy to the injured tissue until 4 or 5 cm in depth in a short time (8-50 sec.).

Validated therapeutic protocols for the treatment of injuries with laser = 1064 nm according to the criteria of Evidence Based Medicine are defined in number of sessions, power density, time of application for spot in function to the depth.

Medical Nd Yag laser devices, without thermal control, can't be used early in presence of intense hematoma, but only after needle drainage and not before third / fifth day from the trauma due to danger of blood clotting.

Today there is a new innovative therapeutic method: laser FP3 SYSTEM. In presence of hematoma and surrounding edema, it is necessary to drain with circular manual scanning with continuous emission at a distance of 10 cm from the skin, draining with high power and low density and many times in a day with breaks of about 30 minutes, divided into mini-sessions (500Joule for session).

The patient should not perceive "heat". The Fp3 System, with Temperature Control System ® detecting T in the first mm deep, respects the absence of heating (T max = 42 ° C).

If the hematoma is over 2,5 cm deep from the skin, laser is set at 4 watt x150-200 joules at mini-session, if it is below 2,5 cm depth from the skin, it is set at 6.5 watt x 150/200 joules at mini-session, giving about a total of 800/1000 joules.

The amount of energy will be a function also of the size of the lesion, but with FP3 it is possible to immediately begin a biostimulating treatment in the first day without fear to clot the hematoma.

Physical therapies must act in the depth of the lesion, neither above nor below, and on that tissue in that precise phase.(M Conforti, 2003).

9.4. Pulsed ultrasound

TPU (Therapeutic Pulsed Ultrasound) presents beneficial effects on the muscular healing process, inducing a reduction in the production of ROS and also the expression of pro-inflammatory molecules (Victor et al., 212). Other authors conclude that, although treatment with pulsed ultrasound can promote the satellite cell proliferation phase of the myoregeneration, it does not seem to have significant effects on the overall morphological manifestations of muscle regeneration (Rantanen et al., 1999).

9.5. ESWT

Extracorporeal Shockwave Therapy (ESWT) is an alternative to surgery in calcific shoulder tendinitis when conservative treatments such as non-steroidal anti-inflammatory drugs, steroidal injections, and physiotherapy fail to relieve symptoms. It has been hypothesized that ESWT is effective in the midterm for reducing pain and improving function for patients with chronic calcific myositis or fibrosis and that a dose-response relationship exists in the treatment parameters for effectiveness (Galasso et al., 2110).

9.6. Rehabilitation programme

The rehabilitation programme should be built around progressive agility and trunk stabilization exercises, as these exercises seem to yield better outcome for injured skeletal muscle than programs based exclusively on stretching and strengthening of the injured muscle. (Järvinen et al., 2007),

In order to assess joint ROM and muscle strength, we used isokinetic dynamometer with concentric contractions (CIBEX Norm) at proposal speeds of each joint, following International accredited protocols. Very important is the dramatic effect of eccentric strength training on muscle strength, both isotonic and isokinetic. It is known that eccentric training reduces the severity of a possible indirectly occurred muscle damage.

The prognosis, returning to the initial concept, is better if the diagnosis is accurate and protocols adequate

Early active exercise in the rehabilitative process is essential for

• Decreased healing time,

• Increased structural strength and stiffness of ligaments,

• Increased collagen synthesis in tendons,

• Increased proteoglycan content in articular cartilage and periosteal expansion of bone tissue.

• Decrease muscle fibrosis.

9.7. Proprioception

Arthrogenic muscle inhibition not only slows strength gains during rehabilitation, it also slows gains in proprioception and increases susceptibility to further injury. Receptors involved in proprioception are located in skin, muscles, and joints. Information about limb position and movement is not generated by individual receptors, but by populations of afferents. Afferent signals generated during a movement are processed to code for endpoint position of a limb. The afferent input is referred to a central body map to determine the location of the limbs in space. A contribution from central feedback mechanisms to the sense of effort is relevant to muscle rehabilitation and prevention re-injuries. Positive feedback is often associated with instability and oscillation, none of which occurs in normal locomotion (Riva, 2013).

10. Complications

A possible complication is chronic organized hematoma, well circumscribed, with mass-related symptoms. It is showed by Computed tomography (CT) like a homogeneous mass with capsule formation with a soft cystic center and a fibrous pseudo-capsule, whereas ultrasound shows it to resemble a multi-locular cyst. CT is unable to discriminate the chronic expanding hematoma from other soft tissue masses.

The mass is surrounded by a rim of hyalinized fibrous tissue with a chronic inflammatory infiltrate and granulation tissue (Nakano et al., 2010). Histologically, the mass is composed of necrotic debris, fibrin and blood clots. The lesion can be treated by hyperthermia, ultrasound therapy or shock waves or, finally, by excision (Silveira et al., 2010)

11. Conclusions

Sport can be resumed when the extensibility, isotonic and isometric and isokinetic stretch tests are balanced and when the contraction is painless.

The recovery of competitiveness is possible when were recovered in field skills specific sport. We think that prevention is the best thing, but it is often difficult to eliminate the risk of intrinsic and extrinsic damage. We recommend an appropriate warm-up, an appropriate training, balancing agonist-antagonist, to recognize stages pre-lesion as contracture or fatigue and do not underestimate the lesion or his scar, do not administer medications inappropriately, do not perform incomplete or too aggressive rehabilitation and especially to properly use the means at our possession like physical therapy.

Muscle hematomas can have a significant impact on an athlete's performance, ranging from short-term performance impairment, muscle deconditioning and compartmental syndromes, to long-term problems, such as myositis ossificans and possibly muscle re-injuries. We recommend the use of protectors, well tolerated by all people, except in hot conditions, when they were uncomfortable (Mitchell,. 2000).

We conclude by suggesting to the physician to better delineate the depth of the lesion on ultrasound imaging, because all high energy treatments require precise localization in depth in order to provide the right energy level.

Author details

Maria Conforti[1,2*]

Address all correspondence to: maria@mariaconforti.it

1 Sports Physician and Physical Therapies Physician, Bergamo, Italy

2 Customer Point INAIL, Milan, Italy

References

[1] Algeri, G, & Conforti, M. Laserterapia-Trattato di Medicina Fisica e Riabilitazione a cura di G.N. Valobra.Vol II Terapia. UTET (Ed). Torino, (2000).

[2] Bailey, D. M, Erith, S. J, Griffin, P. J, Dowson, A, Brewer, D. S, Gant, N, & Williams, C. Influence of cold-water immersion on indices of muscle damage following prolonged intermittent shuttle running. J Sports Sci. (2007). Sep;, 25(11), 1163-70.

[3] Best, T. M, Gharaibeh, B, & Huard, J. Stem cells, angiogenesis and muscle healing: a potential role in massage therapies? Br J Sports Med. (2013). Jun;, 47(9), 556-60.

[4] Castellacci, E, & Ciuti, F. Di Domenica M Conforti M. Il Nd:YAG e la terapia laser ad alta Energia Collana di Medicina Funzionale clinica,biomeccanica,rieducazione e sport. Martina (Ed). Bologna (2003).

[5] Chan, O. Del Buono A, Best TM. Acute muscle strain injuries: a proposed new classification system. Knee Surg Sports Traumatol Arthrosc. (2012). Nov;, 20(11), 2356-62.

[6] Clever, J. L, Sakai, Y, Wang, R. A, & Schneider, D. B. Inefficient skeletal muscle repair in inhibitor of differentiation knockout mice suggests a crucial role for BMP signaling during adult muscle regeneration. Am J Physiol Cell Physiol. (2010). May;298(5):C, 1087-99.

[7] Conforti, M. Laserterapia ad alta versus crioterapia nelle lesioni muscolari. 7° Corso Internazionale "Ortopedia, Biomeccanica, Riabilitazione Sportiva" Assisi November, (2003). , 21-23.

[8] Conforti, M. Riabilitazione Sportiva Titolo: Lesioni muscolari nello sport. Springer Ed. Archivio di Reumatologia (2005 n). pag , 16-17.

[9] Costantino, C, Pogliacomi, F, & Vaienti, E. Cryoultrasound therapy and tendonitis in athletes: a comparative evaluation versus laser CO2 and t.e.ca.r. therapy. Acta Biomed. (2005). Apr;, 76(1), 37-41.

[10] Del Cura JLZabala R, Corta I. Ultrasound-guided interventional procedures in the musculoskeletal system. Radiologia. (2010). Nov-Dec;, 52(6), 525-33.

[11] Fu, F. H, Cen, H. W, & Eston, R. G. The effects of cryotherapy on muscle damage in rats subjected to endurance training. Scand J Med Sci Sports. (1997). Dec;, 7(6), 358-62.

[12] Gabbett, T. J. Incidence, site, and nature of injuries in amateur rugby league over three consecutive seasons. Br J Sports Med. (2000). Apr;, 34(2), 98-103.

[13] Galasso, O, Amelio, E, Riccelli, D. A, & Gasparini, G. Short-term outcomes of extracorporeal shock wave therapy for the treatment of chronic non-calcific tendinopathy of the supraspinatus: a double-blind, randomized, placebo-controlled trial. BMC Musculoskelet Disord. (2012). Jun 6;13:86.

[14] Gharaibeh, B, Chun-lansinger, Y, Hagen, T, Ingham, S. J, Wright, V, Fu, F, & Huard, J. Biological approaches to improve skeletal muscle healing after injury and disease.

[15] Birth Defects Res C Embryo Today(2012). Mar;, 96(1), 82-94.

[16] Järvinen, T. A, Järvinen, T. L, Kääriäinen, M, Aärimaa, V, Vaittinen, S, Kalimo, H, & Järvinen, M. Muscle injuries: optimising recovery. Best Pract Res Clin Rheumatol. (2007). Apr;, 21(2), 317-31.

[17] Järvinen, T. A, Järvinen, T. L, Kääriäinen, M, & Kalimo, H. Muscle injuries: biology and treatment. Am J Sports Med. (2005). May;, 33(5), 745-64.

[18] Junge, A, & Dvorak, J. Injury surveillance in the World Football Tournaments 1998-2012. Br J Sports Med. (2013). Aug;, 47(12), 782-94.

[19] Kaminski, T. W, Wabbersen, C. V, & Murphy, R. M. Concentric versus enhanced eccentric hamstring strength training: clinical implications. J Athl Train. (1998). Jul;, 33(3), 216-21.

[20] Klein, J. H. Muscular hematomas: diagnosis and management. J Manipulative Physiol Ther. (1990). Feb;, 13(2), 96-100.

[21] Lehmann, J. F, Dundore, D. E, Esselman, P. C, & Nelp, W. B. Microwave diathermy: effects on experimental muscle hematoma resolution. Arch Phys Med Rehabil. (1983). Mar;, 64(3), 127-130.

[22] Mayssa, H, Mokalled, A, Johnson, N, Creemers, E, & Olson, E. MASTR directs MyoD-dependent satellite cell differentiation during skeletal muscle regeneration Genes Dev. (2012). January 15;, 26(2), 190-202.

[23] Mesquita-ferrari, R. A, & Martins, M. D. Silva JA Jr, da Silva TD, Piovesan RF, Pavesi VC, Bussadori SK, Fernandes KP Effects of low-level laser therapy on expression of TNF-α and TGF-β in skeletal muscle during the repair process. Wiley Periodicals, Inc.Lasers Med Sci. (2011). May;, 26(3), 335-40.

[24] Mitchell, B. Efficacy of thigh protectors in preventing thigh haematomas.J Sci Med Sport. (2000). Mar;, 3(1), 30-4.

[25] Morris, D, Jones, D, Ryan, H, & Ryan, C. G. The clinical effects of Kinesio® Tex taping: A systematic review.2012 Physiother Theory Pract. (2013). May;, 29(4), 259-70.

[26] Mueller-wohlfahrt, H. M, Haensel, L, Mithoefer, K, Ekstrand, J, English, B, et al. Consensus statement Terminology and classification of muscle injuries in sport: The Munich consensus statement Br J Sports Med (2013). Apr;, 47(6), 342-50.

[27] Nakano, M, Kondoh, T, Igarashi, J, Kadowaki, A, & Arai, E. A case of chronic expanding hematoma in the tensor fascia lata. Dermatol Online J. (2001). Dec;7(2):6.

[28] Nanni, G, Zanobbi, M, & Cattani, A. Congresso Internazionale di Riabilitazione Sportiva e traumatologia Isokinetic (2013). Abstract book Editors G S RoiS Della Villa Calzetti Mariucci , 135.

[29] Parra, P. F. Dal laser all'FP3. Martina (Ed). Bologna, (2007).

[30] Ryan, J. M. Myositis ossificans: a serious complication of a minor injury. CJEM (1999).

[31] Shefer, G, & Benayahu, D. The effect of exercise on IGF-I on muscle fibers and satellite cells.

[32] Front Biosci (Elite Ed)(2012). Jan 1;, 4, 230-9.

[33] Silveira, P. C, Victor, E. G, Schefer, D, Silva, L. A, Streck, E. L, Paula, M. M, & Pinho, R. A. Effects of therapeutic pulsed ultrasound and dimethylsulfoxide (DMSO) phonophoresis on parameters of oxidative stress in traumatized muscle. Ultrasound Med Biol. (2010). Jan;, 36(1), 44-50.

[34] Sofka, C. M, Collins, A. J, & Adler, R. S. Use of ultrasonographic guidance in interventional musculoskeletal procedures: a review from a single institution. J Ultrasound Med. (2001). Jan;, 20(1), 21-6.

[35] Taylor, B. F, Waring, C. A, & Brashear, T. A. The effects of therapeutic application of heat or cold followed by static stretch on hamstring muscle length. J Orthop Sports Phys Ther. (1995). May;, 21(5), 283-6.

[36] Thorsson, O, Lilja, B, Nilsson, P, & Westlin, N. Immediate external compression in the management of an acute muscle injury. Scand J Med Sci Sports. (1997). Jun;, 7(3), 182-90.

Chapter 7

Medical Treatment of Muscle Lesion

Cristiano Eirale and Giannicola Bisciotti

Additional information is available at the end of the chapter

1. Introduction

Though muscular lesions are the most common injuries in sport, there is limited evidence for the majority of management techniques. In particular, treatment aimed at minimizing the risk for recurrent muscle injurieshas progressed little in the past few decades. None of the medical treatment currently used in clinical practice is supported by strong scientific evidence.

In the following chapter we will perform a short analysis of the main medical interventions for cases of muscle strain.

2. Immobilization/Mobilization

Immobilization has been shown to result in beneficial effects in the very early phase of muscle regeneration as it appears to provide the new granulation tissue with the necessary tensile strength to resist the forces created by muscle contractions [1,2]. This can be achieved simply by applying rigid adhesive taping. The use of crutches is also recommended in cases of major lesions. After the first few days, early mobilization should commence. This provokes more rapid and intensive capillary development in the injured area, better regeneration of muscle fibers, and more parallel orientation of the regenerating myofibers in comparison to immobilization, which was the previously preferred treatment for injured muscle [3,4].

3. RICE protocol

The first treatment of a muscle lesion, as with any other injured soft tissue, normally consists of the RICE protocol (Rice, Ice, Compression and Elevation). The rationale behind this treatment is mainly to reduce hemorrhage. However, there are no randomized control trials (RCTs) which have proven the effectiveness of using RICE for soft tissue injury. However there is evidence on the effectiveness of the single components of the RICE regime [3,5].

3.1. Rest

Rest prevents an increase in the lesion gap which can occur as a consequence of the fibrotic tissue that forms with healing of the muscle lesion [4,6]. Rest also reduces the hemorrhage associated with the lesion.

3.2. Ice

There is evidence that ice utilization in the early stages of soft tissue injury is associated with a reduced haematoma and inflammatory process and therefore a quicker regenerative process [7,8].

3.3. Compression

Despite the fact that compression it has been demonstrated to reduce the blood flow in the injured area, its effectiveness is still controversial. In fact, there is no evidence,, that compression may accelerate the healing process in a muscle strain.

However, the clinical recommendations are usually to perform a combination of icing and compression for a period of 15-20 minutes, repeated in 30-60 minute intervals. This protocol has been demonstrated to reduce the intramuscular temperature to between 3° and 7° C, thus decreasing the blood flow by approximately 50% [9,10].

3.4. Elevation

It is advised to elevate the injured body part in order to decrease the hydrostatic pressure and therefore the interstitial fluid within the lesion itself.

4. NSAIDs

Experimental animal models of muscle injury have been used to examine the effect of NSAIDs on healing. These models have mostly demonstrated no effect on muscle healing, no reduction in muscle strength and no altered cytoarchitecture after injury (Jarvinen et al, 1992).

Studies conducted on humans subjects examining the effect of short courses of NSAIDs on acute muscle injury are contradictory [12,13,14,15,16].

While some investigations have not found any effect of NSAID administration on muscle recovery, there are several reports supporting a protective effect of NSAID medication, typically characterized by a lesser degree of muscle damage and functional deficit in the early period after injury.

One research study showed that Diclofenac taken priorto a strenuous exercise program produced lower levels of histological muscle damage in athletes compared with athletes who received placebo medication [17]. In addition, Naproxene has been demonstrated to decrease muscle pain post strenuous exercise [18], while ibuprofen proved to be less effective [19].

However, generally, in patients with acute hamstring muscle injury who were undergoing physiotherapy, the administration of NSAIDs had little effect on pain assessment or muscle performance.

It can be concluded that the short-term use of NSAIDs in muscle injury reduces pain and the time to return to full activity. Conversely, the few studies that have followed the repair process over a longer period of time suggest that any apparent benefit of NSAID treatment in the short term is not maintained in the long term and may result in a higher incidence of GI and CV adverse effects (ref).

An alternative to NSAIDs for analgesia is acetaminophen, which can be considered as effective as NSAIDs for pain reduction after musculoskeletal injury [20].

The prophylactic use of NSAIDs to prevent inflammation and pain that may accompany normal training and activity currently lacks scientific evidence and its use may create harmful collateral effects.

However, it is also worth considering that from a purely clinical viewpoint, the use of NSAIDs' for muscle lesions may possibly predispose to injury recurrence as a result of pain masking.

Finally on a biological level, a number of basic science studies showed that NSAIDs may inhibit muscle regeneration in the first stages of healing, which relies on the inflammatory process.

5. Injective therapy

Many injection protocols have been proposed for the treatment of muscle lesions. Corticosteroid injections, Muller-Wolfart protocol, prolotherapy, classic mesotherapy, mesotherapy with omeophatic products and others have been suggested. However, no protocol has strong scientific evidence, as there are no RCTs supporting their use. Although anecdotal clinical data and expert opinion can be found on each technique and their use in athletes [21], unfortunately, currently there is insufficient scientific evidence to support the use of such protocols..

Further research is required to assess the efficacy of these injection therapies preferably with the integration of various techniques in order to obtain a holistic approach.

5.1. Corticosteroids

The use of corticosteroids in the treatment of muscle injuries is controversial. There are concerns due to the risk of incomplete healing or rupture of the healing tissue. Moreover, any injection carries the risk of introducing infection. Experiments on animal models have been promising. Anaccelerated recovery of contractile tension after a single dose injection of corticosteroids provided soon after a muscle strain, was proven effective in rats, without any major adverse effects recorded [22].

Unfortunately, evidence is lacking on human subjects. To our knowledge, only two studies have been performed on athletes, both of which show promising results. However, neither has been confirmed by other researchers. The first research study [23] retrospectively reviewed American football players treated with corticosteroid intralesional injections for acute hamstring strain. The results demonstrated that the return to play time was reduced and that there were no adverse effects. In the second study [24], baseball pitchers were treated with corticosteroid injection for abdominal strains. This treatment resulted in a quicker recovery and return to play, without any reinjuries. Unfortunately, these studies contained many limitations which warrant further research studies before considering an implementation of such treatment.

5.2. Traumheel®

A frequently used preparation for the symptoms associated with acute musculoskeletal injuries, is Traumeel® (Biologische Heilmittel Heel GmbH, Baden-Baden, Germany). This is an antiinflammatory and analgesic homeopathic remedy combination that contains small amounts of belladonna, arnica montana radix, Aconitum napellus, chamomilla, Symphytum officinale, Calendula officinalis, Hamamelis virginina, millefolium, hepar sulphuris calcareum, and mercurius solubilis,plus a fixed combination of biological and mineral extracts. Its use in sport medicine is based on its effect on pain (Atropa belladonna), inflammation (Echinacea), bruising (Arnica montana), wound healing (Matricaria recutita, Calendula officinalis), bleeding (Achillea millefolium), edema (Mercurius solubilis), and infection (Hepar sulfuris). All these effects may have a positive effect on muscle strain healing, however, its ability to accelerate healing has not yet been demonstrated [25]. Traumeel is described to be well tolerated and without adverse effects, which are important characteristics for a product to be utilized on athletes.

5.3. Actovegin

Actovegin® is a deproteinised haemodialysate produced by Nycomed Austria GmbH. It enhances aerobic oxidation in mammals, which improves absorption of glucose and oxygen uptake in tissue. It does not contain growth factors or hormone-like substances, however, since ithas been thought to be aperformance enhancing agent, Actovegin has been banned for a period by WADA. This is despite the fact that there is evidence in the literature,that oral Actovegin does not have any anabolic or ergogenic activity in terms of muscle development [26]. There is also some scientific evidence that Actovegin may facilitate healing and reduce time of return to play following soft tissue injury [27] However, its use in mainly based on expert opinion, which are reporting good results on the use of Actovegin in athletes.

6. Mesotherapy

Mesotherapy is a term that derives from Greek mesos (middle) and therapeia (therapy). It employs multiple injections of pharmaceutical and homeopathic medications, plant extracts, vitamins, and other ingredients into subcutaneous fat. This technique has been purposed and implemented by Michel Pistor (1924–2003), a French physician which performed the first clinical research on this treatment. Mesotherapy is quite a diffusely used treatment method, especially in the sport medicine field. However there are concerns over its efficacy due to the lack of strong scientific evidence supporting its use.

In particular, there is no scientific research on the use of mesotherapy for muscle strains. However, international guidelines purpose weekly sessions to be started as soon as possible after the lesion. Common substances proposed are an anesthetic, a vasodilator and an anti-inflammatory with deep injection techniques and a miorelaxant with superficial injection techniques in the region of the lesions.

7. Prolotherapy

Prolotherapy derives its name from "proliferation therapy," or "proliferative injection therapy". It has also been called "regenerative injection therapy" ("RIT"), and some contemporary authors name the therapy according to the injected solution. The precise mechanism of action is not known. It involves injecting a non-pharmacological and non-active irritant solution into the body. This is hypothesized to reinitiate the inflammatory process which deposits additional new fibers, thereby repairing lax tendons or ligaments and also possibly promote the release of local growth factors. However, the precise mechanism of action still remains unknown. It has been used for approximately 100 years, however, its modern application can be traced to the 1950s.This was when the prolotherapy injection protocols were formalized by George Hackett, a general surgeon in the U.S.,and were based on his clinical experience of over 30 years. The concept of creating irritation or injury to stimulate healing has been recorded as early as Roman times when hot needles were poked into the shoulders of injured gladiators [28].

There are no trials on the use of prolotherapy in a population with acute muscle tears. There is some evidence for its use in chronic pathologies such as LBP [29], groin pain [30], and knee OA [31]. However, existing evidence is inconclusive. Its actual use is based on "expert opinion" and some practitioners advocate a positive impact of the use of prolotherapy in athletes in term of return to play timeframes.

8. Antifibrotic agents

Many reports indicate that the overproduction of transforming growth factor (TGF)–β in response to injury and disease is a major cause of tissue fibrosis both in animals and humans.

It has been shown that anti-fibrotic agents (suramin which acts as a TGF-β1 inhibitor by competitively binding to the growth factor's receptor) inhibits fibroblast proliferation and neutralizes the stimulating effect of TGF-β1 on the proliferation of fibroblasts in vitro (ref). An in-vivo injection of suramin (5.0 mg) two weeks after strain injury reduced muscle fibrosis and enhanced muscle regeneration, thereby leading to improved muscle strength recovery (ref). The clinical use of suramin has already been approved by the Food and Drug Administration. Although suramin can lead to side effects when administered intravenously, local intramuscular injection may not elicit the same deleterious effects and could be very useful in improving muscle healing. However, further studies are necessary in order to assess the safety and the effectiveness of this treatment [32].

9. Hyperbaric oxygen therapy

Theoreticallys, the restitution of blood supply to the injured area is fundamental for the regeneration process, in particular for the myotubes which depend soley on aerobic metabolism as the source of energy required for their regeneration. This is the basis for the application of Hyperbaric Oxygen Therapy in muscle lesions. Clinical trials are lacking, however a recent experimental study showed positive effects of this treatment on muscle injury. Further research should assess the clinical outcome of Hyperbaric Oxygen Therapy before it may be suggested for this kind of pathology [33].

10. Platelet Rich Plasma (PRP)

Platelet-rich plasma (PRP) is derived from centrifuging whole blood andhas a platelet concentration higher than that of whole blood. It is the cellular component of plasma that settles after centrifugation, which contains various growth factors (GFs). Unfortunately, despite its increasing popularity as a treatment for soft tissue injuries, there remains neither a uniform terminology nor an understanding as to what constitutes PRP. Terminology in common usage includes platelet enriched plasma (PEP) and plasma (preparation) rich in GFs (PRGFs); however, many of these terms are associated with commercial products [34].

Based on a limited number of animal model studies that have shown a positive impact of isolated recombinant GF on muscle regeneration, the application of PRP to an injured muscle is thought to accelerate regeneration, enhance healing and decrease the risk of re-injury. Studies using animal models show a reduction in the recovery time, in particular on the early stages of reparation. Early clinical trials, though mainly consisting of level 3 and level 4 evidence, show an improvement of healing for muscle injury in terms of earlier return to play [35,36].

The use of PRP as a source of GF seems attractive because it is easily obtainable with a simple apparatus and is relatively affordable. Moreover, its use has rapidly gained the support of the popular media as a result of its purported "natural" properties, high level of efficacy, and lack of side effects.

Limited risk of infection is linked to any injective technique but risk may be limited by the use of a correct sterile procedure, Moreover, the utilization of autologus blood guarantees the elimination of the risk of allergic reactions and the possibility to become in contact with infected blood. Previously, bovine derived drugs sometimes led to potentially lethal pathologies of coagulation and they have since been withdrawn from the market.

It seems that PRP does not have a systemic effect, but there is minimal research demonstrating this fact.. Nowadays, there is no evidence that PRP has a carcinogenetic effect. This is also supported by the mechanism of action as growth factors do not penetrate the cellular membrane; therefore they cannot generate DNA mutations. Actually, no other carcinogenetic mechanisms are known, so in general, PRP technique seems to be safe in this respect.

The risk of local complications linked to the use of the PRP technique seems to be more disputed. However, local tissue degeneration, muscular architecture alteration, increasing recurrence rate are all complications which have been taken into consideration in both basic and clinical research. Currently, no studies support such complications.

Different considerations regarding the risk of fibrosis are also of concern. TGF-β1 is the main regulating factor of fibrosis. Thus, it can be speculated that an incorrect use of growth factors may lead to an increase of fibrosis and a potential negative outcome in term of return to play.

From an anti-doping perspective, the topical use of growth factors has been approved. This was probably due to the demonstrable absence of any systemic effect of growth factors.

However, despite its elevated public profile and theoretical benefits, there remains many unanswered questions surrounding the use of these techniques in the management of muscle injuries, and the burden of proof remains with scientists and practitioners to confirm or refute the clinical utility of this technology.

One of the main issues seems to be determining the appropriate PRP concentration to use. Different products are present on the Orthopedics and Sport Medicine market.. However, each product presents different protocols and methods to concentrate the platelets resulting in products with different biological properties. Even if most of the products yield 10% (that means 2ml of PRP for every 20ml of blood withdrawn), their concentration of growth factors is different. It has been estimated that the growth factor concentration may vary from 3 to 27 times blood concentration. Considering that a low concentration of PRP may not give satisfactory clinical results and an excessively elevated concentration may start inhibitory processes, it appears fundamental that the concentration should be carefully monitored and controlled. Some authors indicate that the ideal concentration of PRP is four to six times the normal platelet blood concentration.

Another source of discussion is related to the presence (or absence) of White Blood Cells (WBC) in PRP. It is unclear whether the presence of white cells in PRP is an advantage or an obstacle to healing. In fact, if the anti-infective potentialities of WBC may be of benefit, their proinflammatory nature may actually be counterproductive to healing. This premise is consistent with the current understanding of the potential negative effects of inflammatory mediators on muscle healing.

Currently, it remains unclear what the impact PRP, with or without the presence of WBC, may have on the inflammatory cascade following muscle injury [37] In addition, each muscle has distinct anatomical and physiological characteristics, and as demonstrated in rabbit studies, also has distinct GF response profiles to injury. Thus, each location of injury may theoretically require different PRP preparations.

Another dilemma is the method of PRP subministration. The physiological impact on an acute muscle injury of a bolus infiltration of an unknown concentration of platelets, and thus of GF, and other factors that are found in any PRP preparation is still a mystery. Animal studies suggest that a bolus dose of recombinant GF is not as effective as sustained release. However, with the current utilized technique, all GFs are released within 1 hour from their application and this may potentially reduce their effectiveness.

The timing of application is also a source of discussion. Apparently, the first ten days (inflammatory and regenerative phases) after the lesion may constitute the ideal moment for PRP injection. An application two to three weeks after an injury, with an environment preferentially upregulated by platelet TGF-b a, may actually favor fibrosis over regeneration.

Finally, although the physiological milieu should be sufficient to activate platelets, it is unknown if a preinfiltration activation is necessary [38].

In conclusion, the use of PRP is actually based on anecdotal reports and expert opinion (Level IV evidence). Further research is necessary in order to confirm or deny the effectiveness of PRP in muscle strain. However, the apparent safety and facility of application suggests that sport medicine practitioners should consider PRP when treating elite athletes, for whom such innovative approaches may be fundamental in terms of success.

11. Stem cells

Stem cells are biological cells found in all multi-cellular organisms that can divide (through mitosis) and differentiate into diverse, specialized cell types and can self-renew to produce more stem cells. There are three accessible sources of autologous adult stem cells in humans: bone marrow, adipose tissue (lipid cells) and blood. Scientists believe that stem cell therapy has the potential to significantly revolutionize medicine. A number of adult stem cell therapies already exist, particularly bone marrow transplants that are used to treat leukemia. There is also the potential for a wider variety of diseases to be treated with stem cells (cancer, Parkinson's disease, spinal cord injuries, Amyotrophic Lateral Sclerosis, Multiple sclerosis, and some forms of myopathies). Successful trials on the implantation of stem cells directly on detrusor muscle to treat urinary incontinence have opened the way to their use in muscle pathology. Clinical trials have commenced, but the clinical use of stem cells for the treatment of muscle strains is still for the future. One concern of stem cell treatment is the risk that transplanted stem cells could potentially form tumors [39].

12. Conclusion

Medical treatments of muscle injuries have limited scientific evidence. Their use is often based on level four studies and on personal clinical experience. While /immobilization/mobilization and RICE seem to be established protocols and "classic" treatment (NSAIDs, painkillers) appears to have a limited impact, the effectiveness of any new options for treatment has yet to be demonstrated in sport medicine. While further research is warranted, the sharing of clinical experience amongst sport medicine practitioners seems fundamental in order to perform the best "clinically-based" choices. Our personal experience is that patient reactions to medical treatments are often unpredictable. The same treatment applied to the same kind of lesion in different subjects may have a completely different outcome. However, in our personal clinical experience, oftenthe same patient reacts well to the same treatment when proven successful with a previous injury. The placebo effect component of treatment is undeniable, however there could also be benefits which are highlighted more in some patients and less in others. Our conclusion is that different techniques must be considered when approaching management of a muscle lesion, due to the fact that no one technique has a strong scientific evidence base to its effectiveness. The physician should try to tailor the therapeutic choice on the bases of the lesion's characteristics, the patient needs and expectations, and the subjective reaction to different treatments in the past. Of course, the basic Hippocratic principle of the treatment safety ("Primum, non nocere"), should be always respected, in particular when approaching these kind of lesions which have been proven to heal very well without any therapeutic intervention.

Author details

Cristiano Eirale and Giannicola Bisciotti

Aspetar Hospital, Doha, Qatar

References

[1] Järvinen M., Sorvari T. Healing of a crush injury in rat striated muscle, 1: description and testing of a new method of inducing a standard injury to the calf muscles. Acta Pathol Microbiol Scand. 83A: 259-265, 1975b.

[2] Järvinen M. Healing of a crush injury in rat striated muscle: a microangiographical study of the effect of early mobilization and immobilization on capillary ingrowth. Acta Pathol Microbiol Scand.1976;84A:85-94.

[3] Järvinen TAH., Järvinen TLN., Kääriänen M., Kalimo H., Järvinen M. Muscle injury. Biology and treatment. Am. J Sports Med. 33(5): 745-764, 2005.

[4]   Järvinen M., Letho MUK. The effect of early mobilization and immobilization on the healing process following muscle injury. Sports Med. 15. 78-89, 1993.

[5]   Bleakley C, McDonough S, MacAuley D. The use of ice in the treatment of acute soft tissue injury: a systematic review of randomized controlled trials. Am. J Sports Med. 2004; 34:251-261.

[6]   Buckwalter JA. Should bone, soft tissue, and joint injuries be treated with rest or inactivity. J Orthop Res. 13: 155-156, 1995.

[7]   Hurme T., Rantanen J., Kalimo H. Effects of early cryotherapy in experimental skeletal muscle injury. Scan J Med Sci Sport. 3: 46-51, 1993.

[8]   Deal DN., Lipton J., Rosencrance E. Curl WW. Smith II. Ice reduces edema: a study of microvascular permeability in rats. J Bone Joint Surg Am. 84: 1573-1578, 2002.

[9]   Thorsson O., Lilja B., Ahlgren L., Hemdal B., Westlin N. The effect of local cold application on intramuscular blood flow at rest and after running. Med Sci Sports Exerc. ; 17:710-713, 1985.

[10] Thorsson O., Lilja B., Nilsson P, Westlin N. Immediate external compression in the management of an acute muscle injury. Scand J Med Sci Sports. 7:182-190, 1997.

[11] Järvinen M, Lehto M, Sorvari T. Effect of some anti-inflammatory agents on the healing of ruptured muscle: an experimental study in rats. J Sport Traumatol Rel Res. 1992; 14:19-28.

[12] Mishra DK, Fridén J, Schmitz MC, Lieber RL. Anti-inflammatory medication after muscle injury: a treatment resulting in short-term improvement but subsequent loss of muscle function. J Bone Joint Surg. 1995; 77A:1510-1519.

[13] Reynolds JF, Noakes TD, Schwellnus MP, et al. Non-steroidal anti-inflammatory drugs fail to enhance healing of acute hamstring injuries treated with physiotherapy. S Afr Med J. 1995; 85:517-522.

[14] Moore RA, Tramèr MR, Carroll D, et al. Quantitative systematic review of topically applied non-steroidal anti-inflammatory drugs [published correction appears in BMJ. 1998; 316:1059]. BMJ. 1998;316:333-338.

[15] Shen W, Li Y, Tang Y, et al. NS-398, a cyclooxygenase-2-specific inhibitor, delays skeletal muscle healing by decreasing regeneration and promoting fibrosis. Am J Pathol. 2005; 167:1105-1117.

[16] Warden SJ. Prophylactic use of NSAIDs by athletes; a risk/benefit assessment. Phys Sportsmed. 2010; 38:132-138.

[17] O'Grady M, Hackney AC, Schneider K, et al. Diclofenac sodium (Voltaren) reduced exercise-induced injury in human skeletal muscle. Med Sci Sports Exerc. 2000; 32:1191-1196.

[18] Dudley GA, Czerkawski J, Meinrod A, et al. Efficacy of naproxen sodium for exercise-induced dysfunction muscle injury and soreness. Clin J Sport Med. 1997; 7:3-10.

[19] Rahnama N, Rahmani-Nia F, Ebrahim K. The isolated and combined effects of selected physical activity and ibuprofen on delayed-onset muscle soreness.J Sports Sci. 2005; 23:843-850.

[20] Rahusen FT, Weinhold PS, Almekinders LC. Nonsteroidal anti-inflammatory drugs and acetaminophen in the treatment of an acute muscle injury. Am. J Sports Med. 2004; 32:1856-1859.

[21] Orchard JW, Best TM, Mueller-Wohlfahrt HW, Hunter G, Hamilton BH, Webborn N, Jaques R, Kenneally D, Budgett R, Phillips N, Becker C, Glasgow P. The early management of muscle strains in the elite athlete: best practice in a world with a limited evidence basis. Br J Sports Med 2008;42:158-159.

[22] Hakim M, Hage W, Lovering RM, Moorman CT III, Curl LA, De Deyne PG Dexamethasone and recovery of contractile tension after a muscle injury. Clin Orthop Relat Res. 2005;439:235-242.

[23] Levine WN, Bergfeld JA, Tessendorf W, Moorman CT III Intramuscular corticosteroid injection for hamstring injuries: a 13-year experience in the National Football League. Am J Sports Med. 2000;28(3)297-300.

[24] Conte SA, Thompson MM, Marks MA, Dines JS. Abdominal muscle strains in professional baseball: 1991-2010. Am J Sports Med. 2012 Mar;40(3):650-6.

[25] Schneider C. Traumeel – an emerging option to nonsteroidal anti-inflammatory drugs in the management of acute musculoskeletal injuries. Int J Gen Med. 2011; 4: 225-234.

[26] Ziegler D, Movsesyan L, Mankovsky B, Gurieva I, Abylaiuly Z, Strokov I. Treatment of symptomatic polyneuropathy with Actovegin in type 2 diabetic patients. Diabetes Care 2009 ; 32 : 1479 – 1484

[27] Pfister VA, Koller W. Therapie der frischen Muskelverletzung [Treatment of fresh muscle injury]. Sportverletz Sportschaden 1990 ; 4 : 41 – 44

[28] Hackett GS, Hemwall GA, Montgomery GA. Ligament and tendon relaxation treated by prolotherapy. Oak Park: Gustav A. Hemwall; 1993.

[29] Topol GA, Reeves KD, Hassanein KM. Efficacy of dextrose prolotherapy in elite male kicking-sport athletes with groin pain. Arch Phys Rehabil. 2005;86:697-702.

[30] Yelland M, Glasziou P, Bogduk N, Schluter P, McKernon M. Prolotherapy injections, saline injections, and exercises for chronic low back pain: a randomized trial. Spine. 2004;29(1):9-16.

[31] Reeves KD, Hassanein K. Randomized prospective double-blind placebo-controlled study of dextrose prolotherapy for knee osteoarthritis with or without ACL laxity. Altern Ther Health M. 2000;6(2):68–80.

[32] Negishi S, Li Y, Usas A, Fu FH, Huard J. The effect of relaxin treatment on skeletal muscle injuries. Am J Sports Med. 2005 Dec;33(12):1816-24

[33] Best TM, Loitz-Ramage B, Corr DT, Vanderby R. Hyperbaric oxygen in the treatment of acute muscle stretch injuries. Results in an animal model. Am J Sports Med. 1998 May-Jun; 26(3):367 72.

[34] Creaney L, Hamilton B. Growth factor delivery methods in the management of sports injuries: the state of play. Br J Sports Med. 2008; 42:314-320.

[35] Menetrey J, Kasemkijwattana C, Day CS, et al. Growth factors improve muscle healing in vivo. J Bone Joint Surg Br. 2000; 82:131-137.

[36] Hammond J, Hinton R, Curl L, et al. Use of autologous platelet-rich plasma to treat muscle strain injuries. Am. J Sports Med. 2009; 37:1135–1142.

[37] Weibrich G, Kleis W, Hafner G, et al. Comparison of platelet, leukocyte, and growth factor levels in point-of-care platelet-enriched plasma, prepared using a modified Curasan kit, with preparations received from a local blood bank. Clin Oral Implants Res. 2003; 14:357–362.

[38] Hamilton BH, Best TM. Platelet-enriched plasma and muscle strain injuries: challenges imposed by the burden of proof. Clin J Sport Med. 2011 Jan; 21(1):31-6.

[39] Quintero AJ, Wright VJ, Fu FH, Huard J. Stem cells for the treatment of skeletal muscle injury. Clin Sports Med. 2009 Jan;28(1):1-11

Chapter 8

Surgical Treatment

Giuliano Cerulli, Enrico Sebastiani, Giacomo Placella,
Matteo Maria Tei, Andrea Speziali and
Pierluigi Antinolfi

Additional information is available at the end of the chapter

1. Introduction

Muscular tissue has a good ability to regenerate that promotes the healing of lesions also extended, caused by strains, contusions and muscle lacerations. This characteristic is guaranteed by myogenic precursor cells (satellite cells) that proliferate and fill the structure of the extracellular matrix produced by fibroblasts becoming myoblasts.

Several factors make difficult the healing of the lesion: hematoma, granulation tissue, scar tissue and lesions of nerve bundles. In '84 Garret et al. [1] have shown that the tissue recovery was obstructed by a large percentage of denervated myocytes distal to the lesion.

A well-executed suture could allow early rehabilitation with a lower risk of re-rupture and stitch pullout. The main problem is figuring out which is the best surgical technique, but especially when a surgical repair is necessary and if the benefits outweigh the disadvantages.

In the choice of surgical technique are many points still debated. The surgical indication is very limited and, in most of the muscle injury, conservative treatment is certainly indicated. Location and extent of the lesion are the criteria most examined in the literature.

Some of the few in vivo studies on animals have shown that a surgical suture of the wound can accelerate healing. The myorrhaphy prevents the formation of excess scar tissue, limits the hematoma formation, decreases the infiltration of mononuclear cells, increases the number of regenerating myofibers, decreases the inflammatory response favoring the healing.

For example, lesions of the pectoralis major muscle have wider surgical indication and conservative treatment is recommended only in cases of injury at the sternoclavicular origin, in some partial tears, in older or sedentary individuals.

Some authors tend to wide the indication for surgical treatment to lesions greater than 50% of the thickness of the muscle belly and the debate is still open because of the few tests to date available, but certainly the indication is strengthened by the absence of synergistic muscles that can decrease the workload to the muscle and therefore aid healing.

The aim of this chapter is to perform a review of the literature in order to identify the muscle injury which indicate surgical treatment and its results.

2. Muscle healing

Muscle injuries are debilitating injuries, especially for athletes who risk setbacks in their career. A subcutaneous muscle tear can be caused by direct trauma, such as a contusion from a blunt object or strains, or by indirect trauma such as ischemia or a neurological dysfunction [2]. In any case these injuries are difficult to treat and unfortunately there are no clear and defined guidelines to help the physician [3].

From a biological point of view muscles have been shown to be particularly active and capable of excellent tissue regeneration. The gap between the muscle fibers is filled thanks to the myocyte cell reactivity, the presence of replicative phase cells and the production of connective tissue scar.

The healing process of muscle injury consists of three phases: the degeneration-inflammation phase, the reparative phase and the remodeling-fibrosis phase (Figure 1).

The first phase (first few days post-injury) is characterized by inflammatory stimulation caused by the cellular debris and the pro-inflammatory molecules that are released as a result of necrosis of the injured tissue; also the severed blood vessels release blood within the tissue forming hematoma, which in turn stimulates the inflammatory response. This cascade of events results in the release of cytokines, interleukins, adhesion molecules (e.g., P-selectin, L-selectin, E-selectin), Tumor Necrosis Factor alpha and growth factors (e.g. insulin-like growth factor 1 IGF-1, hepatocyte growth factor HGF, EGF, epidermal growth factor, transforming growth factor alpha and TGF beta, platelet-derived growth factor PDGF) that promote inflammation, cell migration and stimulate progress to the next stage [2 - 3]

The reparation phase (from day 7-10 to week three-four post-injury) begins with the cleaning of the tissue formed in the acute phase by macrophages that engulf the injured tissue and allow the regeneration of tissue within the lesion: it stimulates the proliferation of striated muscle tissue, the neo-angiogenesis within the neo-tissue and stimulates the production of connective scar tissue. The cells that are more active from the point of view of replication (myogenic precursor cells, or satellite cells) are located between the basal lamina and the plasma membranes of each individual myofiber; once they are released by the lesion of the basal lamina and activated by growth factors, they differentiate into myoblast and replicate forming multinucleated myotubes and possibly myofibers.

The final phase, the remodeling-fibrosis, involves the maturation of the neo-muscle tissue and the reorganization of the scar tissue, and is strongly driven by mechanical stress and the stress of the surrounding tissue that drive the neo-tissue to organize in the most functional way possible for contraction. The connective tissue produced is partly demolished, gradually leaving more space for the connections between the myofibers [4].

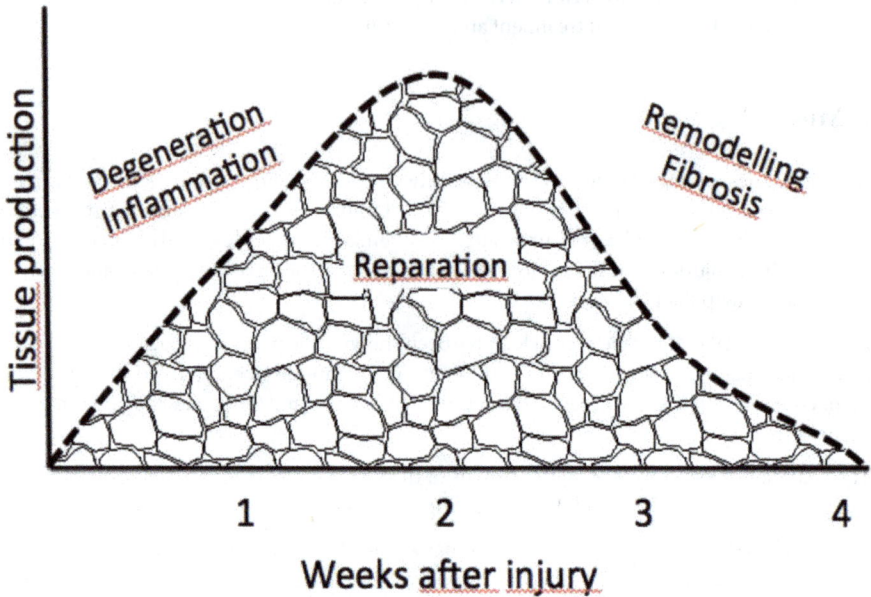

Figure 1. The diagram summarizes the three phases of muscle laceration healing. Note that reparation has a peak around the second week and concludes by the third- fourth week [2].

Fibroblasts that colonize the lesion and produce extracellular matrix play a key role in lesion healing. The connective tissue that is formed fills the gap created by the lesion with a three-dimensional plot that not only guides the proliferation of muscle cells and blood, but allows the transmission and the distribution of mechanical stresses thus acting as a sort of brace and allowing the functional use of the muscle before the lesion is completely healed. It was observed that animal muscles, thanks to this connective tissue, already after 14 days the scar that had formed in complete tears was mechanically more resistant than the surround-ing muscle [4]. It should be kept in mind that in human tissue healing times are longer and recovery is less complete but the sequence and function of the repair steps are the same [5].

This scar tissue is extremely important but it can also be an obstacle to proper healing: in fact, if there is too much of it, instead of promoting, it may prevent tissue proliferation leading to incomplete recovery [3]. A proper healing of muscle tissue is centered on the correct balance between fibroblastic proliferation and myoblast proliferation: the first promote the connective tissue that must act as a scaffold for the repopulation of the lesion by the myoblasts. When the lesion is too large, however, the gap between the proximal and the distal stump is filled with granulation tissue which results in connective tissue scar [6, 7] leaving little room for myoblast proliferation. It is possible that in the final phase (remodeling) structural improvements of the scar may occur but they are only minor [5].

The healing of the lesion depends not only on cell reactivity and the amount of scar tissue, but is closely linked to many other factors. The innervation of the tissue remaining promotes tissue viability: an excessive presence of denervated myocytes downstream of the lesion impairs proper healing [1]. Other aspects to be considered are the supply of oxygen from the surrounding tissue, the vascular proliferation and neo-angiogenesis within the lesion in the post-trauma stage, the percentage and the pattern with which the myoblasts go to form the myotubes and the collagen crosslinking [8].

3. Indication for surgery

Unfortunately very few studies are available in literature that scientifically demonstrate the benefits of one treatment rather than another.

Traditionally muscle injuries are treated conservatively and surgery is frowned upon by many surgeons for this type of lesions of the musculoskeletal system. It is common belief that surgical treatment gives results similar to, or even worse than conservative treatment [9]. Therefore it is not recommended for the fear of causing damage which would lead to further complications. The presence of hematoma and a palpable gap in the muscle belly make surgical suture difficult to perform because it is often impossible to get the fascial ends to close and the muscle fibers are hard to draw back together [5].

However, animal studies have shown that surgically sutured muscle heals more quickly and more functionally. The suture in fact decreases the distance between the muscle stumps allowing a more rapid recovery [10], decreasing major defects in scarring [11], improved healing and a decrease in deep superabundant scar tissue [3].

Obviously, surgery can lead to numerous, although fortunately infrequent, complications; therefore it is a viable option only when it guarantees clear and obvious improvements for the patient or when the lesion cannot heal if treated with the conservative approach.

Generally, surgical treatment is indicated for severe muscle tears [1, 12], in grade 4 lesions on the Ryan classification [13, 14] or when over 50% of the muscle fibers are involved. Grade 1 refers to injuries of a few muscle fibers; grade 2 - injury of a moderate number of muscle fibers; grade 3 - rupture of a moderate number of fibers associated with partial lesion of the fascia; grade 4 -those that involve injury through the full thickness muscle and the fascia (Figure 2).

From the clinical point of view, a massive rupture of the muscle leads to a loss of its strength which may be acceptable in patients with a low functional demand. However, athletes or people with high functional demands need the full recovery of muscle strength which

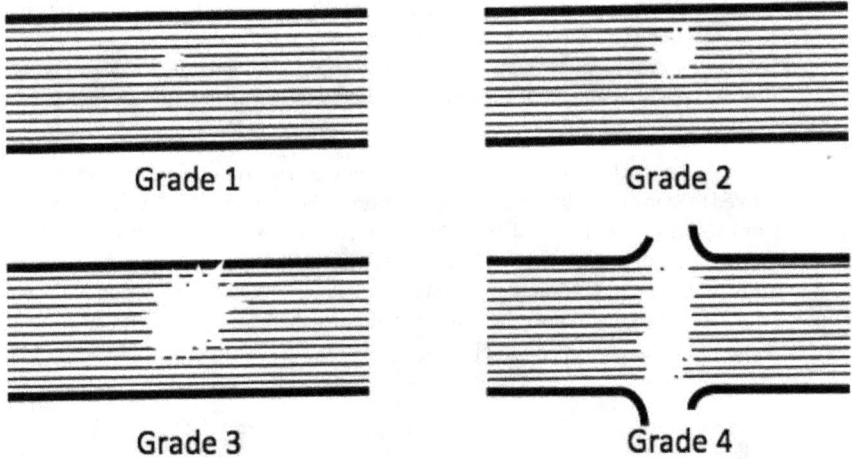

Figure 2. Ryan's Classification for muscle damage. The thin lines represent the muscle fibers, the thick lines represent the fascia.

conservative treatment in some areas and in some types of injury cannot guarantee. In literature, little has been written on myorrhaphy of the skeletal muscle and almost all of the reports focus on injuries of the biceps brachii and petctoralis majors. If these two muscles are severely damaged, a major deficit in strength and the cosmetic damage is not to be underestimated in the case of professional body-builders. The suture of muscle damage is in fact taken into consideration if the action of the muscle is not compensated for by other synergistic muscles or if the hematoma is so large that it compresses the main vessels and determines ischemia of the tissue or overlying skin [15].

The timing of the intervention is not clearly defined in the literature, Kragh et al. [16] recommend to do it the day after the traumatic event because delay it causes the suffering of muscle tissue and of the epimysium.

4. Pectoralis major

A complete lesion of the pectoralis major still allows a normal active mobilization of the shoulder, but will cause an important decrease in strength in adduction and internal rotation of the arm [17] so an early surgical reconstruction is indicated in athletes. In fact, with conservative treatment a significant loss of torque, measured using the isokinetic strength test, has been observed [18, 19] while following surgical treatment a significant increase in isokinetic torque of the muscle has been reported [20, 21]. In addition, the aesthetic damage caused by the gap following injury can cause the end of the career for body-builders and similar professionals for whom the aesthetics of the muscle is essential. Conservative treatment is recommended only in cases of injury at the sternoclavicular origin, in some partial tears, in older or sedentary individuals.

This lesion was classified and reported in literature for the first time by Patissier in 1822 and since then over 200 cases have been reported [22]. The number of these lesions has increased and the increase in the last 30 years is due to the increased participation in heavy physical activity such as weight lifting, weight training, wrestling, rugby and waterskiing. Attributable almost solely to males, these lesions occur in an age range from 16 to 91 years with a peak in athletes aged between 20 and 40 years [22]. The most common mechanism is indirect trauma during bench pressing or other weight lifting movements; less frequent injuries are those following abduction-external rotation, extension-adduction and direct trauma [23].

The lesion of this muscle may occur in different zones. Tietjen [24] used a classification divided into 3 groups: type I consists of muscle contusions and sprains; type II partial tears and type III complete lesions. Each of these groups has a subclassification based on the location of the lesion: A - muscle origin; B - belly muscle; C - myotendinous junction; D - tendon. Statistically, insertion tendon injuries are the most frequent (55%), lesions to the belly or muscular-tendon insertion cover about 35% of these injuries [23].

According to the most recent meta-analysis [23] early surgical treatment achieves significantly better results than conservative treatment with an excellent-good result in 90% of cases, compared with 17% of conservative treatment (P = 0.00000001). When surgery is delayed slightly worse results are obtained, especially after 13 weeks from injury.

While for partial lesions treatment with conservative immobilization for 2-3 weeks is indicated, where surgery is required immobilization should be 4-6 weeks and subsequently a gradual lengthening of the muscle must be performed and only after 6-12 weeks strength training can begin.

5. Biceps brachii

The lesion of the biceps usually involves the tendon portion, more often the long proximal head and to a lesser extent the distal end that inserts into the radial tuberosity. Sometimes biceps muscle tears occur in the belly, especially when the arm remains entangled in ropes during some sports such as skydiving and wakeboarding [25, 26]. Less frequently, the muscle belly can break following direct trauma in a car accident [27].

Complete laceration of the muscle belly of the biceps brachii leads to a loss of muscle strength and unfortunately, few data are available in literature regarding the right choice of treatment. One of the few studies to have compared the effects of a surgical muscle suture with conservative treatment is the one by Kragh and Basamania in 2002 [25]. In a military base in North Carolina with 25,000 paratroopers, the authors performed nine surgeries in a year and compared the results to those of three patients treated conservatively in previous years. The paratroopers treated surgically achieved significantly better results for strength (measured in supination torque) and appearance. Those who had been treated conservatively had a worse appearance, suffered easy fatigue in repetitive movements of pronation and supination (e.g. use of screwdriver), avoided weight-lifting and in two cases the musculocutaneous nerve was in contact with the skin and not covered by muscle tissue thus easily irritated even by the cuffs on the uniform.

The mechanism of injury is important for the occurrence of lacerations. In parachutists, the entrapment of the arm in the static-line during the launch determines a subcutaneous transverse lesion and an almost total one of the muscle belly with the proximal and distal stumps retracted; in this case muscle suture is indicated. In the case of water sports such as water skiing or wakeboarders, the mechanism of injury is similar with the entrapment of the arm in a towline that pulls the athlete at great speed. What differs between the two sports is that the lesion usually reported in water sports causes a tearing injury in the proximal-distal direction of the biceps and is not as clear cut as the paratroopers; this sometimes may preclude the muscle suture and require muscle resection [26].

The injury of the muscle belly of the biceps brachii is rare and closely related to particular sports; the indication for surgery is clear as it prevents functional and aesthetic deficits.

Kragh et al. in [25] with regard to the lesions of the biceps brachii recommend the intervention in the case in which the lesion extend more than 95% of the muscle belly.

6. Quadriceps femoris

No cases of suturing subcutaneous belly lacerations of the quadriceps femoris are described in literature. The only description is in a surgical case report by Straw [28]. The tear had occurred at the proximal musculotendinous junction. With surgery muscular performance improved 151% to concentric power after 6 months compared to preoperative levels.

7. Hamstring muscle

The hamstring is one of the muscle groups most affected by injuries in athletes. They often suffer strains localized in the muscle-tendon junction due to an eccentric contraction. The lesions may occur in different areas: proximal or distal muscle-tendon junction, muscle belly, the proximal and distal tendon insertion [29].

Usually hamstring injurues are treated conservatively with rest, ice, physical therapy, NSAIDs and a gradual return to sport. Rarely a lesion in this anatomical site requires surgical treatment.

One of the rare occasions when the patient may have to undergo surgery is when the hamstring is detached from the ischial tuberosity. This injury is rare but its incidence is increasing, especially in middle-aged patients who continue to be physically active [30]. The triggering mechanism of injury is a sudden flexion of the hip and extension of the knee that causes a contraction of the hamstring. The patient reports feeling a shot in the rear thigh and walks with his leg straight (stiff-legged gait) avoiding flexing hip and knee in order to relieve the pain.

The hamstring avulsion from the ischial tuberosity is not always treated surgically. Presently there is no commonly accepted classification, or any guidelines to be followed for treatment [29]. The current literature recommends conservative treatment if the injury affects only one tendon and the retraction does not exceed 1 - 2 cm. The single damaged tendon tends to heal by adhering to intact neighboring tendons and even professional athletes will be able to return to competitive activity within about 6 weeks from injury.

The rupture of three tendons usually causes a major retraction of the stumps (greater than 5 cm) and in this case surgical treatment is recommended.

When two tendons are completely damaged, the regimen is not clear and depends on the physician's personal experience. Surgery is generally recommended if the patient is less than 50 years old, active and participating in athletic activities. Furthermore, the retraction of the stumps for more than 2 cm may be the indirect sign of injury to the third muscle at the muscle-tendon junction or in the muscle belly; that has gone unseen at diagnosis, making surgery absolutely necessary [30]. It should be remembered that the MRI is difficult to interpret with certainty when multiple tendons are damaged in this region.

Conservative treatment lead to a reduction of strength in the knee flexion and extension of the hip; also a superabundant scar could entrap the sciatic nerve, which runs nearby, giving rise to a "hamstring syndrome". The cause of neurological symptoms in the sciatic nerve is not well defined and remains ambiguous: it is possible that the fibrotic scar tissue generated from the lesion could lead to adhesions with the nerve, it is possible that the detached bone of the tuberosity forms a callus which compresses the nerve, or that the hamstrings during retraction cause the sciatic nerve or one of its branches to stretch [31].

Surgical treatment provides for an incision (longitudinal or transverse) on the posterior side of the proximal thigh, once tendons are isolated, the surface of the ischial tuberosity is debrided, the injured tendons are reinserted with bone anchors and if necessary, the neurolysis of the sciatic nerve is performed to free it from any adhesions.

There is no "one and only" postoperative care in literature; some authors recommend to avoiding using a cast; at least one suggests keeping the knee flexed at 30 ° [29], others recommend a splint at 90 ° for 2 weeks followed by a gradual lengthening of the knee [31], others advise protecting the affected hip with a cast to be worn for 6 weeks that allows only movements between 15 ° and 30 ° of flexion [30]. This is followed by a a gradual recovery of the joint's ROM and muscle strength during which time it is important to avoid too much tension on the insertion of the proximal hamstring in the first post-operative period. In particular, passive aggressive stretching should be avoided in the first 3 months post-op [29]. The return to sports-specific conditioning is expected between 6-9 months after surgery. It should be kept in mind that the full recovery of muscle strength requires a long time; often more than a year is needed to obtain an equal force in both legs. Residual muscle atrophy is common, especially in the long head of the biceps which results in a compensatory hypertrophy of the short head [32].

In the preoperative period hamstring stretching exercises should be avoided to prevent further distancing of the ends of the lesion; instead isometric contractions of the quadriceps and gluteal muscles should be encouraged to reduce muscle atrophy as well as ankle pumps to prevent deep vein thrombosis [30].

The results of surgical treatment reported in literature appear to be satisfactory with 62 -90% of patients satisfied with return to sporting activity levels the same as before the injury [33, 34, 35, 36]. A recent review of the literature [37] shows that early surgical treatment guarantees a better performance in terms of rate of return to sports, patient subjective satisfaction, recovery of strength and performance compared to conservative treatment. Unfortunately the results presented in literature are not easy to interpret because the techniques used are varied and, being a rather rare lesion, the cases analyzed are few.

The results of the operation depend on many factors. The timing of surgery seems crucial as after 14 days from injury there is a higher risk of adhesions between the lesion and the sciatic nerve [38] so surgery should be performed before this limit. If surgery is performed after five weeks, the post-operative cast must be worn for a longer perid of time [39]. It is not clear how the retraction of the tendon influences the treatment decisions : while in children retraction is an important factor in avulsion fractures, in skeletally mature subjects the importance of retraction has not yet been demonstrated. It has been shown how the level of retraction changes if observed on MRI or intra-operatively and it is closely related to hip and knee flexion and muscle activation [29].

Another rare lesion that can take place to the hamstring is a lesion to the distal insertion. In literature this injury is briefly described and the need for surgery is indicated although no more than 10 case reports and one case series with only a few patients enrolled, have been published.

The most common in the distal region is the avulsion of the biceps femoris associated with a multiligamentous lesion of the knee with a trauma in varus and hyperextension [40]. This muscle is an important and strong flexor and an active stabilizer of the knee and its injury can cause weakness and instability of the knee, especially in athletes [41]. Moreover, in the case of partial tears, the haphazard rearrangement of scar tissue and the formation of adhesions may jeopardize competitive sport activity because it causes pain. From an analysis of the 19 cases present in literature [41], it can be concluded that this type of injury, both complete and incomplete, allows the return to competition and that sometimes conservative treatment of partial tears may eventually require surgery to stop the painful symptoms.

The semimembranosus muscle has a role in flexion and internal rotation of the tibia. An injury to its distal portion determines a worse prognosis for players than the biceps femoris. There are fewer reports in literature (6 cases) [41], and it seems that the early reconstruction of total lesions lead to good results (2 cases). However, in the case of partial lesions, despite late reconstruction (4 cases), the subjects were unable to return to the same level of sporting activity as performed before previous to the injury. Biopsies performed on the unhealed muscles showed a severe denervation of muscle fibers. We can therefore suppose that a partial tear of the distal myotendinous junction of this muscle can cause serious nerve damage and determine a worse prognosis [41].

The semitendinosus muscle contributes to flexion strength at high degrees of knee flexion and intrarotation of the tibia. The tendon of this muscle is often harvested for use as a graft for reconstruction of the anterior cruciate ligament, so in theory it is an "expendable" tendon. Indeed it has been shown that athletes who have had removed their semitendinosus tendon were able to return to the previous level of activity without the harvest causing an important deficit in the competitive performance [42]. A traumatic injury of this region, however, can result in a partial or total lesion that causes pain, and interferes with the physical activity of the patient. Also in this case few articles are available in literature and it is not clear when it is advisable to choose conservative treatment and when to opt for surgical treatment. From our literature search we found 25 cases described [40, 41, 43, 44], 14 patients had been treated conservatively and 11 surgically. The surgery in all cases was a tenotomy with eventual release of adhesions, in no case was a suture performed to restore the damaged anatomical structure. In 5 of the 14 cases (35%) treated conservatively there was a treatment failure and the patient needed surgery that subsequently gave good results. Of the 11 patients treated surgically al returned to their previous level of athletic activities.

The study with the largest case series [40] emphasized that early surgical treatment (within 4 weeks from injury) leads to a much earlier return to sports: with conservative treatment (7 cases) return to sport occurs at an average of 18.4 weeks, with surgery (5 cases) at 6.8 weeks, while if conservative treatment fails and surgery is needed (5 cases), return to the field is much later, at 29.6 weeks on average. Unfortunately, however, the results are not statistically significant because of the small sample number.

8. Adductor muscle

A lesion at the proximal end of the abductor complex is not a common injury. There are few articles in literature about it, and those few are of a low level of evidence and with a few selected cases. An eccentric contraction during a movement of forced abduction of the lower limb may cause this type of acute injury. The most common mechanism is bilateral abduction of the lower limbs with a hip flexion and internal rotation of the other hip [45]. Usually the acute injury is preceded by painful symptoms previous to the accident that express an acute injury on a chronic disease in the area. In fact, histological studies [46, 47] have shown that in the area near the lesion there are degenerative tissue alterations. For this reason the first therapeutic approach to acute injuries of proximal abductor insertion was based on the results of treatment of the chronic lesion. Tenotomy, often used for chronic pain resistant to conservative therapies, had not guaranteed excellent results: 40% of patients were unable to return to competitive activity after surgery and the strength of the adductors reported a significant decrease at the isokinetic test [48]. These results led to the surgical reconstruction of the injured tendon / muscle to prevent the loss of strength and try to increase the percentage of athletes who could return to their previous level of competitive activity [46].

It was later shown that about 60% of the athletes complained of an aspecific symptom, especially abdominal or inguinal pain in the period prior to the injury [49]. However, the importance of the integrity of these anatomical structures has decreased. Studies on the conservative treatment of these lesions have shown that the anatomical continuity of these structures is not essential for a high athletic performance and electromyographical studies support the idea that the abductor muscles do not play a key role in sprinting and cutting movements [50, 51].

The most recent study with the largest series includes 19 players of the American National Football League (NFL) [49], 14 were treated conservatively and 5 surgically. The authors conclude that although all the players returned to play in the top league, those who received conservative treatment returned to the field sooner (6.1 + / - 3.1 weeks) than those treated surgically (12.0 + / - 2.5 weeks). Moreover, besides the risk of complications with surgery, the operation is not easy to perform if the lesion is at the level of the muscle-tendon junction [45].

The information available in the literature on this subject is scarce, with a low level of evidence and often conflicting. Some authors recommend surgery to suture / reinsert in the case of acute injuries occurring in athletes and excision / tenotomy in the case of inveterate injuries; other authors do not recommend surgery because it extends recovery time and does not guarantee better results than conservative treatment, considering also the non fundamental function of this muscle group in sport activities. Much still needs to be understood in this regards and future studies should be conducted with better methods and possibly with a larger number of patients.

9. Suture versus immobilization

Few studies in the literature have compared muscle suture and immobilization. Animal studies, usually in the Sprague-Dawley rat, have shown that lesions performed for experimental purposes heal better if sutured. Almekinders [52] has shown that the benefits obtained by suturing muscles are significant at one week after injury, while at two weeks surgical treatment or treatment with simple immobilization bring the same results in terms of maximum failure load, active force generation as well as from the histological point of view. Menetrey [3] instead found significant improvements with suturing muscle in respect to not suturing and immobilization; in fact one month after the injury the sutured muscle produced 81% of the tetanus strength misured in the intact muscle, while the non sutured muscle produced 35% and the immobilized muscle 18%. It is evident how the overabundance of connective tissue in the scar tissue inhibits the formation of myofibers at 12 weeks [1] whereas the suture prevents the formation of scar tissue in depth; it restricts the formation of hematoma by decreasing the gap of the lesion and the infiltration of mononuclear cells is limited to the surface region only. Desmin's detection has proved that the greatest number of regenerating myofibers is in the sutured muscle already at 2 days after injury, this is not because it limits the inflammatory phase or cellular necrosis (that occurs anyway) but probably because it produces a microenvironment favorable to repair, keeping the muscle stumps together [3].

Clearly the results of the animal tests should be interpreted with caution for several reasons: the lesion that is created is a surgical one, metabolism and healing of the lesion are different between humans and rats. In humans, the only studies comparing surgery and conservative treatment are about lesions of the biceps brachii [25, 53] where the best results are had in patients treated with the myorrhaphy. However, these articles have a poor methodology and take into account only a small number of patients; obviously future larger and better conducted studies are required in order to determine more specifically which type of treatment is most suitable in humans. It remains clear, however, that surgical treatment is rarely necessary, only for certain types of injuries, and only with a specific indication. We perform surgery only when strictly necessary.

10. Types of sutures

Once you choose a surgical approach it is important to decide the surgical technique and how to suture the muscle.

The suture of a muscle belly is easier in its proximal third and distal third, whereas only in some muscles in the middle third; this is because the tendon fibers flatten and extend into the muscle belly giving the stitches a greater support [54].

Literature describes many types of knots and sutures, such as the conventional Kessler, the modified Kessler and the figure-eight horiziontal mattress and more complex ones, such as the Mason-Allen, the Modified Mason-Allen and suturing the perimeter of the lesion.

The integrity and viability of the remaining muscle tissue is important and indicative for a good prognosis; furthermore the preservation of the epimiysium and the possibility of suturing it to the muscle makes the suture more resistant. From an in vitro study on pig muscles [55], it has been shown that suturing the epimysium gives the suture greater resistance to tensile stress compared to sutures made only on he muscle tissue and perimysium. This is because the epimysium consists of more connective tissue and is composed of two layers, hence much more resistant to tension compared to the perimysium [56].

The Kessler stitch would seem to be more resistant to pull-out suturing than simple stitch or simple suturing with a tendon graft [57].

Kragh [16] compared the Kessler stitch and a stitch combinations (Mason-Allen stitch and stitch around perimeter) in pig muscle. These two types of sutures were considered the strongest in a pilot study carried out before the main study where 9 different types of suturing were compared: simple stitch, running simple (epimysium based, non-core) stitch, the figure of eight stitch, the modifed Kessler stitch, a vertical mattress stitch, a horizontal mattres stitch (core), a horizontal mattress stitch (inverted, epimysium based, non-core), a double right angle stitch, a combination (Modified Mason-Allen and perimeter) stitch. At the tensile tests carried out, the Kessler stitch achieved a maximum load of 35 N, whereas the combined suture achieved 74 N. Not only did the combined suture achieve a greater tensile load, but also the Kessler stitch failed because the sutures were pulled away from the muscle tissue, whereas in the combined suturing, the better distribution of the forces induced a gradual lengthening of the muscle fibers and the stitches were not torn away from the tissue at the 35 mm lengthening.

Similar results were obtained on fresh frozen cadaveric human tissue [58]. Comparing Kessler, figure eight, mattress, Mason-Allen, perimeter and perimeter-Mason-Allen on different muscles of human cadaver, Kessler stitch was the least resistant and tore the muscle with an average load of 1.65 kg; the strongest suture, as was observed in other studies, was the combined suture, Mason-Allen plus perimeter stitch, that withstood a weight of 6.4 kg on average. It was also observed that the simple sutures tend to tear the tissue and the epimysium longitudinally, whereas the more complex sutures failure involves more the transversal tissue. In fact, the epimysium is the key to a robust suture, it is more robust in the tissue where the suture can adhere firmly, the complex sutures involve a greater surface area than the simple ones.

It should also be noted that the simple sutures close the epimysium flaps but in the deep layers, fibers are free and when subsequent contraction of the muscle flaps occur, although held together at the extremity by the suture, deep below the surface tend to form a gap that favors the formation of hematomas, prolong the period of healing and promote excessive fibrosis which may in turn lead to exuberant scar tissue. Hence, the complex suture allows the surgeon to pull together the edges of the tear both at the extremes and deep in the muscle enhancing a greater biological performance [58].

The muscle tissue, due to its physical characteristics, does not offer a solid anchor for sutures which, if positioned improperly, tend to tear the fibers and are pulled from the muscle. When the suturing encompasses multiple points on the injured muscle and the correct technique is used, it can sustain heavy loads and prevent further injuries and ineffective sutures. In theory a stronger suture and one that is less damaging to the muscle tissue should allow earlier mobilization without the risk of failure; therefore improving the healing, shortening the period of immobility and in turn decreasing muscle atrophy.

These in vitro tests demonstrate how to make the most of myorrhaphy. In vivo, however, there are no significant differences between the stitches used Even when comparing a Kessler stitch with a simple suture in a tendon graft, Chien et al. [57] found no difference in terms of muscle healing in rabbits.

Some authors have proposed the use of grafts to reinforce the suture, but It is still unclear whether the use of an augmentation graft suture, as performed by Botte et al. [59] on a case series of 58 patients, is useful to make improvements in clinical and functional outcomes.

11. Conclusions

The indication for surgical treatment applies to a small number of muscle lacerations. The tearing of the muscle belly is a common occurrence in athletes and nowadays are difficult to predict or prevent. There is no clear indication for surgical suture for these lesions and there is no real guide line to follow. The majority of the authors in literature consider performing surgery when the lesion affects more than 50% of the total of muscle fibers. Such an extensive injury would provoke a massive scar reaction making it difficult to achieve efficient and functional tissue leading to an excess of collagen and fibrotic tissue which would change the muscle mechanics and facilitate the onset of new lesions. It has also been evaluated and demonstrated that large lesions also present decreased strength, especially in those cases where the affected muscle is not assisted by other agonist muscles. The best results were obtained in patients treated with surgery compared to those treated conservatively with splinting.

In addition, such an extensive lesion would also be very disfiguring in appearance for those who make fitness and muscle shape their job such as body builders. These lacerations leave the muscle anatomy altered, and conservative treatment fails to restore the geometric lines and shapes of the muscle.

The muscles most affected by these injuries in sports are the pectoralis major (in lifters), the biceps brachii (in the paratroopers and water sportsmen who are pulled by ropes) and the rectus femoris.

Surgery brings the margins of the lesion together thus decreasing the hematoma and reducing the reactive fibrous reaction which in turn leads to smaller scars. The approach also enhances a faster return to mobilization of the affected segment and an earlier recovery of muscle tone.

The muscle belly tissue is not a robust structure for anchoring the stitches to, therefore the choice of method, anchor points and suture type must be made carefully.

It is evident how few publications there are in literature that deal with the management of massive muscle injuries; only a few studies comparing the therapeutic options have been conducted and the majority of articles available concern in vitro studies or animal studies. It is necessary that further studies are conducted in order to obtain enough scientific evidence to guide the treatment and management of these patients.

Author details

Giuliano Cerulli[1,2,3,4], Enrico Sebastiani[5], Giacomo Placella[5], Matteo Maria Tei[5], Andrea Speziali[5] and Pierluigi Antinolfi[6]

1 University of Perugia, Perugia, Italy

2 Nicola's Foundation ONLUS Arezzo, Italy

3 Let People Move Research Institute Arezzo, Perugia, Italy

4 International Orthopedic and Traumatologic Institute Arezzo, Italy

5 Residency program in Orthopedics and Traumatology, University of Perugia, Perugia, Italy

6 "Santa Maria della Misericordia" Hospital, Orthopedic and traumatology department, Perugia, Italy

References

[1] Garret WE Jr, Seaber AV, Boswick J, Recovery of a skeletal muscle after laceration and repair. J Hand Surg 1984;9A: 683-692

[2] Huard J, Li Y, Fu FH, Muscle injuries and repair: current trends in research. Journal of Bone and Joint Surgery. 2002:84A(5):822-832

[3] Menetrey J, Kasemkijwattana C, Fu FH, Moreland MS, Huard J, Suturing cersus immobilization of a muscle laceration, Am j Sports Med 1999;27(2): 222-229

[4] Kaariainen M, Kaariainen J, Jarvinen TLN, Sievanen H, Kalimo H, Jarvinen M. Journal of Orthopaedic Research. 1998;16:197-206

[5] Beiner JM, Jokl P. Muscle contusion injuries: current treatment options. Journal of American Academy of Orthopedic Surgeon. 2011;9:227-237

[6] Jarvinen M, Healing of a crush injury in rat striated muscle: 2. A histological study of the effect of early mobilization and immobilization on the repair processes. Acta Pathologica et Microbiologica Scandinavica. 1975;83:269-282

[7] Lehto M, Duance VC, Restall D. Collagen and fibronectin in a healing skeletal muscle injury: An immunohistological study of the effects of physical activity on the repair of injured gastrocnemius muscle in the rat. Journal of Bone and Joint Surgery. 1985;67:820-828

[8] Lehto MUK, Jarvinen MJ, Muscle injuries, their healing process and treatment. Ann Chir Gynaecol. 1991;80:102-108

[9] Noonan TJ, Garrett WE Jr. Muscle strain injury: diagnosis and treatment. Journal of American Academy of Orthopaedic Surgeon. 1999;7:262-269

[10] Aspelin P, Ekberg O, Thorsson O, Wilhelmsson M, Westlin N. Ultrasound examination of soft tissue injury of the lower limb in athletes. American Journal of Sport Medicine. 1192;20:601-603

[11] Mellerowicz H, Lubash A, Dulce MC, Dulce K, Wagner S, Wolf KJ. Diagnosis and follow-up of muscle injuries by means of plain and contrast-enhanced MRI: Experimental and clinical studies. Rofo Fortshr Geb Rontgenstr Neuen Bildgeb Verfahr. 1997;166:437-445

[12] Jarvinen TAH, Kaarianen M. Muscle strain injuries. Curr Opin Rheum. 2000;12:155-161

[13] Ryan AJ. Quadriceps strain, rupture and charlie horse. Med Sci Sports 1969;1:106-111

[14] Miller WA, Rupture of the musculotendinosus juncture of the medialhead of the gastrocnemius muscle. American Journal of Soprt Medicine 1977;5:191-193

[15] Ferrario A, Monti GB, Jelmoni GP. Traumatologia dello sport, clinica e terapia. Edi-Ermes. 2005

[16] Kragh JF Jr, Svoboda SJ, Wenke JC, Ward JA, Walters TJ. Suturing of lacerations of skeletal muscle. J Bone Joint Srug Br. 2005;87B:1303-5

[17] Kretzler HH Jr, Richardson AB. Rupture of the pectoralis muscle. American Journal of Sports Medicine. 1989;17:453-458

[18] McEntire JE, Hess WE, Coleman SS. Rupture of the pectoralis major muscle. Journal of Bone and Joint Surgery. 1972;54:1040-1045

[19] Scott BW, Wallace WA, Barton MAJ. Diagnosis and assessment of pectoralis major rupture by dynamometry. Journal of Bone and Joint Surgery. 1992;74:111-113

[20] Liu J, Wu JJ, Chang CY, Chou YH, Lo WH. Avulsion of the pectoralis major tendon. Journal of American Soprt Medicine. 1992;20:366-367

[21] Pavlik A, Csepai D, Berkes I. Surgical treatment of pectoralis major rupture in athletes. Knee Surgery Sports and Traumatology Arthroscopy. 1998;6:129-133

[22] Petilon J, Carr DR, Sekiya JK, Unger DV. Pectoralis major muscle injuries: evaluation and management

[23] Bak K, Cameron EA, Henderson IJP. Rupture of the pectoralis major: a meta-analysis of 112 cases. Knee Surgery Sports and Traumatology Arthroscopy. 2000;8:113-119

[24] Titjen R. Closed injuries of the pectoralis major muscle. J Trauma. 1980;20:262-264

[25] Kragh JF, Basamania CJ. Surgical repair of acute traumatic closed transection of the biceps brachii. Journal of Bone and Joint Surgery. 2002;84°(6):992-998

[26] Pascual-Garrido C, Swanson BL, Bannar SM. Closed proximal muscle rupture of the biceps brachii in wakeborders. Knee Surgery Sports Traumatology Arthroscopy. 2012;20:1019-1021

[27] Shah AK, Pruzansky ME. Ruptured biceps brachii short head muscle belly: a case report. Journal of Shoulder and Elbow Surgery. 2004;13(5):362-365

[28] Straw R, Colclough K, Geutjens. Surgical repair of a chronic rupture of the rectus femoris muscle at the proximal musculotendinous junction in a soccer player. Br Journal of Sports Medicine. 2003;37:182-184

[29] Askling CM, Koulouris G, Saartok T, Werner S, Best TM. Total proximal hamstring ruptures: clinical and MRI aspects including guidelines for postoperative rehabilitation. Knee Surg Sports Traumatol Arthrosc. 21:515-533. 2013

[30] Cohen S, Bradley J. Acute proximal hamstring rupture. J Am Acad Orthop Surg. 15:350-355, 2007

[31] Chakravarthy J, Ramisetty N, Pimpalnerkar A, Mohtadi N. Surgical repair of complete proximal hamstring tendon ruptures in water skiers and bull riders: a report of four cases and review of the literature. Br J Sports Med. 39:569-572. 2005

[32] Silder A, Heiderscheit BC, Thelen DG, Enright T, Tuite MJ. MR observations of long term musculotendon remodeling following a hamstring strain injury. Skeletal Radiol. 37:1101-1109. 2008

[33] Klingele KE, Sallay PI. Surgical repair of complete proximal hamstring tendon rupture. Am J Sports Med. 30:742-747, 2002

[34] Chakravarthy J, Ramisetty N, Pimpalnerkar A, Mohtadi N. Surgical repair of complete proximal hamstring ruptures in water skiers and bull riders: a report of four cases and review of the literature. Br J Sports Med. 39:569-572. 2005

[35] Brucker PU, Imhoff AB. Functional assessment after acute and chronic complete ruptures of the proximal hamstring tendons. Knee Surg Sports Traumatol Arthrosc. 13:411-418. 2005

[36] Orava S, Kujala UM. Rupture of the ischial origin of the hamstring muscles. Am J Sports Med. 23:702-705. 1995

[37] Harris JD, Griesser MJ, Best TM, Ellis TJ. Treatment of proximal hamstring ruptures – a systematic review. Int J Sports Med. 32:490-495. 2011

[38] Konan S, Haddad F. Successful return to high level sports following early surgical repair of complete tears of the proximal hamstring tendons. Int Orthop. 34:119-123. 2010

[39] Chamichael J, Packham I, Trikha SP. Avulsion of the proximal hamstring origin: surgical technique. J Bone Joint Surg Am. 15:350-355. 2007

[40] Cooper DE, Conway JE. Distal semitendinosus ruptures in elite-level athletes: low success rates of nonoperative treatment. Am Journal Sports Med. 38(6):1174-8. 2010

[41] Lempainene L, Sarimo J, Kimmo M, Heikkila J, Orava S. Distal tears of the hamstrin muscles: review of the literature ans our results of surgical treatment. Br J Sports Med. 41:80-83. 2007

[42] Smith FW. Rousenlund EA, Aune AK. Subjective functional assessments and the return to competitive sport after anterior cruciate ligament reconstruction. Br J Sports Med. 38:279-284. 2004

[43] Schilders E, Bismil Q, Sidham S. Partial rupture of the distal semitendinosus tendon treated by tenotomy - a previously underscribed entity. Knee. 13:45-7. 2006

[44] Adejuwon A, McCourt P, Hamilton B, Haddad F. Distal semitendinosus tendon nrupture: is there any benefit of surgical intervention?. Clin J Sports Med. 19:502-504. 2009

[45] Campbell. Canale ST. Chirurgia ortopedica. X edizione. Verducci Editore. 2005

[46] Rizio L, Salvo JP, Schurhoff MR, Uribe JW. Adductor longus rupture in professional football players: acute repait with suture anchors - a report of two cases. Am J Sports Med. 32(1):243-245. 2004

[47] Ippolito E, Postacchini F. Rupture and disinsertion of the proximal attachment of the adductor longus tendon: case report with histochemical and ultrastructural study. Ital J Orthop Traumatol. 7:79-85. 1981

[48] Akermark C, Johansson C. Tenotomy of the adductor longus tendon in the treatment of chronic groin pain in athletes. Am J Sports Med. 20:640-643. 1992

[49] Schlegel TF, Bushnell BD, Godfrey J, Boublik M. Success of nonoperative management of adductor longus tendon ruptures in national football league athletes. Am J Sports Med. 37(7):13941399. 2009

[50] Mann RRMoran GT, Dougherty SE. Comparative electromyography of the lower extremity in jogging, running, and sprinting. Am J Sports Med. 14(6):501-510. 1986

[51] Neptune RR, Wright IA, Van Den Bogert AJ. Muscle coordination and function during cutting movements. Med Sci Sports Exerc. 31(2):294-302. 1999

[52] Almekinders LC. Results of surgical repair versus splinting of experimentally transected muscle. Journal of Orthopaedic Trauma. 1991;5(2):173-176

[53] Heckman JD, Levine MI. Traumatic closed transection of the biceps brachii in the military parachutist. Journal of Bone and Joint Surgery. 1978;60-A:369-72

[54] Chammout MO, Skinner HB. The clinical anatomy of commonly injured muscle bellies. J Trauma. 1986;26:549-552

[55] Kragh JF, Svoboda SJ, Wenke JC, Ward JA, Walters TJ. Epimysium and perimysium in suturing in skeletal muscle lacerations. The Journal of Trauma Injury, Infection, and Clinical Care. 2005;59(1):209-212

[56] Nishimura T, Hattori A, Takahashi K. Ultrastructure of the intramuscular connective tissue in bovine skeletal muscle: a demonstration using cell-maceration/scanning electron miscroscope method. Acta Anatomica. 1994;151:250-257

[57] Chien SH, Chen SK, Lin SY, Chen SS, Wu HS. Repair method and healing of skeletal muscle injury. The Kaohsiung Journal of Medical Schiences. 1991;7(9):481-488

[58] Chance JR, Kragh JF, Agrawal M, Basamania CJ. Pulout forces of sutures in muscle lacerations. Orthopedics. 2005;28(10):1187-90

[59] Botte MJ, Gelberman RH, Smith DG, Silver MA, Gellman H. Repair of severe muscle belly lacerations using a tendon graft. J Hand Surg Am. 12(3):406-412, 1987

Prevention

Chapter 9

Prevention of Muscle Injuries — The Soccer Model

M. Giacchino and G. Stesina

Additional information is available at the end of the chapter

1. Introduction

Muscle injuries are frequent in sports, and represent about 30% of all time-loss injuries in men's professional football (soccer) [1-8] and almost 20% in men's amateur level [9].

Four muscle groups of the lower limbs account for 92% of muscle injuries (hamstrings 37%, adductors 23%, quadriceps 19%, and calf 13%) [1].

In sports such as soccer, but also in athletics, basketball, volleyball etc, muscle indirect injuries and overuse injuries are more common (about 96% in soccer [1]) than direct injuries (contusions). Contact situations are more frequently involved in muscle injuries in other sports like rugby, American football, ice hockey [10,11]. In elite soccer 16% of muscle injuries are re-injuries and cause 30% longer absence from competitions than first injury [1].

Muscle injuries result from a complex interaction of multiple risk factors and events.

Several parameters are usually identified as risk factors. These are usually classified as either intrinsic, athlete-related, or extrinsic, environmental risk factors.

Gender [1,12], age [2,13-21,45], skill level [12,23,24], body size and composition [14,25,26], previous injury history [2,3,8,13,15,16,19,21,27,28,43-45], anatomy or biomechanics abnormality [19], joints ROM and flexibility [29,30], muscle strength, imbalance and tightness [2,21,22,29], limb dominance [14], training errors such as poor technique, or errors in training program, warm-up or cooling down [33-35], aerobic fitness [25], fatigue [16,26,32,45], are included among intrinsic risk factors. Footwear, climatic conditions and turf type [36-42] are examples of extrinsic risk factors. Some of these risk factors can be modified.

Muscle injury prevention is advocated both by athletes and coaches. Yet, most of techniques for muscle injury prevention used by athletes or taught by coaches are entirely based on their own experience, but without supporting scientific evidence.

The aim of this chapter is to present current concepts about the prevention of the muscular injuries and to test which strategies are best supported by scientific evidence, both with respect to primary prevention (prevention of the first injury) and secondary prevention (re-injury prevention).

In this chapter are also proposed some practical suggestions, dedicated to the members of soccer's team, that are involved in the management of muscle injuries risk factors (coaches, fitness trainers, physiotherapists, team doctors).

When muscle injuries occur, the safe return to competition is often difficult, both in order to get prior level of performance and to avoid re-injury.

The anatomical healing of a muscle injury is a primary condition for safe return to sport, but it is not enough to manage re-injury risk. Thus, anatomical healing is not synonymous of "athletic healing".

A database of aerobic fitness, muscle strength, and other performance related parameters, is also proposed in this paper, to get a reference for the muscle injury rehabilitation program and the full return to competition.

These parameters have to be registered by laboratory and field tests, performed by the healthy athlete, during pre-season and competition period and then, in case of muscle injury, these have to be used as a reference, to programme his return to prior level of competition.

In relation to the authors' personal experience, this chapter will be set on the prevention of muscles injuries in a male professional soccer team: the suggestions and observations here described are, however, applicable to lower levels soccer teams and most others sports.

2. Analysis of risk factors for muscle injuries

2.1. Intrinsic risk factors

- Gender

There is not sound evidence on the impact of gender on muscle injury risk in soccer, mainly because women's soccer has become very popular in the last years and most scientific studies have been carried out using as reference point the data of male players (Figure 1).

In a review [12] seven studies showed that female athletes had a higher incidence of injury, two reported that male athletes showed a higher incidence of injury, five studies found no association between sex and injury, and one found that the rate of ankle and knee specific injuries differed with gender. There is no evidence of difference in the incidence of muscle injuries between males and females. It is also well documented that female athletes have more knee injuries than male athletes, specifically ACL sprains. Within intercollegiate sports, female soccer players were 9 times more likely to sustain an ACL tear than male soccer players [1].

In conclusion, although it is clear that female athletes are at increased risk of suffering ACL injuries, the relation between gender and other types of lower extremity injury is unclear.

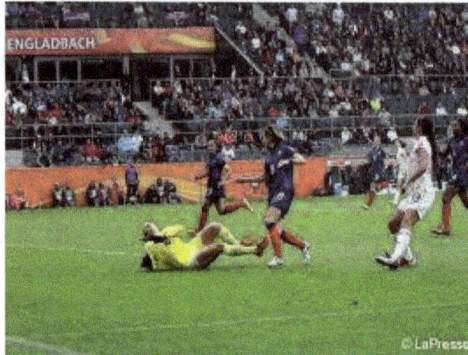

Figure 1. Female soccer is today very popular.

• **Age**

Age is a widely studied risk factor for muscle injuries, particularly in recent years, with the increase in the average age of players, especially at the amateur level (Figure 2). In available literature, there are conflicting data about age as a predisposing factor to muscle injuries. Some studies have identified increasing age as an independent risk factor for muscle injuries in Australian footballers [14-16] and soccer players [2,45]. These authors found increased risk in Australian footballers and soccer players older than 23 years [14,45]. Furthermore each year of age has been reported to increase the risk of muscle injuries by as much as 1.3 times in Australian footballers [15] and by 1.8 times in soccer players [17]. In a study on 123 female soccer players (age range 14–39 years), the authors found a significantly increased risk of overall injury in athletes older than 25 years compared with younger athletes [18]. In a study on professional soccer players the incidence of global muscle injuries increases with age, but an increased incidence with age has been found for calf muscle injuries only, and not for hamstring, quadriceps or hip/groin injuries [19]. During training sessions, players in the oldest age group (over 30 years) had a significantly higher incidence than young (below 22 years) players, while there were no differences compared to the intermediate (22-30 years) age group. During matches, young players had a lower incidence than the intermediate and older age groups [19]. All studies that report age as significant risk factor conclude that age increases hamstring injury risk independently of other variables such as previous injury.

The explanation for increased muscle injury risk, with age is quite controversial. Some authors maintain that it is due to an increase of weight and a reduction of the flexibility of the hip flexors in athletes 25 years or older [20]; others indicate the cause in the reduction of lean body mass and strength [21].

Other hypotheses are age-related changes in muscle structure [13] and entrapment of L5/S1 nerve root due to hypertrophy of the lumbo-sacral ligament [22].

However, there are also some studies that found no correlation between aging and increase of muscle injuries [12,22,23].

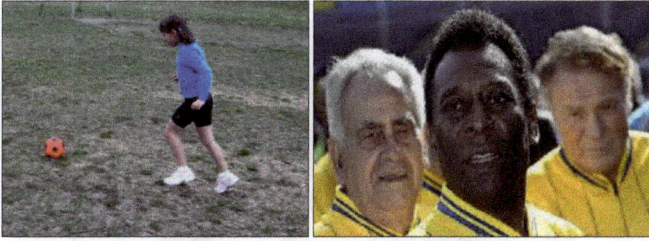

Figure 2. Soccer: a passion all over the world, for babies and old players.

In consideration of data available in literature further studies of longer duration are required to determine the effective importance of aging on muscle injuries.

- Skill level

Several study analysed the relation between skill level and injury and results in this respect appear contradictory (Figure 3). A study found that young soccer players with low skill level had a twofold increased incidence of all injuries, compared to a group with more skilled athletes. More than 79% of all injuries were in the lower extremity [24].

Similarly another study on soccer players, found a twofold increased incidence of all severe injuries in lower skill level players [23].

However, some data are difficult to interpret: in a review [12], it is evident that two studies have shown that low skill level groups have an increased risk of muscle injury while two report that athletes in high skill level groups are at increased risk.

This discrepancy is due to the difficulty to compare different sports without unique criteria for assessing the skill level.

Also, less skilled athletes may not compete as long as those in higher skill level groups. So they may have the same number of injuries, but show higher incidence rate based on less exposure. Finally, higher skill level groups may play at a higher level of intensity and aggressiveness than lower skill level, thereby increasing the risk of injury.

- Body size

Body size has been analysed in risk factor studies in different ways, including height, weight, lean muscle mass, body fat content, body mass index (BMI). These variables have been considered as risk factors for injury because an increase in any one of the indicators above produces a proportional increase in the forces that stress articular, ligamentous and muscular structures; however, the relation between body size and injury is unclear (Figure 4).

A recent study [25] reported an increased incidence of injury among boys taller than 165 cm in a prospective study of youth soccer players, but body size was not a risk factor for girls. Another author [14] reported an increased incidence of quadriceps injury among Australian football players of height less than 182 cm compared with taller athletes; however, height was

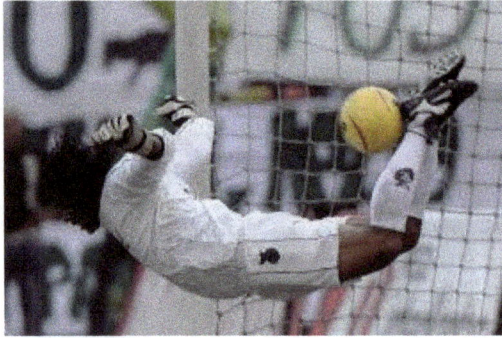

Figure 3. Importance of skill level as muscle injury risk factor is quite controversial.

not associated with hamstring or calf muscle strains. The evidence for weight and body mass index (BMI) as risk for muscle injury is conflicting.

A review [26] shows that five study found no significant association between weight and hamstring injury and only two identified a significant relationship.

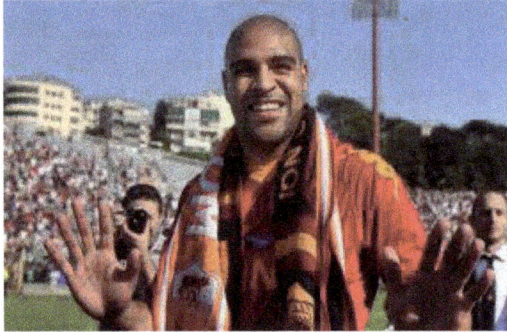

Figure 4. Body weight may be a functional stress.

- Previous injury

A detailed clinical history represents the starting point for setting up an adequate prevention program. Soccer team physicians have to investigate previous muscle injuries of each new player recruited during the pre-season training camp: all information available about all previous injuries (anatomic site, degree, time-loss, etc.) have to be registered (Figure 5). Several authors have shown that previous injuries represent a significant risk factor for new injuries, both in male soccer [2-44] and among male athletes in other sports [13,21]. A study [29] shows that the injury risk is doubled among previously injured players and although the results were not significant, the risk seems to increase gradually with the number of previous injuries and decrease with time since the previous injury. A recent study [19] shows that players with a muscle injury in the previous season have increased injury rates of up to threefold compared with uninjured players. In addition to this, a re-injury tends to cause longer absence than the first injury [3,16]. Improvements in controlled rehabilitation with functional tests before returning to full training and matches might reduce the risk of re-injury [27].

The specific risk factors involved in the recurrence of muscle injury have not been clearly established, but these may be related to the same extrinsic and intrinsic factors that were involved with the original injury. In addition, factors related to modifications after the original muscle injury (tightness or weakness, scar tissue, biomechanical alterations, neuromuscular inhibition, etc), as well as questionable treatment options (incomplete or aggressive rehabilitation, underestimation of an extensive injury, etc), may further predispose an athlete to re-injury [8,28].

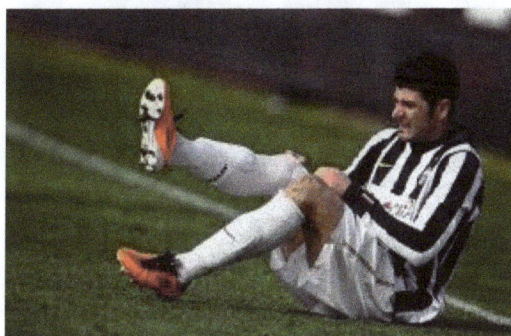

Figure 5. Detailed informations about all previous injuries have to be registered.

The presence of scar tissue can alter muscle transmission pathway, decrease tendon/aponeurosis complex compliance and lead to a modification of functional response in the muscle tissue around the fibrous scar.

Similarly, a study [15] found that a history of knee or groin injury increased the risk of hamstring muscle injuries, and the authors postulated that the biomechanical properties of the lower extremities may change, increasing the risk of further injury.

For this reason, athletes must be aware of the importance of adequate rehabilitation before returning to full competition.

The team medical staff, early in pre-season, must plan a working program to influence properly the functional response of the scars. This work, involving doctors, physiotherapists, fitness coach, field rehabilitator, is focused on the aim of improving the elasticity of scars and make them, as much as possible, functionally similar to the surrounding healthy muscle tissue.

- Anatomical alignment

The joint forces and the structures that must resist them (articular surfaces, menisci, ligaments, tendons and muscles) are related through anatomical alignment (Figure 6) of the joints and skeletal system. For this reason, alignment of the hip, knee, and ankle has been suspected to be a potential risk factor for lower extremity injuries.

Several studies reported no association between anatomical alignment and subsequent muscle injury. There are only a few studies that associate anatomical alignment with injuries to joints, ankles and knees [19].

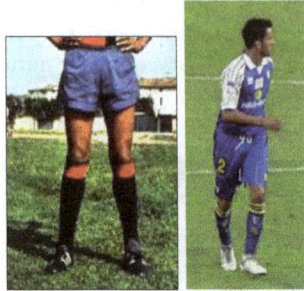

Figure 6. Anatomical mal-alignment of knee.

- Flexibility

Muscle flexibility is the ability of a muscle to lengthen, allowing the joint (or more than one joint in a series) to move through a range of motions (Figure 7). Good muscle flexibility allows muscle tissue to tolerate stress more easily and allow efficient and effective movement.

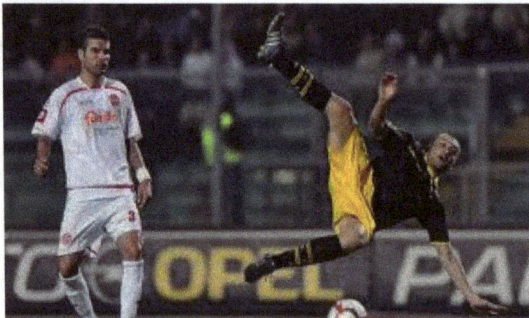

Figure 7. Soccer players need a good muscle flexibility

It is proposed that greater flexibility may reduce the risk of strain injury, due to an improved ability of the passive components of the muscle-tendon unit to absorb energy as a result of a better compliance [29].

However, this point is disputed in the literature. A recent review [30] shows that seven prospective studies demonstrated no relationship between flexibility of knee flexor and hamstring injury, while three studies showed an association, in professional European soccer players, between flexibility values obtained in pre-season and injuries suffered during the season. This discrepancy of results is due mainly to the use of different tests to assess muscle flexibility, which are not always comparable. The flexibility is, however, a parameter that sports physician should carefully consider, especially for soccer players affected by hamstring injury.

In the next sections of this chapter the usefulness of stretching to improve flexibility and reduce muscle injury risk will be considered.

- Muscle strength, imbalance and tightness

Strength deficits or imbalances have been suggested to increase muscle injury risk, above all for hamstring [29].

The relationship between muscle injury and strength deficit (Figure 8) is controversial. More specifically, it is unclear when strength imbalances were only the consequence of the original injury or a risk factor for re-injury, or both. Strength deficits between the two limbs or between agonist and antagonist have been reported in sports with asymmetric kinetic pattern like soccer [2]. In soccer strength imbalance has been involved in injuries of the lower limbs [22], because the players usually use, when kicking, nearly always the same side of their lower limbs. This alters the strength balance between the two leg or between antagonist muscle groups.

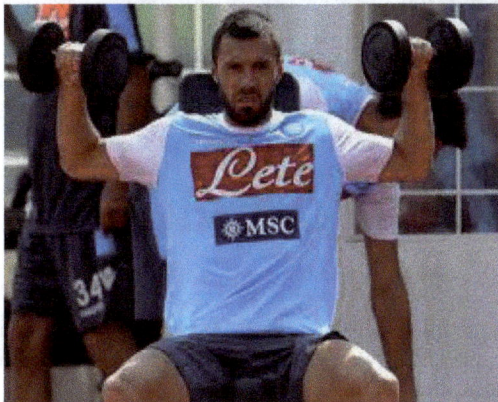

Figure 8. Training of muscle strength

The development of muscle strength symmetry and balanced ratio in the function of knee flexors and extensors can reduce muscle injuries in soccer [32]. The players with untreated strength imbalances were found to be 4 to 5 times more likely to sustain a hamstring injury. Some authors have shown that in football players is important to compare the strength of the flexor and extensor muscles of the thigh, of the two limbs, where differences over 15% can be predictive for flexor injuries [32]. A lower hamstring to quadriceps (H:Q) ratio suggests a relatively poor capacity for the hamstring to act as a "brake" at the flexing hip and extending knee joints during the terminal swing phase of running. An author [29] shows a significant association between pre-season hamstring muscle tightness and subsequent development of a hamstring muscle injury. The same relationship was also found for quadriceps muscle tightness and for the development of quadriceps muscle injuries. Another study [21] confirmed that a simple program of eccentric exercise could reduce the incidence of hamstring injuries in Australian football. For this reason it is essential to work to get a correct balance between the two leg and especially between hamstrings and quadriceps.

- Limb dominance

In some sports, the dominant leg may be at increased risk of injury because it is preferentially used for kicking (figure 9), pushing off, jumping. However, the association between limb dominance and injury is controversial. Several risk factor studies have reported that limb dominance has an effect on injury.

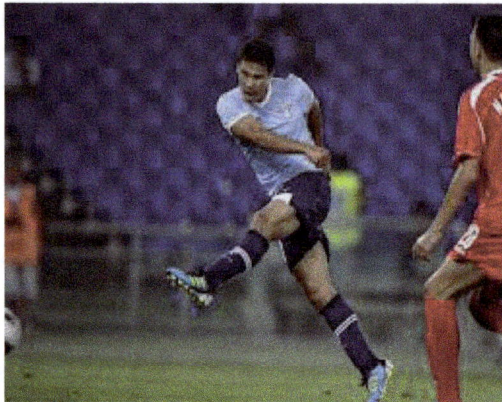

Figure 9. Soccer players have usually a dominant kicking leg

A study [14] reported that quadriceps strains were more commonly sustained by the dominant leg than the non-dominant side but there was no association between limb dominance and injury of the hamstrings or calf muscles.

Quadriceps and adductor injuries were more common in the kicking leg, most probably due to a greater volume of shooting and passing/crossing actions with the dominant leg. These cause a greater exposure to high-risk movements and can affect the correct balance of the whole kinetic chain. However, it has also been suggested that specific limb dominance in soccer players may result in lingering muscle imbalances that could lead to an increased predisposition for injury.

- Poor technique, errors in training program, warm up, cooling down

Every sport, at any level of practice, involves knowledge and mastery of technical movements, which are both sport- and role-specific. Soccer teams' technical and medical staff knows from experience that even top level players can make errors when performing specific technical movements. Poor technique, errors in training program, carelessness in warm up or cooling down modalities are suspected to be involved in the pathogenesis of muscle injuries. The importance of stretching exercises (Figure 10) and the modality of warm up and cooling down are also controversial. Stretching and warm up are commonly practiced before sport activity, but there are conflicting opinions regarding methods of reducing muscular injury through warm-up and stretching techniques [33-35]. The effects of following athletic performance and injury prevention are not fully understood. A recent review examined the available literature on the effects of stretching on sports injury and performance [34]. The conclusions of this study are, in opinion of this paper's authors, widely acceptable. It is well known that a single session of stretching impairs acutely muscle strength and power (even if on power the effect is lower). These effects are less evident when stretching is associated with other pre-participation activities performed in warm-up, such as practice drills and low intensity movements. With respect to the effect of pre-participation stretching on injury risk, the studies reviewed show that pre-participation stretching in addition to warm-up has no impact on injury risk during activities with preponderance of overuse injuries (such as military recruits or recreational runners). However, the stretching interventions applied in these studies may have been insufficient to induce an acute change in the viscoelastic properties of the muscles stretched. There is some evidence to indicate that pre-participation stretching does reduce the risk of muscle strains. However, further research is needed in this area.

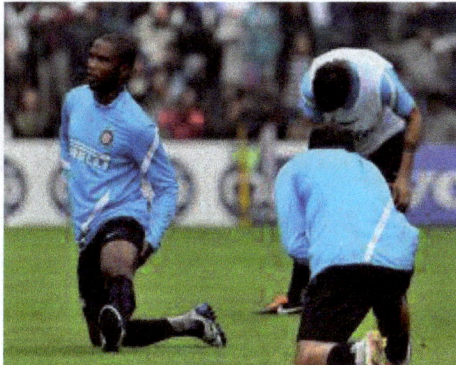

Figure 10. Stretching exercise

The first step in assessing any potential effect of pre-participation stretching on muscle injury is to plan the optimal stretching prescription. The following stretching recommendations for injury prevention are suggested by authors [34]:

- target pre-participation stretching to muscle groups known to be at risk for a particular sport, e.g. hamstring strains in soccer;
- apply at least four to five 60-s stretches to pain tolerance to the target muscle groups and perform bilaterally, in order to be confident of decreasing passive resistance to stretch;
- in order to avoid any persistent stretch-induced stretch loss, perform some dynamic pre-participation drills before actual performance, e.g. sub-maximal ball kicking and dribbling drills in soccer.

- Aerobic fitness

Soccer teams physicians sometimes observe re-injuries when players come back to team training and competition, apparently full healed by muscle injuries. This situation sometimes occurs in athletes that have perfectly passed all clinical, imaging, functional assessment. It is likely that a poor level of aerobic fitness (Figure 11) in early period of return to competition may be involved in re-injury. So it seems reasonable that poor level of aerobic fitness could be a risk factor also for first injury, because athletes fatigued can change their muscle recruitment patterns and this event may impair the distribution of forces loading on the articular, ligamentous and muscular structure. At the beginning of the season and before the come-back after an injury, it is important to assess the level of physical condition. A study on severe injury in male soccer players [25] found poor physical condition to be a risk factor for all injuries.

For the same reason it is extremely important that our athlete achieves a good aerobic condition before starting technical and tactical work, sports- and role-specific.

Even after an injury that does not involve muscles, the achievement of a good aerobic fitness is strictly required in order to operate a safe return to competition.

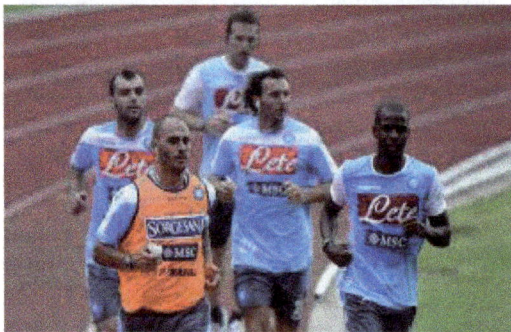

Figure 11. Aerobic fitness care

- Fatigue

Closely linked to aerobic fitness, fatigue (Figure 12) and its associated performance failures are an important risk factor for injuries. Some studies have shown that a greater rate of muscle injuries occur in the later stages of matches and training sessions [16,32,45]. Some studies have evaluated the effects of fatigue on muscles, especially on the hamstring. The data showed a decrease in hip and knee flexion during sprinting [26] and a significant reduction in combined hip flexion and knee extension angles, with reduced hamstring length and consequent increased risk of injury.

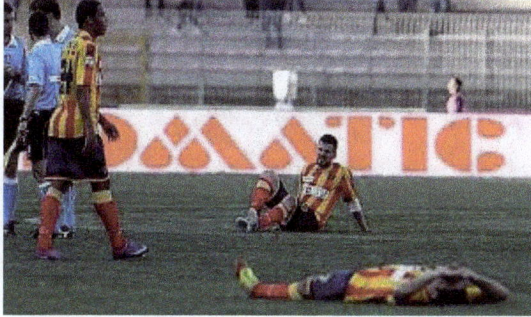

Figure 12. Fatigue is a not-negligible risk factor.

2.2. Extrinsic risk factors

- Shoe type

In available scientific literature, there are not studies based on relationship between soccer footwear and muscle injuries. The majority of the studies are performed on articular (ankle and knee) footwear related risk injury.

- Playing surface

Natural grass has always been the traditional surface for playing soccer, both for matches and training. Nevertheless, in countries with extremely cold or dry climate, it is difficult to develop a pitch of adequate quality accessible all year round. Furthermore, this would also involve high maintenance costs. The use of artificial surfaces has thus been introduced in order to solve these problems.

Since the appearance of artificial grass playing surfaces, athletes, coaches, fitness trainers, physiotherapists and doctors have suspected a relationship between this type of surface and injuries in soccer, rugby, American or Australian football.

Certainly there has been an evolution of the quality of surfaces over the years. Artificial turf first gained considerable attention in the 1960's, when it was used in the construction of Houston Astrodome stadium, in Houston, Texas (Figure 13).

The specific product used was called Astroturf. This surface was known for its abrasive properties, and the risk of carpet burn injuries was experienced by anyone who tried to make a slide tackle on this surface. In addition to this disadvantage, playing soccer on first- and second-generation artificial turf had the problem of a distorted bounce and roll of the ball, which appeared to make control more difficult for the players and was suspected to lead to an increased risk of injury. Carpet burns were not the only injuries suspected to have a relation to early artificial surfaces, and some studies analyzed the risk of other injuries on these pitches [36-39].

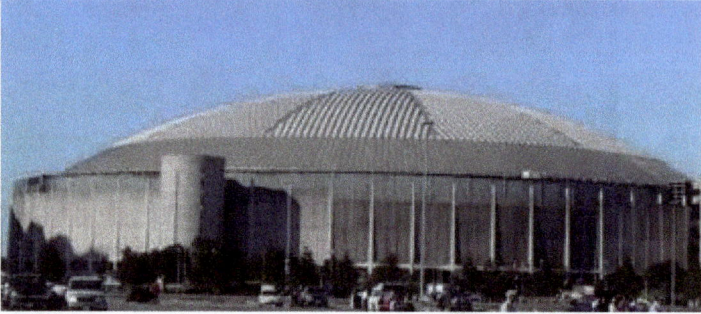

Figure 13. Houston Astrodome Stadium, Houston, Texas.

Some of the studies observed an increased injury rate on artificial turf, but these were not statistically significant, probably in reason of small numbers.

Another study [40] found a significantly higher injury risk on artificial turf versus natural grass (25 v 10 injuries/1000 hours of exposure, p<0.01).

The development of new technologies, has led to the production of new surfaces, specifically dedicated to soccer. The use of the term "football turf" without any reference to generation is now the official terminology recommended by FIFA for artificial turf devoted to soccer.

In 2001 FIFA introduced the FIFA Quality Concept for Football Turf to ensure the quality of football turf pitches. Today within the FIFA quality program, a certification and licensing programme that guarantees the quality of turfs based on uniform criteria has been created. The certification is named "FIFA RECOMMENDED" as described in the following official FIFA classification (table 1).

FIFA Recommended 1 Star	Dedicated football turf standard for amateur and grassroots football
FIFA Recommended 2 Star	Turf standard that meets the very highest demands of professional and elite football.

Table 1. "FIFA RECOMMENDED" certification for football turfs (FIFA Quality Program).

The modern third and fourth generation surfaces are very different respect to early surfaces and often these are promoted as possessing the same properties and injury-risk profiles as grass (Figure 14).

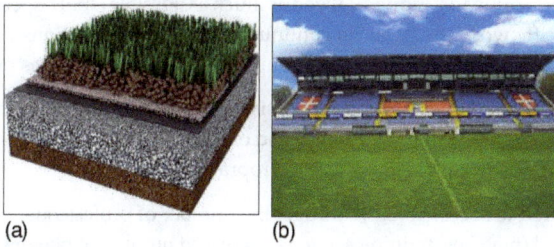

(a)   (b)

Figure 14. a) Modern artificial grass b) Silvio Piola Stadium - Novara - Italy

Recent reviews evaluated the effect of playing surface of third-generation [41] and of third- and fourth-generation [42] on injury rate.

The studies reviewed provide a few specific data about these pitches and muscle injuries.

The first review reported that the effect of these synthetic surfaces on injury rates has not been clearly established because the available literature is largely limited to football and soccer data with a majority of short-term studies. In their conclusions the authors reported that many peer-reviewed studies cite a higher overall rate of injury on first- and second-generation artificial turf surfaces compared with natural grass, but despite differences in injury type, the rate of injury on third-generation and natural grass surfaces appears to be comparable.

In the second review, the purpose of the authors was to compare the incidence, nature and mechanisms of injuries on last generation artificial turfs and natural turfs about football codes (rugby union, soccer, American football). The authors searched in electronic databases using the keywords 'artificial turf', 'natural turf', 'grass' and 'inj*'. Delimitation of all articles sourced, resulted in 11 experimental papers. These 11 papers provided 20 cohorts that were assessed and statistically analyzed. Analysis demonstrated that 16 of the 20 cohorts showed no significant effects for overall incidence rate ratios between artificial and natural surfaces. About muscle injuries, two cohorts showed beneficial inferences for effects of artificial surface on muscle injuries for soccer players, even if there were also two harmful, four unclear and five trivial inferences across the three football codes.

In conclusion the authors stated that new studies of effects of artificial surfaces on muscle injuries are required given inconsistencies in incidence rate ratios depending on the football code, athlete, gender or match versus training evaluation.

3. Management of risk factors

- Team medical organisation

In modern soccer, both at professional top level and at lower levels, an optimal link between the functions of technical staff and medical staff is essential.

Proper planning of workloads, individualized as much as possible (sport-specific, role-specific, single player-specific work load), and a continuous flow of informations between technical and medicals staff are required. These two groups of staff have to work as one big team.

Technical staff mainly includes head coach, assistant coach, fitness coach or athletic trainer, goalkeeper coach. Medical staff includes the head of medical department who coordinates the work of a group of doctors, physioterapists, chiropractors.

Currently, compared to soccer 15-20 years ago, the number of professional duties of the head coach has increased (matches, training sessions, increased number of players to train in teams' ranks, media sessions, trips). With such an organisation of soccer teams, the head coach and his staff cannot be directly engaged, daily and with the appropriate continuity, in the field training program of the injured player.

According to the authors' experience, a new professional figure, linking between the two staff, is taking on increasing importance: the field rehabilitator.

The field rehabilitator, in the authors' opinion, is the key professional link, necessary for the proper management of re-injury risk factor. He must possess the professional skills of both the physiotherapist and the fitness coach (Figure 15).

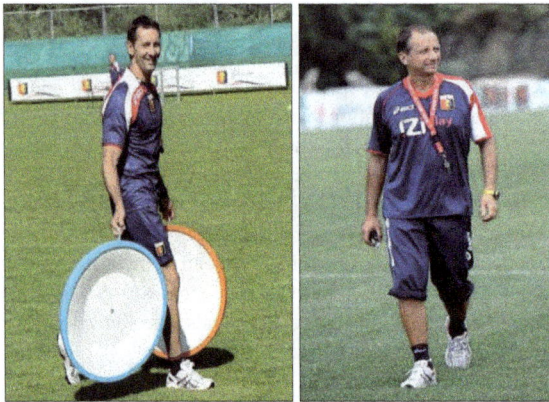

Figure 15. Fitness coach (l) and field rehabilitator (r)– Genoa C.F.C. 2012-13

He begins his work when the injured player ends the rehabilitation program and starts the reconditioning work on the field. In case of muscle injury (or other injury), the aim of his work is to take the player to a level of physical fitness and technical training comparable to his usual standard, ready to rejoin the group of healthy players to normal training sessions.

To achieve this goal, it is imperative to set the field rehabilitation program on a scientific basis, thus referring to well known parameters of physical fitness, which are specific to each player.

The setting up of a database with these parameters will be presented in a later section.

With respect to muscle injury prevention program, all components of technical and medical staff are involved in the management of risk factors.

Team's doctors have to plan examinations for detecting any previous muscle injury, scars, anatomical malalignment, poor flexibility, muscle strength deficit, or imbalance and tightness.

Each member of the medical and technical staff, according to his competence, works to correct, where possible, any anatomical, biomechanical, functional abnormality.

For this reason, it is necessary that all staff members are fully informed about the risk factors related to each player.

In the following sections all steps involved in the management of risk factors are discussed.

- Medical history and clinical evaluation of the athlete

In this section we aim to suggest some guidelines to set up an appropriate prevention program, available to use "on the field".

The following suggestions are referred to each new player recruited in the team ranks. Obviously, in case of a "veteran" player, a large part of the work is ready since the first incorporation. All the information provided should be linked to the personal experience of medical staff, the club organization, the quality and compliance of the athletes and, not least, to the economic availability of the soccer club. We start with simple evaluations, applicable also to recreational athletes, to enter tests progressively more complex, some of which are more expensive and mainly dedicated to professional clubs and high level players. As it is not strictly related to the subject of present chapter, we will skip the details about the cardiological and clinical checkup for eligibility to competitive sports, compulsory in Italy. According to Italian laws, the athlete can neither play nor train without the certificate of eligibility to competitive sport, main guarantee for the athlete, the medical team and the club.

The first step is to perform a complete and accurate medical history. All information will help the medical team to obtain a full view of the athlete's physical characteristics, his strengths and weaknesses and a better knowledge of his previous problems. The prevention program must be simultaneously a training and rehabilitation/physiotherapy program, and must follow the athlete through the season in collaboration with medical and technical staff. Simple and targeted questions must be placed, if possible in the same language of the player (in case of foreign player), if necessary with the help of a translator.

To get the best collaboration and compliance, our experience shows that it is useful to avoid the topic "previous injury" before having established some feeling with the athlete, who often initially "forgets" to report some previous injuries, especially muscular ones.

A good approach would be providing the athlete full information about the medical staff and physiotherapy organization of the new team, the modalities and equipment available in physiotherapy service, the role of the field rehabilitator, before training (preventive work) and/ or in recovery after injury. Then we get information on the player's knowledge and habits about prevention work.

After this first approach, we analyze the intrinsic risk factors identified in medical history: focus on the characteristics of joints (ankles, knees, back and shoulders - especially in case of a goalkeeper) and then we proceed to the past problems, therapeutic interventions (conservative and surgery), recovery time and the use of bandages, orthotics, bite that must always be checked carefully.

Finally, we evaluate the muscular structure. It is important to review every single muscle, making specific questions about past trouble, in particular relating to hamstring and quadriceps, heavily stressed in soccer players. It is necessary to dwell on the dynamics of accidents, the diagnosis, the treatments carried out and the period of absence from competitions, and any discomfort felt by the athlete after his full return to competition.

After performing a detailed history, we go on by physical examination, which must start with the postural control on podoscope to evaluate plantar stance, knee and column alignment and check for any length imbalance.

The assessment of main joints stability is the following step, as well as the verification of the joints ROM (range of movement), in particular of hip, knee and ankle.

Then we evaluate some additional intrinsic risk factors involving the muscles: check for possible strength imbalances or muscle stiffness - especially for hamstrings - and with manual evaluation of the muscles, "feel" the presence of scars that may lead to changes in contraction. These are important functional outcomes for the preventive program assessment, both for physiotherapy, with manual treatment of stiffness areas, and rehabilitation, with correct work for muscle flexibility improvement.

The final doctor report should emphasize every aspect of the clinical examination that can be useful for planning the prevention program, also through the creation of a database easily accessible, for instance using a graphic model of immediate interpretation (Figure 16).

These evaluations are easy to perform and cheap, and can be used with both professional and amateur athletes. After medical history and clinical evaluation, a full muscles and tendons ultrasound examination - the importance of which is emphasized in a special section - should be performed. Finally, in case of a new athlete's evaluation protocol, the MRI evaluation of lumbar spine can be added, to check for possible structural failures related to muscle injuries, and knee MRI, to highlight ligament, meniscus or cartilage damages. These last evaluations, more expensive, will be set according to the economic budget of each club.

In our experience, two more points are to be considered for a good preventive program drawing up: -1 clinical or functional simple and repeatable tests, that must be performed several times during the season both to get new medical information and to check the effectiveness of our program -2 weekly collegial meeting with all the members of the team medical staff, to present the problems found, organize and discuss the preventive program and give each ones specific tasks, to ensure that athletes follow strictly their personal prevention program.

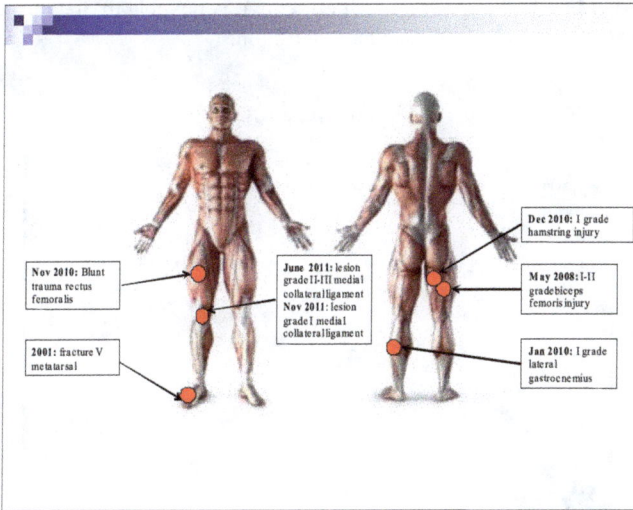

Figure 16. Graphical model to remind sites of previous injuries.

To make the preventive program easy to use and apply by athlete, medical and technical staff guidelines have to be written in a simple way, printed together with images that show the correct execution of the field and gym exercises.

There are several tests that can be used to predict the risk of injuries, to identify the muscles to work on and to evaluate the effectiveness of our strategies.

We suggest two tests that we normally use, and that are giving effective responses: further investigations are, however needed in this area.

One, named Functional Movement Screen (FMS™), simple and easy to use, and the other, based on use of tensiomiography (TMG), more technological, expensive and not easy to use but which allows to evaluate the individual muscles of the lower limbs.

3.1. FMS: Functional Movement Screen

This is a test based on the execution of a series of simple exercises that allow the assessment of postural balance and symmetry of the different muscle chains [46,47].

For each exercise is given a score from 0 (impossible to carry out the proposed exercise) to 3 (perfect exercise). The maximum score is 21(Figure 17).

The exercises are the following:

Deep Squat, Hurdle Step In-Line Lunge, Shoulder Mobility, Active Straight Leg Raises, Trunk Stability Push Up, Rotary Stability [46,47].

In addition, according to the scores in each exercise, it is possible to draw up a preventive exercise program to improve movement harmonization.

Scoring Sheet FMS

NAME:			AGE:	HEIGHT:	
WEIGHT:		M/F:	PHONE:		
ADRESS					
SPORT:					
HAND DOMIN:	R)	L	LEG DOMINANCE: R)	L	

TEST	RAW SC	FINAL	COMMENTS
Deep Squat		O	
Hurdle STEP.L		O	
Hurdle STEP.R			
In-Line LUNGE.L		O	
In-Line LUNGE.R			
Sho.Mob.L		O	
Sho.Mob.R			
Active IMP.L			
Active IMP.R			
ASLR.L		O	
ASLR.R			
TSPU		O	
EXT			
Rot.STAB.L		O	
Rot.STAB.R			
FLX			
TOTAL		O	

Figure 17. FMS score schedule

This test should be repeated periodically to assess the effectiveness of our work protocol, and before the return to the field after an injury to check if functional alterations still persist.

3.2. TMG or tensiomiography: (In our practice we use TMG SYSTEM 100 ® TMG-BMC Ltd)

This is a device provided with a special sensor which, positioned on the muscle to be analyzed, records the muscle contraction induced artificially by electric pulse.

The sensor measures the radial enlargement of the muscle: the values are detected at different stimulation intensities and the results are placed in a time/displacement chart (Figure 18). The processing of these data through a specific software provides a measure of possible muscle imbalances, directing the work on strengthening exercises or, if muscle show an excessive tightness, on flexibility improvement protocols. In addition, this test gives us information on the balance between agonists/antagonists muscles and between the muscle groups of the two legs.

The test should be performed systematically to check the effectiveness of the preventive program, to improve the quality of the muscle contraction, and it should be performed also before full return to the field, in case of injury.

There is no safe scientific evidence that prove efficiency of this test in preventing injuries, but it is now used by some professional soccer teams, and can represent an opportunity for further investigations.

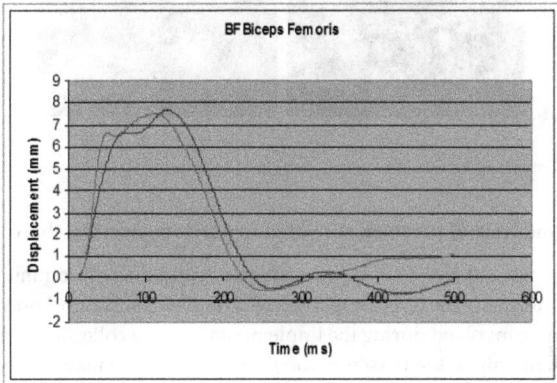

Figure 18. Displacement/time biceps femoris chart

- Ultrasound evaluation

Several studies report that a previous muscle injury is an important risk factor for muscle injury [2,3,8,13,15,16,19,21,27,28,43-45]. Ultrasound and MRI are the reference modalities of imaging for the diagnosis and monitoring of muscle injuries (Figure 19).

At the beginning of each season new players are recruited in the ranks of soccer teams. A detailed medical history sometimes cannot detect all previous muscle injuries, mainly due to two reasons. First of all, the reluctance of some players to report all previous injuries (i.e.: fear to be considered a player with a high injury risk). Secondly, the possible forgetfulness of long standing muscle injuries.

Ultrasound may be the preferred primary modality to complete medical history and clinical evaluation of previous muscle injuries, because of its portability, ease of use and decreased costs. Ultrasound also, compared to MRI, allows a rapid and complete examination of all muscle compartments, both under rest standard condition and real-time functional and dynamic assessment. MRI must be used as a second step, to increase the information on the outcomes of some injuries.

All information collected by ultrasound (muscle scars and calcifications, their site, size, orientation, dynamic response) have to be related to what is reported by the player (comfort, discomfort, pain, tightness).

The knowledge of these anatomical outcomes represents a basic step, both for the technical and medical staff, in order to plan a correct prevention work on these non-negligible risk factors.

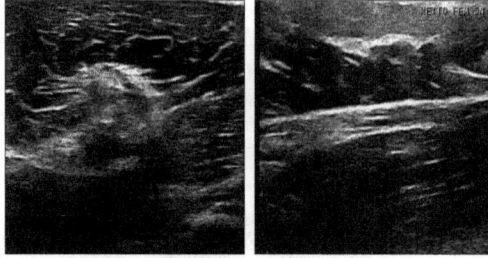

Figure 19. Ultrasound images of scares: biceps femoris (left), rectus femoris (right).

- Evaluation and analysis of parameters related to performance: Database

A good medical, rehab and physiotherapy organization and the best communication between all members of the team are the basic properties required for a successful prevention program. The other component involved during the implementation and collection of additional data is the technical staff, mainly in the person of the fitness coach who takes care of physical work in the gym and on the field.

A continuous dialogue between medical staff and fitness coach is important in order to provide information on players' health, and to liaise on the problems that some exercises or excessive loads can cause. For this reason it is important to set a database where the team staff can enter medical, physiological and functional data, always respecting the privacy of the athlete.

All the parameters of the test to which the athlete has been subjected have to be placed, to monitor constantly the psychophysical condition of the athlete.

Blood tests and all examinations required by law for the eligibility of professional athletes must be entered in the database.

Other parameters that we would suggest to insert in the database include: how much time the athlete passes in the massage room, the number of manual treatments that he runs during the week and the fatigue perception experienced in training or game, assessed by the CR-10 Borg scale [48] (Table 2). These data allows us to understand when an athlete's fatigue is dispro-portionate to the workload and when he feels the need to be processed manually in order to reduce stiffness. When these two parameters begin to rise over the standard average values the risk of possible muscle injuries increases.

In addition to the FMS e TMG results, we also recommend to enter in the work program some field and laboratory tests that provide information on some of the intrinsic factors listed above: aerobic fitness, strength imbalance, body size.

To assess body size, we are interested in monitoring the weight, lean body mass and body fat percentage as well as the state of hydration. These can be evaluated in a simple way with the use of a scale, a caliper and, if available, a machine for bio-impedance body composition analysis (BIA).

Rating	Perceived Exertion
0	Nothing at all
0,5	Very very light
1	Very light
2	Fairly Light
3	Moderate
4	Somewhat hard
5/6	Hard
7	Very hard
8	
9	Very very hard
10	

Table 2. CR-10 Borg scale.

For the aerobic fitness evaluation many field tests have been proposed. According to our experience we prefer submaximal test, as the Mognoni test, in place of the maximal test used a few years ago, because the latter is highly dependent on the compliance of the athlete.

While to assess the maximal frequency and fatigue we use the yo-yo intermittent recovery test, to evaluate the strength imbalance we prefer an isokinetic test and for a rapid measurement of the explosive force we use the jump test.

Mognoni test. This is a test that allows to determine the speed and, consequently, the frequency of the anaerobic threshold and consists in allowing the player to travel the distance of 1,350 meters in 6 minutes while maintaining a constant speed of 13.5 km/h. To facilitate the correct execution, we should put on the path signals at regular intervals (50 meters), and make the athletes follow a call sound that indicates when they have to come to the signal.

At the end of the test, the concentration of blood lactate is measured through a sample and the threshold speed and consequently the threshold frequency are extrapolated through a mathematical formula (Table 3).

Moreover, we also assess the fatigue perception by the CR-10 Borg scale.

The periodical execution of the test allows on the one hand the technical staff to verify the aerobic capacity of the athlete and to modulate the workload during the season, and on the other hand the medical staff to monitor his state of health. Furthermore, testing the athlete also before his return to the field after a long muscle injury allows us check if he has found a good physical condition, an aspect that reduces the risk of re-injury.

blood lactate (mmol/l⁻¹)	threshold speed (Km/h)
1,5	15,55
2,0	15,04
2,5	14,55
3,0	14,11
3,5	13,70
4,0	13,26
4,5	12,98
5,0	12,66
5,5	12,38
6,0	12,33

Table 3. Correlation between concentration of lactate in the blood and threshold speed (Source: "Il libro dei test" Marella-Risaliti ed. Correre 1999)

Yo-Yo intermittent recovery test (Bansgbo, 1997): assesses the subject ability to recover during progressively increasing exercise. The test involves running a shuttle between two cones placed 20 meters away from each other, performing at the end of each fraction of 40 meters, 10 seconds of active recovery. The running speed and the recovery time are dictated by a pre-recorded sound signal.

The initial speed is 10 km/h and increases progressively. When the athlete is unable to maintain the suggested speed for two consecutive step, the test ends. The meters run and final speed are included in the database.

This test is useful for performance evaluation in sports involving the alternation of high and low intensity phases, as in soccer. This test periodically repeated allows an evaluation of the improvements determined from training through the distance travelled. In addition, the test performed after long muscle injuries evaluates fitness to fatigue, which is another intrinsic risk factor for muscle injury.

Jump tests: these tests that are performed with the use of a force platform. We recommend to perform two exercises:

Squat Jump: the athlete with hands on hips reaches the position of semisquat (90°) and jump as high as possible. In the database we record the best performance of the three that we usually ask to carry out. The results are measured in cm or msec and give us an indication of the explosive force

Countermovement jump: the athlete with free arms turns quickly to reach the semisquat position (90°) and jump as high as possible. In the database we record the best performance of the three that we usually ask to carry out. The results are measured in cm or msec and give us indication of the explosive elastic force.

Isokinetic tests: the isokinetic devices are tools which allow to perform muscle exercises with constant angular velocity throughout the range of movement; after a determined angular velocity is reached during an acceleration phase, the device does not allow this speed to be overcome. In this way, the resistance that the athlete meets is equal to his effort, allowing him to perform a safer and less traumatic exercise for muscle than an isotonic one. The isokinetic test should not be considered useful to evaluate only the maximum force but also to evaluate muscle functionality throughout the whole range of movement.

The most important parameter to consider is the peak force, the maximum force that the athlete is able to express during the exercise, followed by the work done and the power developed. It is essential to compare the values obtained in the two legs to evaluate possible imbalances and work to correct them.

Another important parameter is the muscle agonists/antagonists strength ratio because, as we have previously pointed out, muscle imbalances are an intrinsic risk factor for muscle injury.

The battery of all the tests listed above should be performed at the same time, in order to integrate the results and obtain a complete picture of the health state of the athlete and his fitness. These results are then processed by the team doctor to detect possible situations of risk and to provide information both to therapists and rehabilitators for immediate action. Moreover, they should be repeated several times (4-5) during the season and entered into the database to assess how the indices change with training.

Once again, it is important to emphasize that all these tests should also be performed before returning to the field from a long injury and values should be similar to those obtained when the athlete was in a good physical condition

In fact a good physical condition, a proper adaptation to fatigue, a good balance of strength between the two limbs are the key parameters to minimize the risk of muscle injury.

- **Other practical suggestions**

In the available scientific literature, there are many conflicting data about the significance of different risk factors on incidence of muscle injuries, and therefore it is difficult to organize a prevention program universally recognized and validated. We can suggest performing a work protocol, which is developed in relation to the availability of medical structures and the compliance of the athlete. The protocol must be modified and improved over time, according to further scientific evidence.

As suggested above, a careful history and physical examination are essential to detect, since the first control, all intrinsic and extrinsic factors (shoes, orthotics, etc.) that may increase the risk of injury.

Then the data must be processed and shown to all medical staff, especially doctors, physio-therapists and rehabilitators.

The physiotherapists need to focus on the manual treatments that have been agreed and programmed. In fact, the possible muscle scars or areas of stiffness need special care and must be systematically monitored and managed. We prefer to avoid deep manual treatments and massage before and after strength session, and close to the matches, as in some athletes these treatments can cause a feeling of discomfort on match day.

It is recommended that scar treatments, with technique of deep transverse massage, are performed earlier in the week, especially after the aerobic session and at least 24 hours before the next training session. For the following days, our advice is to treat the antagonist muscles and the other muscles involved in the same kinetic chain.

We also recommend the assessment of the lumbar and dorsal muscles, strictly related to hamstring. In athletes with previous hamstring injuries we suggest to treat them, manually at least once a week.

The other important figure for the preventive work is the field rehabilitator. For this reason, the advice is to select a person with a degree allowing him/her to serve as both physical therapist and fitness coach. This figure must be placed in the medical staff and should be accountable to the doctor.

His work should be set in order to dedicate to each athlete 3 session a week, 45-60 minutes before training and 10-15 minutes during cooling-down.

In fact, we should not insert extra workload after the physical and tactical training, because usually the attention and compliance of the player are lower at the end of the session. After training, simple postures or exercises of muscle compensation are well tolerated.

To assess the degree of fatigue, as described above we use the Borg CR-10 scale, that shows us if the results are consistent with the athlete workloads, compared to the average values of the team and the typical values of the athlete.

We also suggest to set a good warm-up program, using different exercises according to the problems of the single athlete such as exercise bike 10-15 min, varying seat height, number of revolution/min and intensity of exercise, or walking/running on the treadmill. Finally, continue with mobilization exercises focusing on the mobilization of the spine, hips and knees.

As a result we recommend that proprioceptive exercises are carried out using traditional tablets or skimmy, setting circuits with different proprioceptive stimuli. According to our experience, it is better to plan proprioceptive exercise early in the week and then reduce it with the approach of the match.

Other exercises in preparation to the match can be performed by bouncer and trampoline equipment, to enhance the work of propulsion and thrust by the limbs.

As a final step it is important to introduce some muscles strengthening exercises. We think it is important to give different stimuli to the muscles and for this reason it is better to vary the types of exercises, especially in order to improve muscular balance and strength.

We propose to perform eccentric exercise especially on the hamstring and quadriceps, if possible manual and managed by the rehabilitator that can modulate the loads. These exercises can be associated with working sessions with elastic bands. Finally, we suggest exercises with isoinertial equipment, which allow us to work on different eccentric muscle chains and allow an excellent simulation of the field work.

These three methods: manual eccentric, working with elastic bands, isoinertial works can be combined successfully, both within the same session and alternating during the week.

At the end of the training session, we can propose 5-6 minutes of postural exercises to relax the posterior chain and the column or through 10-15 min of relaxing work in the pool.

Last useful advice is to use cryotherapy after training to reduce possible overload inflammation affecting the tendons, joints and muscles

There are several ways to perform cryotherapy, the simplest of which is to use cold water (10-12 degrees) for a period of time ranging from 5 to 7 min. After cryotherapy it is recommended to avoid manual treatment.

4. Conclusion

Muscle injuries are frequent in soccer and involve mainly four muscle groups of the lower limbs (hamstrings, quadriceps, adductors and calf). Re-injuries risk represents a serious problem in order to plan safe return to full training and competitions. Some factors are suspected to be related to the onset of muscle injuries in soccer players and are described as intrinsic and extrinsic risk factors. The relationship between these risk factors and muscle injuries is currently not completely understood. Nevertheless, the management of risk factors involves medical and technical staff of soccer teams, in order to plan a muscle injury prevention program. The program has to be performed both for general prevention (dedicated to all players) and personal prevention (player-specific). Several prevention programs have been proposed by some authors and are experimented by coaches, medical staffs and athletes. The effectiveness of these programs on many occasions is not corroborated by scientific evidence. This is probably due to the large number of factors that affect the neuromuscular performance in soccer. The assessment of the athlete, however, represents the first step to program the prevention work. Personal history and clinical evaluation, imaging evaluation, laboratory and field tests are needed for all new players recruited in the team's ranks. The setting up of a database with many parameters of healthy athletes is also proposed, with the aim of evaluating each single player in pre-season and competition period. In case of injury this will be used as a reference to plan return to competition. Finally, we offer some practical suggestions to be used in prevention programs of football teams.

The wide border between empiricism and scientific evidence is often an obstacle to the realization of practical proposals. It should not become an excuse for inaction. We cannot ignore the experience accumulated in years of work by medical and technical staff of soccer teams. For this reason, while we are aware that the development of new studies is certainly desirable, we hope in a growing collaboration between all the components involved in the management of the players, in order to improve current knowledge and direct future guidelines about the prevention of muscle injuries in soccer.

Author details

M. Giacchino[1*] and G. Stesina[2]

*Address all correspondence to: calcki@alice.it

1 Istituto di Medicina dello Sport F.M.S.I. Torino, Italy

2 FC Juventus, Turin, Italy

References

[1] Ekstrand, J, Hagglund, M, & Waldén, M. Epidemiology of muscle injuries in professional football (soccer). Am J Sports Med. (2011). Jun;, 39(6), 1226-32.

[2] Arnason, A, Sigurdsson, S. B, Gudmundsson, A, Holme, I, Engebretsen, L, & Bahr, R. Risk factors for injuries in football. Am J Sports Med. (2004). Jan-Feb;32 (Suppl 1):SS16., 5.

[3] Ekstrand, J, Hagglund, M, & Waldén, M. Injury incidence and injury patterns in professional football- the UEFA injury study. Br J Sport Med. (2011). , 45, 553-8.

[4] Hawkins, R. D, Hulse, M. A, Wilkinson, C, Hodson, A, & Gibson, M. The association football medical research programme: an audit of injuries in professional football. Br J Sport Med. (2001). , 35, 43-7.

[5] Hagglund, M, Waldén, M, & Ekstrand, J. Injury incidence and distribution in elite football- a prospective study of the Danish and the Swedish top divisions. Scand J Med Sci Sports. (2005). , 15, 21-28.

[6] Junge, A, Dvorak, J, Graf-baumann, T, & Peterson, L. Football injuries during FIFA tournaments and the Olympic Games, (1998). development and implementation of an injury-reporting system. Am J Sports Med. 2004 Jan-Feb;32(Suppl 1):SS89, 80.

[7] Waldén, M, Hagglund, M, & Ekstrand, J. Injuries in Swedish elite football- a prospective study on injury definitions, risk for injury and injury pattern during 2001. Scand J Med Sci Sports. (2005). , 15, 118-25.

[8] Waldén, M, Hagglund, M, & Ekstrand, J. UEFA Champions League study: a prospective study of injuries in professional football during the 2001-2002 season. Br J Sport Med. (2005). , 39, 542-6.

[9] Inklaar, H. Soccer injuries. I: Incidence and severity. Sports Med. (1994). , 18(1), 55-73.

[10] Lopez V JrGalano GJ, Black CM, Gupta AT, James DE, Kelleher KM, Allen AA. Profile of an American amateur rugby union seven series. Am J Sports Med. (2012). Jan;, 40(1), 179-84.

[11] Feeley, B. T, Kennelly, S, Barnes, R. P, Muller, M. S, Kelly, B. T, Rodeo, S. A, & Warren, R. F. Epidemiology of National Football League Training Camp Injuries From 1998 to 2007. Am J Sports Med. (2008Aug). , 36(8), 1597-603.

[12] Stevenson, M. R, Hamer, P, Finch, C. F, Elliot, B, & Kresnow, M. Sport, age, and sex specific incidence of sports injuries in Western Australia. Br J Sports Med (2000). , 34, 188-94.

[13] Hagglund, M, Waldén, M, & Ekstrand, J. Previous injury as a risk factor for injury in elite football: a prospective study over two consecutive seasons. Br J Sport Med. (2006). , 40(9), 767-72.

[14] Orchard, J. W. Intrinsic and extrinsic risk factors for muscle strains in Australian football. Am J Sports Med (2001). , 29, 300-3.

[15] Opar, D. A, Williams, M. D, & Shield, A. J. Hamstring strains injuries: factors that lead to injury and re-injury. Sports Med. (2012). , 42(3), 209-26.

[16] Gabbe, B. J, Finch, C. F, Bennell, K. L, & Wajswelner, H. Risk factors for hamstring injuries in community level Australian football. Br J Sports Med. (2005). , 39, 106-11.

[17] Woods, C, Hawkins, R. D, Maltby, S, Hulse, M, Thomas, A, & Hodson, A. The Football Association Medical Research Programme: an audit of injuries in professional football. Analysis of hamstring injuries. Br J Sport Med (2004). Feb; , 38(1), 36-41.

[18] Ostenberg, A, & Roos, H. Injury risk factors in female European football. A prospective study of 123 players during one season. Scand J Med Sci Sports (2000). , 10(5), 279-85.

[19] Murphy, D F, Connolly, D, & Beynnon, J. B D. Risk factors for lower extremity injury: a review of the literature Br J Sports Med (2003). , 37, 13-29.

[20] Henderson, G, Barnes, C. A, & Portas, M. D. Factors associated with increased propensity for hamstring injury in English Premier League Soccer Players. J Sci Med Sport (2010). Jul;, 13(4), 397-402.

[21] Gabbe, B. J, Bennell, K. L, Finch, C. F, Wajswelner, H, & Orchard, J. W. Predictors of hamstring injury at the elite level of Australian football. Scand J Med Sci Sports. (2006). , 16, 7-13.

[22] Orchard, J. W, Farhart, P, & Leopold, C. Lumbar spine region pathology and hamstring and calf injuries in athletes: is there a connection? Br J Sports Med. (2004). Aug; , 38(4), 502-4.

[23] Verrall, G. M, Slavotinek, J. P, & Barnes, P. G. Fon GT, Spriggins AJ. Clinical risk factors for hamstring muscle strain injury: a prospective study with correlation of injury by magnetic resonance imaging. Br J Sports Med. (2001). , 35(6), 435-439.

[24] Mundiguchia, J, Alentorn-geli, E, & Brughelli, M. Hamstring strain injuries: are we heading in the right direction? Br J Sports Med Feb (2012). , 46(2), 81-85.

[25] Chomiak, J, Junge, A, Peterson, L, & Dvorak, J. Severe injuries in football players. Influencing factors. Am J Sports Med (2000). S5):SS68., 58.

[26] Brooks JHMFuller CW, Kemp SPT, Reddin DB. Incidence, risk, and prevention of hamstring muscle injuries in professional rugby union. Am J Sports Med (2006). Aug;, 34(8), 1297-306.

[27] Van Mechelen, W, Hlobil, H, & Kemper, H. C. Incidence, severity, aetiology and prevention of sport injuries: a review of concepts. Sports Med (1992). , 14(2), 82-99.

[28] Lehance, C, Binet, J, Bury, T, & Croisier, J. L. Muscular strength, functional performances and injury risk in professional and junior elite soccer players. Scand J Med Sci Sports. (2009). , 19(2), 243-251.

[29] Engebretsen, A. H, Myklebust, G, Holme, I, Engebretsen, L, & Bahr, R. Intrinsic risk factors for hamstring injuries among male soccer players: a prospective cohort study. Am J Sports Med. (2010). Jun;, 38(6), 1147-53.

[30] Prior, M, Guerin, M, & Grimmer, K. An evidence-based approach to hamstring strain injury. Sport Health (2009). March;, 1(2), 154-164.

[31] Meeuwisse, W, Tyreman, H, Hagel, B, et al. Dynamic model of etiology in sport injury: the recursive nature of risk and causation. Clin J Sport Med (2007). , 17(3), 215-19.

[32] Croiser, J. L, Ganteaume, S, Binet, J, Genty, M, & Ferret, J. M. Strength imbalances and prevention of hamstring injury in professional soccer players: a prospective study. Am J Sports Med (2008). Aug;, 36(8), 1469-75.

[33] Woods, K, Bishop, P, & Jones, E. Warm-up and stretching in the prevention of muscular injury. Sports Med. (2007). , 37(12), 1089-99.

[34] Mc Hugh, M. P, & Cosgrave, C. H. To stretch or not to stretch: the role of stretching in injury prevention and performance. Scand J Med Sci Sports. (2010). , 20, 169-81.

[35] Safran, M. R, Garrett, W. E, Seaber, A. V, Glisson, R. R, & Ribbeck, B. M. The role of warmup in muscular injury prevention. Am J Sports Med. (1988). Mar;, 16(2), 123-129.

[36] Renstrom, P, Peterson, L, & Edberg, B. Valhalla artificial pitch at Gathenburg a two-years evaluation. Sweden: Rapport Naturvandsverket, (1977). , 1975-1977.

[37] Engebretsen, L, & Kase, T. Soccer injuries and artificial turf]. Tidsskr Nor Laegeforen (1987). , 107, 2215-7.

[38] Nigg, B. M, & Segesser, B. The influence of playing surfaces on the load on the loco-motor system and on football and tennis injuries. Sports Med. (1988). , 5(6), 375-85.

[39] Ekstrand, J, & Nigg, B. M. Surface related injuries in soccer. Sports Med. (1989). , 8(1), 56-62.

[40] Arnason, A, Gudmundsson, A, Dahl, H. A, & Johansson, E. Soccer injuries in Iceland. Scand J Med Sci Sports (1996). , 6(1), 40-5.

[41] Dragoo, J. L, & Braun, H. J. The effect of playing surface on injury rate: a review of the current literature. Sports Med. (2010). , 40(11), 981-90.

[42] Williams, S, Hume, P. A, & Kara, S. A Review of Football Injuries on Third and Fourth Generation Artificial Turfs Compared with Natural Turf. Sports Med. (2011). , 41(11), 903-23.

[43] Dvorak, J, Junge, A, Chomiak, J, Graf-baumann, T, Peterson, L, Rosch, D, & Hodgson, R. Risk factor analysis for injuries in players. Possibilities for a prevention program. Am J Sports Med. (2000). Sep;28(5 Suppl):SS74., 69.

[44] Witvrouw, E, Danneels, L, Asselman, P, Have, D, & Cambier, T. D. Muscle flexibility as a risk factor for developing muscle injuries in male professional soccer players: a prospective study. Am J Sports Med. (2003). Jan;, 31(1), 41-6.

[45] Hagglund, M, Waldén, M, & Ekstrand, J. Risk factors for lower extremity muscle injury in professional soccer. The UEFA injury study. Published online before print December 21,2012, doi:10.1177/0363546512470634.Am J Sports Med. December 21, (2012).

[46] Cook, G, Burton, L, & Hoogenboom, B. Pre-Participation Screening: The Use of Fundamental Movements as an Assessment of Function- Part 1. N Am J Sports Phys Ther. (2006). May;, 1(2), 62-72.

[47] Cook, G, Burton, L, & Hoogenboom, B. Pre-Participation Screening: The Use of Fundamental Movements as an Assessment of Function- Part 2. N Am J Sports Phys Ther. (2006). Aug;, 1(3), 132-9.

[48] Borg's Perceived Exertion and Pain ScalesChampaign, IL: Human Kinetics; (1998).

Chapter 10

How and When to Use an Injury Prevention Intervention in Soccer

Alexandre Dellal, Karim Chamari and Adam Owen

Additional information is available at the end of the chapter

1. Introduction

Soccer is a high intensity intermittent contact sport exposing elite level players to contin‐ual physical, technical, tactical, psychological, and physiological demands (Owen et al, 2011; Dellal et al, 2011). Due to the huge financial rewards of being successful at the elite level of the sport, the demands placed upon the players are ever growing because of increased fixture schedules that generally include less recovery periods between train‐ing and competitive match play, disposing players to a greater risk of injury (Dellal at al, 2013; Dupont et al, 2010; Rey et al, 2010; Morgan and Oberlander 2001; Junge and Dvorak 2004). The number of competitive matches played by elite European soccer play‐ers (Table 1) during one season can be >80, with 1.6 to 2 matches per week throughout its entirety (excluding friendly games) (Figure 1). It should be noted that, a player com‐peting at the higher echelons of world soccer such as Lionel Messi has accumulated be‐tween 64 to 69 official competitive games throughout seasons 2011-2012, 2010-2011, and 2009-2010 as shown in Table 2. As reported in this context, modern day soccer involves a continued, intensive cycle and predisposes players to greater injury risks due to accu‐mulative fatigue or overload. Previous research has already found a correlation between low training and match availability due to injury, with decreased team success (Arnason et al, 2004). This is of particular importance for teams unable to replace players due to limited funds or resources, and subsequently highlights the need for all clubs irrespec‐tive of budgets, resources and funding potential to minimize injury risk of players in or‐der to be more successful. After all, there seems to be no point in pushing players constantly to be physically, technically and tactically better if they are consistently un‐available to play.

Country	Match played in 1st League	Match played in League cup	Match played in National cup	Match played in UEFA Champions League or Europa League	Other games (National or European super cup, champions cup, etc)	National team	Minimal rate of match per years	Maximal rate of match per years	Summer holidays
Spain, La Liga	38	1 to 10	0	6 to 15	2 to 4	4 to 11	51	78	30 to 41 days
England, Premier League	38	1 to 9	1 to 9	6 to 15	2	4 to 11	52	84	40 to 55 days
Germany Bundesliga	34	1 to 5	1 to 6	6 to 15	1	4 to 11	47	72	41 to 53 days
France Ligue 1	38	1 to 5	1 to 6	6 to 15	2	4 to 11	50	77	25 to 35 days
Italy Calcio	38	2 to 11	0	6 to 15	1	4 to 11	51	76	41 to 53 days

Table 1. Official match played by elite soccer players from European teams.

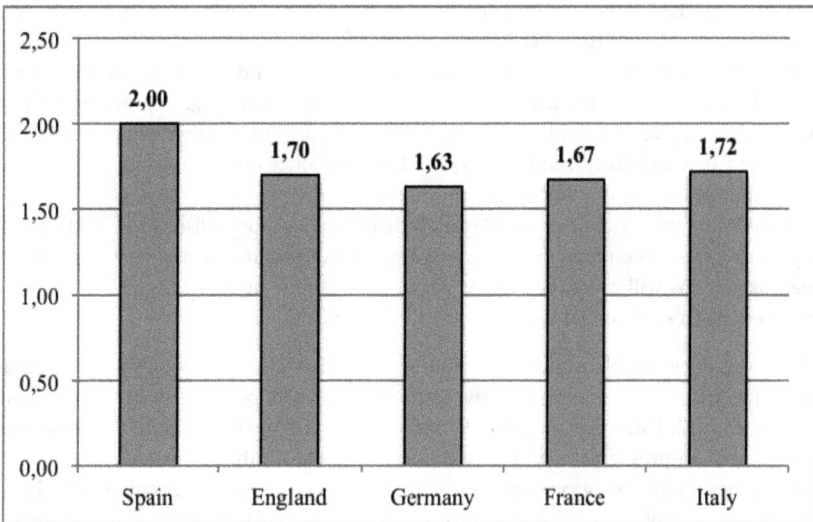

Figure 1. Mean number of official matches per week played across the 5 best European Leagues (excluding the friendly games).

	Players	Season 2011-2012	Season 2010-2011	Season 2009-2010
1	Messi Lionel	69	66	64
2	Ronaldo Cristiano	69	59	46
3	Iniesta Andres	47	50	41
4	Xavi	51	50	53
5	Falcao Radamel	52	42	43
6	Pirlo Andrea	56	36	51
7	Drogba Didier	47	49	57
8	Van Persie Robin	60	38	34
9	Ibrahimovic Zlatan	55	49	49
10	Alonso Xabi	54	63	56
11	Yaya Touré	49	52	37
12	Neymar	59	67	62
13	Osil Mesut	62	64	62
14	Rooney Wayne	50	48	49

Table 2. Official matches played by the 14 best players during the 3 last seasons (according to the official "Ballon d'Or" ranking).

The financial outlay clubs make season upon season in order to gain success is well into the high percentages of club turnover (wages, transfer fees and contractual terms agreed). The expense of a player being out through a non-contact injury could be substantial and seen as a negative investment or non-efficient with every game missed through a preventable injury. Consequently, the need to implement a sport-specific injury prevention structure within the organization that technical, conditioning coaches and other individuals involved with the player training status is of paramount importance. According to previous research the most significant injury predictor of soccer players is their injury history (Olsen et al, 2004). The fact that players have some type of chronic problem or low training or match availability over numerous seasons will more than likely manifest itself moving forward unless appropriate injury prevention steps are taken.

It is however, questionable whether some types of exercise-based injury prevention programs actually facilitate true learning of new biomechanical and neuromuscular characteristics (Padua et al, 2012; Paterno et al, 2004). Whereas the effects of short duration exercise-based injury prevention programs may induce transient changes in the performance of functional tasks that regress following cessation of the program. In order to experience biomechanical and/or neuromuscular changes it is likely that extended-duration training periods are necessary to facilitate long-term retention of movement control (Padua et al, 2012). Yet, performing injury prevention drills over a prolonged period, as performed by Owen et al (2013b), may still be insufficient to induce large reductions in the incidence of specific injuries.

Essentially, players may respond differently to intervention programs and this should be a consideration for further detailed investigations. Alternatively, despite certain programs being performed during the entirety of the season, it is possible that specific prevention sessions or individual exercises may have been insufficient in terms of longevity and duration required to elicit large training adaptations. This is pertinent to elite level athletes who generally possess relatively high levels of general fitness and would unlikely experience gains similar to lesser skilled individuals despite being at a greater risk of injury (Ekstrand et al, 1983).

The incidence of injuries among elite adult male soccer players during competitive match-play was described to be approximately between 24.6 and 34.8 per 1000 match hours (Walden et al, 2005; Arnason et al, 2008; Parry and Drust, 2006), and training injuries ranging between 5.8 to 7.6 per 1000 training hours (Walden et al, 2005; Arnason et al, 2008) even if some studies report values outside these ranges. Walden et al (2005) revealed that the risk of injury in European professional soccer is high with the most common injury being the posterior thigh strain. Hawkins et al (2001) reported an average of 1.3 injuries per player per season in English professional soccer, with the propensity of injuries occurring in the final 15min period of each half. Comparatively, fewer injuries occur during the first half of matches compared to the second (Hoy et al, 1992; Hawkins and Fuller 1996, 1999). The stressors encountered during actual match play have been suggested to show no detrimental effect of consecutive games on physical performance, but a greater injury risk (Carling et al, 2012; Dupont et al, 2010; Rey et al, 2010).

Almost one third of all soccer related injuries are muscle related and the majority (92%) affect the major muscle groups of the lower extremity: hamstrings, 37%; adductors, 23%; quadriceps, 19%; and calf muscles, 13% (Ekstrand, 2011). Over a period of two seasons, the Football Association Audit of Injuries also showed the hamstrings to be the most commonly injured muscles, constituting 12% of all strains (Hawkins et al, 2001). The implications manifesting in players being 2.5 times more likely to sustain a hamstring strain than a quadriceps strain during a game (Hawkins et al, 2001). This is clear evidence as to why clubs invest heavily in time and resources of injury prevention in an attempt to reduce the prevalence of injuries (injury rate). However, eagerness to return to play resulting in an incomplete rehabilitation has shown the increase the re-injury rate for hamstring injuries thus, questioning the success of current injury prevention programs (Croisier, 2004; Hagglund et al, 2005).

Previous research has suggested that muscle strains may occur due to insufficient warm-up (Kujala et al, 1997; Worrell, 1994), poor flexibility (Kujala et al, 1997; Worrell, 1994; Hartig and Henderson, 1999) even if some recent research are conflicting in this regard, muscle imbalances (Worrell, 1994), muscle weakness (Croisier et al, 2002), neural tension (Turl and George, 1998), fatigue (Kujala et al, 1997; Worrell, 1994), previous injury (Engebretsen et al, 2008), increasing age and poor running technique although the evidence to represent these findings are both minimal and conflicting. Chamari et al (2012) has recently showed Ramadan Intermittent Fasting to induce higher injury rates in Muslim elite soccer players with a higher number of contractures for muscles themselves, and some tendinosis for tendons. Over-emphasis on one-sided activities, such as kicking, lateral movements and single-leg jumping, may also lead to asymmetry and dominance of one leg, which in turn may cause greater than normal differences in strength between compared to contra-lateral muscle groups. Further-more, an unfavorable difference between agonist and antagonist muscle groups is considered to leave the weaker muscle group at a disadvantage and such an example, hypertrophy of the quadriceps at the expense of the hamstring may lead to hamstring injuries. Indeed, Croisier et al (2008) and Knapik et al (1991) suggested that players with a strength imbalance greater than 15% were 2.6 times more likely to suffer injury in the weaker leg.

Ekstrand and Gillquist (1984) have showed that intervention prevention strategies allowed players to have 75% fewer injuries than a control group (ankle, sprain, strain). **In this context, the aim of the present book chapter will be to present the literature review showing how different prevention methods and strategies appear to result in the reduction of injuries to soccer players both during training and matches.** However, the combination of concurrent prevention programs could further positively affect the injury rate, especially the high incidence of lower extremity non-contact muscle injuries. Therefore, based on all the previous research findings and suggestions, the importance of injury prevention at the elite level of professional soccer led to the development of this review. The current review aims to examine the impact a 4-part structured injury prevention intervention would have on injuries occurring within elite level professional soccer clubs.

2. Prevention techniques used in soccer

The majority of injury prevention training studies have generally examined the effects of individual components on injury incidence. However, this is not representative of a soccer specific environment where the time constraints dealt necessitates the development of a mixed conditioning approach that allows for the simultaneous development of several fitness qualities. From a practical perspective, injury prevention programs are implemented with the expectation that they will elicit improvements in performance (through increasing players' availability and reducing lay-off durations when injury occur) and reduce the incidence of injury, however, this is not always representative of research findings. Recently, it has been suggested that a multicomponent injury prevention intervention may increase motivation through an integrated approach within a team sport environment (Owen et al, 2013b). This particular investigation recently reported that significantly less muscle injuries were observed during integration of a 4-part injury prevention program concomitant with a bigger squad size (large effect, p<0.001) when compared to a control season (Owen et al, 2013). It was reported during this investigation that high levels of contusion injuries were apparent within this study, which led the author to suggest that the multicomponent prevention technique is beneficial when integrated in order to reduce muscle injuries but may not be able to prevent other types of injuries (contact injuries). Prevention exercise is commonly included before, during or/and after the training sessions and matches. Within this chapter, we are going to describe the most common prevention technique used in soccer specific, especially by fitness coach. Sometimes one out of these is enough to reduce the injury occurrence, sometimes it is the combination of 2 or more that appears necessary.

2.1. Functional strength

Muscular strength is an important component of physical performance in sport, in terms of both performance and injury prevention (Fousekis et al, 2010). As a factor contributing to success in soccer, the quadriceps muscle plays a fundamental role in jumping, ball-kicking, and to a lesser extend, in sprinting, whereas hamstring contributes to the knee flexion, which is a major factor in stride power (sprinting or accelerate and decelerate). In addition to their direct contribution to athletic performance, the hamstring muscles are of paramount importance during running and stability activities (Zakas et al, 1995), which are continually required in intermittent team play such as soccer, which induces many short, explosive actions, directional changes and decelerations. Impairments in the eccentric muscle contractions involved in explosive phases of elite level soccer such as accelerations and the aforementioned decelerations may be linked to an increased risk of joint and muscle injury (Greig and Siegler, 2009). As a result, training interventions are continuously evolving in order to address this issue, for example Askling et al (2002) suggested that the addition of pre-season strength training for the hamstrings through eccentric overloading brings significant benefits for elite soccer players, both from an injury prevention and performance enhancement viewpoints.

A recent large scaled randomized controlled trial by Petersen et al (2011) addressed the efficacy of the Nordic hamstring exercise program (NHE, see more details here under in the eccentric strength section of the present chapter) for preventing acute hamstring injuries in soccer players. They found that introducing this ten-weeks program to reduce eccentric weakness, a common intrinsic factor associated with hamstring injuries, reduced the incidence of these injuries by 70%. This backed-up previous findings by Arnason et al (2008). Using a larger sample size Arnason's study looked at a total of 24 teams, with over 650 soccer players, over a four years period. These players professional belonged from soccer teams in the Icelandic and Norwegian leagues. The study showed that teams combining the Nordic eccentric exercise protocol and the stretching program were on average undergoing 65% fewer hamstring injuries. When discussing functional strength within a preventative structure it is important that a gradual overload with the primary aim of increasing muscle strength through soccer specific movements is adhered to. Consequently, it is reasonable to suggest that a multicomponent approach to function strength is followed as a closer analysis of the Nordic hamstring exercise that only involves movement at the knee joint. The fact that the hamstring involves work over two joints (hip and knee), the Nordic hamstring exercise clearly doesn't replicate any of the functional activities used in football specific training and therefore should not be used in isolation, but as part of a preventative strength program. In this context, Owen et al (2013b) had suggested that implementing a functional strength program as part of a multicomponent injury prevention structure may significantly reduce muscle strains/tears.

Since the physiological demands of soccer combine repetitive high-speed bouts with constant change of directions as well as physical contact with opposition players on a continuous basis, the fact that muscle injuries are accounted for a significantly high percentage of all injuries should not be unexpected. The hamstring muscle groups are responsible for accelerating and decelerating during high-speed running and sprints. Previous research has suggested that several reports from European elite soccer leagues revealed how hamstring strains are the most

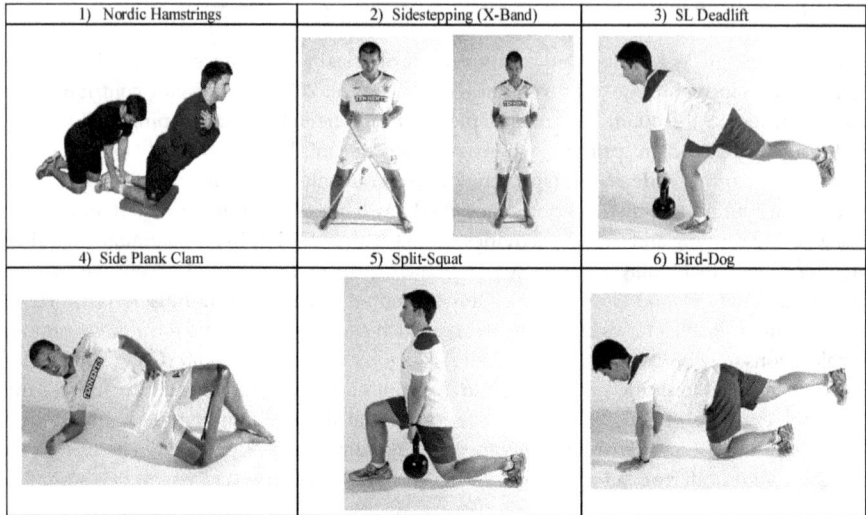

1) Nordic Hamstrings	2) Sidestepping (X-Band)	3) SL Deadlift
4) Side Plank Clam	5) Split-Squat	6) Bird-Dog

Figure 2. Functional strength program (from Owen et al, 2013b)

common type of injury in male soccer players (Junge and Dvorak, 2004). This is the reason for the functional strength aspect of prevention programs to include unilateral exercises that stress the hamstring and gluteal muscle groups through various ranges of lengthening. Figure 2 provides different possibilities of functional strength exercising.

2.2. Eccentric strength

Eccentric strength is considered as an important component of muscular strengthening. Despite complex eccentric strengthening protocols do exist, some simple on-field exercises have been implemented and proposed as a means to reduce injury risks. One of these is the famous "Nordic Hamstring Exercise (NHE)" (mentioned above in the functional strength section of the chapter) that have been proposed to deal with the high injury and re-injury rates of soccer players' hamstrings. The reasons of this muscular group for getting injured has been proposed by Proske and Morgan (2001), with the heterogeneous arrangement of individual muscle sarcomeres inducing microscopic damage coming from non-uniform stretching during eccentric actions. If eccentric movements are repeatedly performed, such as in soccer, this might provide a weak point at the level of muscle architecture, inducing a higher injury risk. Hamstrings are susceptible to injury during terminal swing phase of the leg while sprinting (Schache et al, 2009) because firstly, peak hamstring musculo-tendinuous stretch seems to occur during the swing phase before the foot contact with the ground; and secondly, hamstrings are undergoing an active lengthening contraction during late swing, producing the potential conditions or a strain injury to occur.

The interest of the NHE lies in the fact that it has been shown that it elicits higher activation of the hamstrings compared to a selection of exercises that are routinely used in classical "strength training" or injury rehabilitation (Ebben et al, 2006). In this context, it has been suggested that an eccentric peak torque increase could improve the capability of the hamstrings to absorb energy prior to failure, therefore, reducing the risk of injury (Stanton and Purdham, 1989). Therefore, Arnasson et al (2008), have prospectively investigated over four consecutive soccer seasons (1999-2002) the number of hamstring strains vs. players' exposure for 17 to 30 elite soccer teams from Iceland and Norway. They reported a lower incidence of hamstring strains amongst teams utilizing the eccentric training program vs. the controlled group of players. It was revealed that NHE combined with warm-up stretching appeared to significantly reduce the risk of hamstring strains. Additionally, the authors reported that no effect was observed from flexibility training alone. Arnasson et al (2008) have provided a detailed explanation of the NHE exercise (mentioning Bahr and Maehlum 2004): NHE is a partner based exercise that involves the one partner stabilizing the performer legs and can be easily performed with soccer players performing it alternatively by couples of players (Figure 3). The goal of the performer is to hold as long as possible while achieving maximum loading of the hamstring during the descending eccentric phase. Throughout the movement the player leans forward while keeping his back and hips extended, working towards resisting the forward fall through engaging the hamstring muscles as long as possible until he lands on his hands. Upon landing, players touch-down with their hands moving to touch the ground with his chest. Following on, players forcefully push-off back to the kneeling position with minimal concentric load on the hamstrings. The load is progressively increased through the training program by attempting to withstand the forward fall longer. When the performer can withstand the whole range of motion for 12 repetitions, the load can be increased by adding speed to the starting phase of the motion. Finally, the initial speed and, thus initial load can be developed further by having a partner pushing the performer at the back at the moment of the motion start. More functionally though, players may increase loads through weighted vests or light dumbells being held.

Recently, Iga et al (2012) investigated the neuromuscular activation characteristics of the hamstrings during NHE in soccer players combined with the associated alterations in the eccentric strength of the knee flexors.. The NHE exercise is easily performed amongst soccer players, with them performing it alternatively in pairs pre-game or training. The study of Iga et al (2012) investigated the isokinetic eccentric peak torques of the dominant and non-dominant limbs of a training and a control group isokinetically at 60, 120, and 240 °/s, pre- and post-training. The study comprised of four weeks NHE training as shown in Table 3. No difference was observed when both limbs were compared for EMG activity, showing that some authors were wrong to suggest that the dominant limb of soccer players were activated to a higher degree compared to the non-dominant limb during NHE (Brughelli and Cronin 2007). This study also showed that the EMG activity was greater at more extended knee positions during NHE, highlighting the importance of performing the NHE on the whole range of motion of the movement. Specific training significantly improved peak torque by up to 21% in all assessment conditions and data showed that both hamstrings of dominant and non-dominant limbs were engaged identically during the NHE pre- and post-training. Therefore, training induced significant gains in the eccentric peak torque of both soccer players' limbs. In accordance, this study showed that the NHE exercise is a simple exercise that can be easily implemented in the soccer players' training routine inducing eccentric hamstring force in order to allow hamstring muscles to withstand high levels of force and eccentric movements throughout various lengthening movements, consequently reducing the risk of injury. The NHE, also called the "YoYo Hamstring Curl" or "Nordic Hamstring Lowers", even if mono-articular when the trunk remains in-line with the thighs, can be easily implemented during soccer training sessions, up to 3 times per week. These exercises are suggested to not only improve eccentric hamstring peak torque, but will probably impact on sprint performance which will provide a good basis for injury prevention. In this context, it has been shown amongst French soccer players, that professionals revealed higher eccentric hamstring torques than amateurs, and were also faster on short sprints (10m), emphasizing the possible role of hamstring force on sprint performance (Cometti et al, 2001). Moreover, Saliba and Hrysomallis (2001) showed that isokinetic assessment of lower limbs showed low to moderate significant correlations with vertical jump height of Autralian footballers. Nevertheless, given the paucity of well-controlled studies dealing with eccentric strength and athletic performance, further research is still needed in this area (Brughelli and Cronin 2007).

Another possible role of eccentric exercise lies on the fact that it has been suggested that after certain types of eccentric exercise, the optimal length of tension development in muscle shifted to longer muscle lengths. In their review, Brughelli and Cronin (2007) suggest that the latter adaptation may result in greater structural stability at longer muscle lengths, therefore presenting interesting implications for injury prevention and athletic performance.

In this context, it has been suggested that optimum length may be a greater risk factor for muscle strain injuries than classical isokinetic strength ratios warranting future research in this area (Brughelli and Cronin 2007). In the context of injury prevention, with particular emphasis on eccentric training, Malliaropoulos et al (2012) have recently published a review on hamstring injury prevention. They introduced exercise classification criteria for guiding clinicians in designing and implementing strengthening programs adapted to track and field athletes. The various types of exercises presented and the principles exposed may serve as a foundation for future applications of new eccentric programs aiming at decreasing the high incidence of hamstring injury in other sports such as soccer. O'Sullivan et al (2012) have also showed the effect of eccentric exercise on musculo-tendinous flexibility (see "stretching" section of the present chapter).

Finally, evidence has suggested that eccentric strengthening is a way of potentially treating patellar tendinopathy, achile tendinopathy and hamstring strains (Fields et al, 2010), while it could also increase the strength (Potier et al, 2009; Clark et al, 2005) and the angle where the peak torque occurs (Brughelli et al, 2009).

Hamstrings have the higher risk of re-injury (Maliliaropoulos et al, 2011; Alonso et al, 2009), which cause significant problems within soccer. Although players participate regularly within a NHE program, hamstring injuries are possible due to the effects of previous injury history. Players who present hamstring injury histories, maintain a level of scar-tissue (cicatrix) deep

Week	Session per week	Sets and Repetitions
1	1	2x5
2	2	2x6
3	3	3x6
4	3	3x8

Table 3. NHE training protocol in soccer players (adapted from Iga et al, 2012)

within the injury location which has the potential to reinjure continually. The work of prevention begins also when players get injured because if it is not immediately well treat, reinjury is risk is high. The role of the technical staff and fitness coach is to use the physiologic delay that the injury requires to be totally treated and to propose progressive exercise to the players in order to lead him to an official game. Individuals involved with the rehabilitation phase (e.g. technical, medical and fitness staff) must then use the physiological delay due to injury in order to treat and to implement a progressive exercise structure aimed at bringing the player to the correct physical, injury free state leading up to an official game.

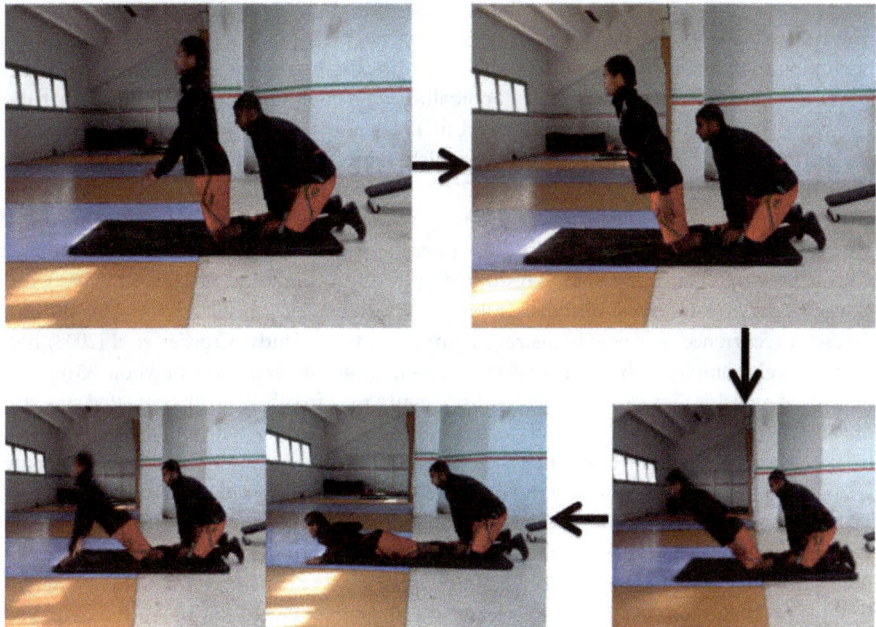

Figure 3. Illustration of a Nordic Hamstring Exercise repetition (NHE).

2.3. Isokinetic testing

Initial research have used isokinetic testing evaluation to study the "balance" of the main body joints, as the knee for example, by comparing the force and power of the agonists (knee flexors) to those of the antagonists (knee extensors). This comparison was achieved by the calculation of the Hamstring/Quadriceps ratio (HQ). For a long period of time the suggested ratio was provided as Hconcentric / Qconcentric forces and "balanced knees" were considered for ratios ranges of 0.48 to 0.66 when measured at low (60°/s) or fast (240°/s) angular velocities (Croisier, 2004). In this context, Aagaard et al (1995) have then presented a functional H/Q ratio that was defined by calculating eccentric hamstring strength relative to concentric quadriceps strength (Hecc/Qconc representative for knee extension). They also calculated the opposite ratio, i.e., hamstring strength relative to eccentric quadriceps strength (Hconc/Qecc representative for knee flexion). The ratio was obtained at 50° (with 0° representing full extension) at angular velocities of 30, 120, and 240 °/s. They also corrected the measured values on the basis of gravity which had high influence on the change in H/Q ratio. A ratio of 1:1 H/Q strength relationship was demonstrated for fast knee extension, showing the functional capacity of the hamstrings for providing knee-joint/muscular stability at such high-speed movements. Thus, this study showed that conventional H/Q (both concentric) ratios had to be interpreted with caution as not functional. Later, Impellizzeri et al (2008), demonstrated that the isokinetic variables and ratios measured were reliable allowing their use in clinical follow-up.

In early isokinetic studies, Bennell et al (1998) suggested that isokinetic muscle strength testing (including functional H/Q ratios) was unable to directly discriminate between higher hamstring risk players of Autralian Rules Football. In this context, it has to be noted that the assessments of that study were performed in 102 senior male Autralian Rules footballers assessed isokinetically at 60 and 180°/s, which represents relatively low-speed angular velocities. In a further study, Dauty et al (2003) have investigated the relationship between knee isokinetic assessment and injuries in 28 elite soccer players on a one-year follow-up basis. They showed that a mixed ratio: Hecc/Qconc (measured at 60°/s) lower than 0.6 was associated with a previous hamstring injury history despite the resumption of competitive soccer. Nevertheless, this ratio and all other isokinetic measured and calculated variables did not predict a recurrence or a new hamstring injury. In a wider study, Croisier et al (2008) had prospectively completed the entire season follow-up in 462 soccer players, of whom 35 injured hamstring muscles. Significantly higher muscle injury risks in subjects with untreated strength imbalances compared to players with no imbalances in pre-season with a relative risk of 4.66 have been found. Nevertheless, when the isokinetic variables got normalized by appropriate strength training, the risk of injury did decrease to that of players without imbalances in pre-season (relative risk =1,43). The authors concluded that (1) the isokinetic evaluation is of great importance in pre-season for the detection of strength imbalances, as a factor that increases the risk of hamstring injury and (2) when the imbalances got restored to a normal strength profile, this induced a decrease of muscle injury risk to normal values. This study, completed on a wide sample of soccer players, showed that isokinetic assessment could be used before, and during the season, in order to detect potential at-risk players, and thereafter, work to correct the eventual observed imbalances, inducing a decrease of the hamstrings injury risk.

In the same context, Yeung et al (2009) have investigated 44 sprinters from Hong-Kong that reporting the eight of them sustained hamstring injuries during the season. The injury rate was of 0,87 per 1000-h of exposure, being higher at the beginning of the season with 58,3% of injuries occurring in the first 100-h of exposure. Statistical analysis showed that athletes with a low the H/Q peak torque ratio of less than 0.60 assessed at an angular velocity of 180°/s have a 17-fold increased risk of hamstring injury. The authors concluded that pre-season H/Q peak torque ratio assessments should be performed in order to identify the sprinters prone to hamstring injury.

Furthermore, Fousekis et al (2011) recently studied 100 soccer players from four professional teams undergoing a composite musculoskeletal assessment at pre-season with numerous associated injury-risk factors that have been controlled. Thirty-eight of the players did sustain one or several lower-limb muscle strains. Sixteen and seven of the players were clinically diagnosed for non-contact muscle strains in their hamstrings and quadriceps, respectively. For hamstrings: players with eccentric hamstring strength asymmetries, functional leg length asymmetries, and no previous hamstring injuries were at a greater risk of sustaining a hamstring muscle strain. For quadriceps: players with eccentric strength and flexibility asymmetries in their quadriceps muscles as well as the heavier and shorter players were at greater risk of sustaining a quadriceps strain. These authors concluded that soccer players showing functional asymmetries displayed a higher risk of hamstring strain. In this context, they suggested that the systematic isokinetic evaluation of the soccer players' lower limbs during pre-season can provide therapists and coaches data about the predictive elements of non-contact hamstring strains and therefore allow for eventual implementation of preventive training programs. Overall, although isokinetic exercise is widely used in rehabilitation in order to prevent injuries, apart from some situations, isokinetic assessment does does not fully predict functional measurements associated with on-field performances and injury occurrence. In this context, Rochcongar (2004) suggested that for optimal use, isokinetic assessment should be used in association with other techniques of evaluation as clinical methods and imagery to improve the quality of diagnosis.

2.4. Core stability

Within many sports, especially the team-contact sports, the need to develop the players' capacity in order to maintain possession of the ball either in rugby, hockey, or soccer for example is fundamental to the outcome of the game. Due to the nature of these contact sports, the coming contact of players when competing for the ball is part of the game and happens continually throughout the duration of the match (e.g. tackles, set-pieces). In order to be able to compete and deal with physical contact in trying to maintain possession, players must have a solid, stable, balanced core/foundation on which to produce moments of strength. Stability of the 'core' commonly referred to as the lumbar-pelvic hip complex, is crucial in providing a foundation for movement of the upper and lower extremities, to support loads, and to protect the spinal cord and nerve roots (Willson et al, 2005).

Core stability is achieved by the muscular system of the trunk providing the majority of the dynamic restraint coupled with passive stiffness from the vertebrae, fascia, and ligaments of the spine. It is believed that the core is made up of the paraspinals, quadratus lumborum muscle, abdominal muscles, hip girdle musculature, diaphragm and the pelvic floor muscles. Core stability is defined as the ability to control the position and motion of the trunk over the pelvis to allow optimum production, transfer and control of force and motion to the terminal segment in integrated athletic activities (Borghuis et al, 2011). Indeed, the central role of the body core for stabilization and force generation in all sporting activities is being increasingly recognized. Indeed, core stability training is seen as being pivotal for efficient biomechanical function necessary to maximize force generation, and minimize joint loads in all types of activities (Hibbs et al, 2008) ranging from running to throwing and subsequently decrease the incidence of injury (Willson et al, 2005). The player's capacity to be strong and to resist to opponents could also allow avoiding bad movement and involuntary sprain.

According to Goodstein (2011) it is important to have a strong, stable core as this impacts on all functional soccer related movements. The primary function of the core is to maintain dynamic stability of the body's center of gravity as indicated earlier. The diagrams included in Figure 4, as well as pelvic tilts and dead bugs, show different preventive exercises for reach the different aim of the core stability training. Due to the repetitive forward flexion of the core region, it is of paramount importance to strengthen the lower hip and upper extensors (Owen et al, 2013b). It is also vitally important to increase strength levels through multi-plane diagonal and rotational exercises such as those shown within Figure 4.

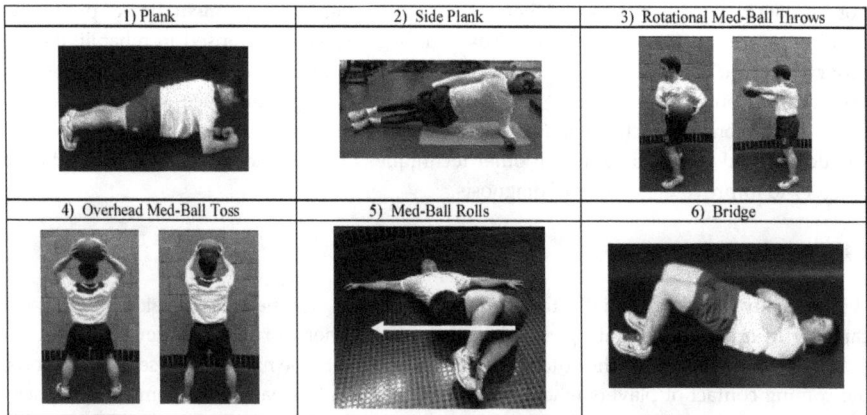

1) Plank	2) Side Plank	3) Rotational Med-Ball Throws
4) Overhead Med-Ball Toss	5) Med-Ball Rolls	6) Bridge

Figure 4. Core stability program (from Owen et al, 2013b)

2.5. Balance and proprioception training

The importance of training stability, balance and coordination skills are becoming more important in many disciplines (Hrysomallis, 2011; DiStefano et al, 2010). This type of training is considered to be an efficient strategy for the prevention of injury by improving functional postural activation. The support for this training method is further substantiated by their cost effectiveness and ease to administer nature, making it accessible to clubs of all levels/status, statures and totally independent of resources and available finances. Proprioception can be defined as a specialized variation of sensory modality of touch that encompasses the sensation of joint movement and joint position (Lephart et al, 1997). Proprioception is a key component of the body physiology as it allows the neuromuscular system to maintain balance, stability and mobility while activated muscle stabilize a joint (Laskowski et al, 1997). Proprioceptors are found within joint capsules, ligaments, muscles, and tendons, and in the skin. Their main function is to make sure body joints are kept in stable avoiding damaging unstable positions.

Recent research has postulated the significant positive effect of balance training in its attempts to reduce the risk of ankle sprains in competitive team sports players and its benefits for the prevention of ankle sprain recurrences (Verhagen et al 2004). Stasinopoulos (2004) performed a research study investigating the effects of preventative interventions on the incidence of ankle inversion sprains among team sports players. It was revealed that proprioceptive training is an effective method that led to a reduced rate of ankle sprains. More specifically, ankle-strengthening exercises have been indicated to improve strength and joint position sense, in subjects with a history of ankle sprains. In this context, the implementation of balance training within elite level sport has been suggested to decrease injury rates for hamstring, patellar tendinopathy, gastrocnemius strains, and overall lower extremity issues (Willardson, 2007; Kraemer and Knobloch, 2009).

Soccer players may be predisposed to injuries due to the dynamics involved within the sport. Single leg dominance is a fundamental issue within elite level soccer and this dominance may lead to imbalances within players and predispose them to an increased risk of injury. According to Goodstein (2011) it is vitally important that soccer injury prevention programs focus on strengthening the posterior chain on the dominant side including the hip extensors, abductors, and external rotators, while strengthening the adductors and hip flexors of the non-dominant side. Indeed, these muscles are suggested to frequently become tight and weak as the antagonists of the continuing kicking motion. Balance and coordination are the basics for every sports movement, but vitally important within training and competitive soccer match-play due to the fact that the key soccer specific skills are produced from a single-leg stance. Soccer player's balance involves the entire kinetic chain (knee, pelvis, torso, and head). Earlier research involved a study following 600 male soccer players over three seasons (Cerilli et al., 2001) with half the group was placed within the proprioceptive and balance training group consisting of 20min per day for a minimum of 6 weeks training, and results showed a significant decrease of ACL injuries when compared to the control. More precisely, Caraffa et al (1996) revealed that this training program induce sevenfold lower incidence in ACL injuries both in amateur and semi-professional players. However, there were differences according to the age (adult vs. youth soccer players) and gender (male vs. female). Indeed, it was clearly showed that female players presented between 2 and 3 times higher risks of ACL injuries than male soccer male players (Vescovi and Van Heest, 2010; Walden et al, 2011). This has been shown to be caused by different morphology with especially an impaired alignment.

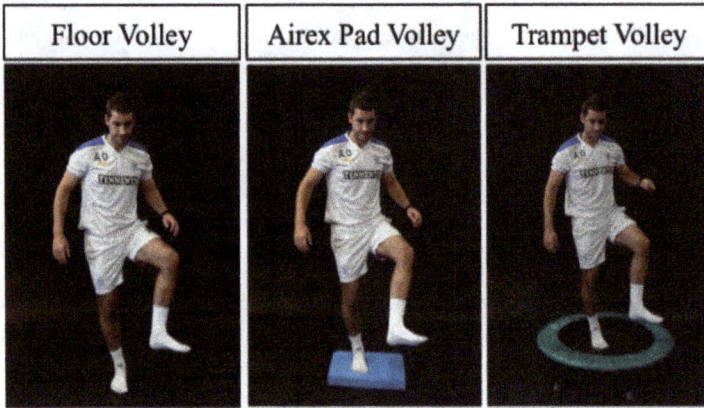

Figure 5. Proprioception program (from Owen et al, 2013b)

2.6. Plyometric and proprioceptive exercise on sand

Exercise on sand is commonly used in rehabilitation and in order to prevent injuries. Moreover, knowing that plyometric is considered as a method allowing reducing the severity of injuries (Heidt et al, 2000, Chimera et al, 2004; Miyama et Nosaka, 2004), several technical staff and fitness coaches use the combination of plyometric and proprioception on the sand in order to reduce the risk of lower limb's joints sprain and to increase the proprioceptive capacity. Impellizzeri et al (2010), have showed that plyometric training on sand improved squat jump height, and sprint performance (10 and 20m) while the muscle soreness was lower as compared to plyometric training applied on grass. This was probably due to effects on neuro-muscular factors related to the stretch-shortening cycle. Unfortunately, no studies have demonstrated that this prevention training reduces the risk on injury. Future studies are needed to work on this field.

2.7. Stretching

There are several types of stretching, nevertheless, static stretching is the most common form used worldwide (Fields et al, 2010). Passive static stretching consists of an athlete lengthening a muscle group and holding the position for a set duration ranging from 10 to 60-s. For a long period of time it was believed that static stretching had many potential positive benefits, of which one was the prevention of muscle injury. Thus, despite the data reported in the scientific literature, the consensus among sports coaches and practitioners still leans in favor of the use of stretching in each training session (Fields et al, 2010). In this context, Shehab et al (2006) have published a survey showing how strong belief in stretching remains among coaches. They showed that 95% of coaches believed that pre-exercise stretching decreases injury risks and 73% of them felt that there were no drawbacks at all with the use of stretching during training.

Nevertheless, despite its large use among sport practitioners, stretching does not seem to clearly prevent muscle injuries.

In this context, two large meta-analyses came with strong evidence to question the value of pre-exercise stretching as a part of training routine of runners. A review of 12 major studies including 8806 runners investigated the role of passive stretching in possibly preventing lower limbs muscle injuries. The results showed that were no trends showing any beneficial effect of stretching in preventing running injury. In their comprehensive meta-analysis of articles spanning 1997-2002, Thacker et al (2004) examined the role of pre-exercise passive stretching to prevent sports injuries showing that there was no evidence at all for any reduction in the injuries in general, and muscle injuries in particular. These two large meta-analyses reinforced the findings of original investigations that had rather surprisingly showed a trend toward a small increase in injuries among runners who stretched compared to control groups, going against the intuition of many sports practitioners. In this context, Van Mechelen et al (1993), conducted a randomized trial with 421 runners with stretching, warm-up, and cool-down performed before and after running. The results showed a slightly lower injury rate in the control group compared to the one that used static stretching as a pre-running intervention. Later, Pope et al (2000) studied 1538 military recruits assigned to either static stretching or a no-intervention control group also showing no difference between groups for the injury rate. Twellar et al (1997) reported a 4-years prospective trial results, showing no evidence that flexibility decreased sports injuries, suggesting again, that flexibility from stretching was not necessarily a beneficial attribute to runners. Accordingly, in their review, Herbert and Gabriel (2002) concluded that static stretching had no effect on delayed muscle soreness or injury rate. In the same context, Andersen et al (2005) published a meta-analysis of original studies. The main results showed that with respect to injury risk, the combined risk reduction of 5% indicates that the stretching protocols used in these investigations do not meaningfully reduce lower limbs injury risks of army recruits undergoing military training. Later, in their original investigation, Arnasson et al (2008) reported hamstring strains and player exposure prospectively collected during four consecutive soccer seasons (1999 to 2002) for 17-30 elite soccer teams from Iceland and Norway. These authors clearly showed that there was no difference in the incidence of hamstring strains when comparing the teams that used flexibility training program and those who did not.

Conversely, the study of Hartig et al (1999) reports conflicting results. These authors studied two different military companies undergoing basic training at the same time. Hamstring flexibility was assessed at the start and end of the 13-weeks infantry basic training program. The control group was composed of 148 subjects that proceeded through normal basic training, i.e., not including any stretching. The intervention group composed of 150 members underwent the same program but added three hamstring stretching sessions per week. The results showed that hamstring flexibility significantly increased in the intervention group vs. the control group. Along, with flexibility, the number of injuries was also significantly reduced in the intervention group. Forty-three injuries were reported for the control group giving an incidence rate of 29.1% compared to the 25 injuries in the "stretching" group for an incidence of 16.7%. In this particular study, the number of lower limbs overuse injuries was significantly lower in the infantry basic trainees that achieved increased hamstring flexibility at the end of the training intervention. Nevertheless, these authors did not categorize the types of the reported injuries, and therefore, data about muscle injuries can not be extracted from this study. Of interest, is the fact that this study data have suggested that flexibility demonstrates a significant U-shaped relationship with the incidence of injury; subjects at both extremes of flexibility are at more risk than the average group. This raises the need to study flexibility and injury rates in the "normal" range of flexibility, as both, too stiff or too flexible subjects might flaw the investigations' results. Therefore, unless a need for an extreme range of motion as needed for some rare sports as gymnatics, it seems not necessary to reach very wide ranges of flexibility, as this might be linked to an augmented risk of injury.

In this context, it is also of interest to note that whether stretching has a potential but discussed role in the prevention of muscle injuries might also depend on the type of sport practiced (Witrouw et al, 2004). Indeed, these latter authors believe that part of the contradictions that are reported by the literature regarding the effects of stretching on injury prevention can be explained by considering the type of sports practiced. They state that sports involving bouncing and jumping activities with a high intensity of stretch-shortening cycles (SSCs) as soccer require a muscle-tendon unit that is compliant enough for being able to storing and release the high amount of elastic energy that will therefore benefit performance. If the athletes of such sports have non-compliant muscle-tendon units (MTU), the energy absorption and release could exceed the capacity of the MTU, leading to increased risk of injury. Consequently, the rationale for injury prevention in these sports is to check for non-compliant (stiff) athletes and train them for flexibility. In contrast, in the sports containing low-intensity SSCs as for jogging, cycling, or swimming, there is no special need for a very compliant MTU. Indeed, in such sports, most of the power generation comes from active muscle activity which is directly transferred through the tendons to the articular system in order to generate motion. Therefore, flexibility training inducing very compliant MTU may not be advantageous. This conjecture is supported by the literature about runners (see above) where strong evidence exists of no beneficial effect of static stretching on injury rates in these sports.

Another consideration about flexibility training is the "timing" of stretching for optimal injury prevention (Fields et al, 2010). In this context, many athletes have adopted the strategy of stretching post-activity rather than before. Indeed, one investigation provides data showing that this might offer injury protection. Verrall et al (2005) have published a prospective study in which they followed hamstring injuries in a single soccer team through four playing seasons. The intervention program consisted of the athletes stretching after practicing and while fatigued (end of session). The intervention also comprised sport-specific training drills with an emphasis on augmenting the amount of high intensity interval training. The results favored the intervention in that in pre-intervention 9 and 11 players sustained hamstring injury compared with 2 and 4 after intervention. In addition there has also been an effect on the severity of injuries. Indeed, competition days missed were reduced from 31 and 38 to 5 and 16 after intervention (Verrall et al, 2005). Therefore, it seems safer to stretch in post-sessions rather than before.

In the context of flexibility training, it is of interest to stress that a good (normal) flexibility might be achieved not only by static stretching, but also by other means as eccentric exercise. Indeed, O'Sullivan et al (2012) have recently systematically checked six electronic databases to identify the randomized clinical trials having compared the effectiveness of eccentric training to either a different intervention, or a no-intervention group on flexibility. Both studies assessing flexibility using range of motion and muscle fascicle length were included. This meta-analysis individualized six studies that met the inclusion/exclusion criteria showing consistent, strong evidence in all the six investigations in three different muscle groups that eccentric training improves lower extremity flexibility. Therefore, obtaining a "normal" range of motion can not only be achieved by post-session static stretching, but also by eccentric exercise.

Static stretching has been questioned not only for its potential role in slightly increasing injury risk, but also for its' detrimental effect on sport performance. In this context, Behm and Chaouachi (2011) have provided recommendations as to the use of stretching in sports. There are clear differences of the effects of static or dynamic stretching on sport performance. Thus, the latter authors have suggested that a warm-up to minimize impairments and enhance performance should not include static stretching and rather be composed of a submaximal intensity aerobic activity followed by large amplitude dynamic stretching followed by sport-specific dynamic activities. For the sports that necessitate a high degree of static flexibility, warm-ups should include short duration static stretches with lower intensity stretches in a trained population to minimize the possibilities of sports performance impairments. Indeed, Chaouachi et al (2008) have shown that the detrimental effects of static stretching on performance are less pronounced in subjects use to such static stretching. In this context, future studies should investigate the effects of dynamic stretching on injury prevention, since recent literature have shown that dynamic stretching should be used rather than static stretching, increasing number of practitioners have replaced the static stretching in their training programs, by active dynamic stretching.

Therefore, the present chapter authors do believe that intense static stretching should be avoided during warm-up and training sessions and should rather be performed at the end of the sessions for flexibility training purposes. The latter, could also be achieved through other means, as eccentric exercise which has also many potential positive effects muscle injury prevention (see the "*Eccentric exercise*" section of the present chapter).

2.8. Training load (intensity & volume) — The training approach

Periodization, and the capacity to plan and design a schedule with the appropriate training load (intensity, volume, and frequency) is a key factor in attempt to avoid injury. In this this context, the term 'advanced planning' or 'periodization' should be considered as a functional injury prevention strategy. Every individual involved with the physical development of players (e.g. technical, medical and conditioning staff) have their own views on the planning, design and execution of training programs but whatever the method is planned and used, the final target is to manage and manipulate the players fatigue and level of performance whilst minimizing injury risk. More often than not, the technical staff spend more time exerting the players through technical drills and SSGs, however, the conditioning or medical staff are held responsible for injuries. This section of this book chapter aims to highlight the role of the technical staff in injury prevention techniques and through advanced planning or periodization of training, they will limit the risk of imposing accumulated fatigue upon their players which lead to muscle strains or overuse injuries.

As indicated previously, hamstring injuries are the most prevalent muscle injury in professional soccer. Due to the multifactorial nature of these injuries it's becoming increasingly apparent that the interplay between these factors has a significant role to play when we consider how we should best attempt to prevent these injuries. The game has significantly evolved over these last two decades and performance data provided each season is showing significant increases in position specific performance markers (Di Salvo et al, 2007). Coaches are considered to have the greatest influence on player development; the next generation of professional coaches needs to be able to deliver quality sessions that can achieve multiple outcomes. This would include a coaching curriculum that stretches the players over a season whilst ensuring injury rates are maintained at an acceptable and hopefully low rate with an optimal performance. In this context, it is of interest to note that the RPE (rating of perceived exertion) method has been validated for training load monitoring purposes in numerous sports, of which soccer (Impellizzeri et al, 2004). Only rare scientific studies have reported training load manipulation and injury rates measures. In this context, Gabett (2004) have showed in rugby league Australian players, using the RPE-method to monitor training load, that the manipulation of the latter variable induced alterations in the injury rate. Indeed, when pre-season training load was set at high standards, this induced higher muscular injury rates compared to seasons when the training load was reduced. It is of interest to note that high pre-season loads were not only detrimental for injuries in general, and muscle injuries in particular, but also had a negative effect on aerobic fitness. Therefore, in order to achieve good endurance fitness and low injury rates, the training load has to be monitored and maintained at relatively low standards. In this context, it is the opinion of the present chapter authors, that team sports as soccer do not need very high levels of physical training loads. Rather, the technical staff should monitor the latter training variable and emphasize on optimal fitness training while insisting on technical and tactical training which is of paramount importance of the outcome of the games.

According to recent research by Owen et al, (2013a) due to the varying physical and technical demands of particular sided game formats (3vs3 to 11vs11), in elite professional soccer, performing the correct type of sided-game at specific times of the training week may enable technical, sports science and conditioning staff to maximally prepare players physically, technically and tactically thus increasing the efficiency of their training sessions and weekly schedule. This may be beneficial to the players from an injury prevention perspective as well as performance enhancement in relation to applying an overload of different energy systems and inducing higher speeds at the correct time in order to minimize the fatigue risk effect moving towards competitive match-play. Arguably, this strategy of 'advanced planning' may be the most important factor influencing injury prevention due to the fact that the technical staff implement and dictate most of the pitch based training sessions. Advanced planning between technical, conditioning and medical staff is vital in order to elicit the correct volume, duration, and intensity of training and ensure maximum player freshness pre-game (Owen et al, 2013a).

3. Which prevention program should be used?

The previous review of literature presented in this book chapter and describing the different methods of prevention strategies, should help the coach, the technical staff and the medical staff to reduce the injury occurrence. They have to adapt the prevention program according to the sport, the athletes' morphology, age, gender, their injury history, and the period of the season.

First of all, all players should to be tested at the beginning of the pre-season in order to detect what prevention program they eventually need. They should be tested in isokinetic, functional strength, mobility (lumbar-pelvic, ankle, knee, hip), flexibility, balance and theirs morphologies. These results have to be combined to their injury history. All of these information will allow to draw the needs for each player, and therefore designing individual specific prevention programs.

A Cochrane review by Goldman and Jones (2010) on such interventions concluded that there was insufficient evidence from randomized controlled trials to draw conclusions as to the effectiveness of interventions used to prevent injuries. This current lack of evidence for interventions and the current high incidence of injuries seen in the game could also suggest that injuries should be considered multifactorial in their etiology. Therefore, we have yet to understand how works the interplay between all of the intrinsic and extrinsic factors that may contribute to each specific injury. It could also be suggested that there is some element, be it intrinsic or extrinsic, in the day to day management of the players that maybe a significant contributing factor in the aetiology of these injuries and we have yet to establish what this might be.

For example, a recent large scaled randomized controlled trial by Petersen et al (2011) addressed the efficacy of the Nordic hamstring exercise program for preventing acute hamstring injuries in soccer players. They found that introducing this ten weeks program to reduce eccentric weakness, a common intrinsic factor associated with hamstring injuries, reduced the incident of these injuries by 70%. This backed up previous findings by Arnason et al (2008). Using a larger sample size Arnason's study looked at a total of 24 teams, with over 650 soccer players, over a four years period. These players were from professional soccer teams in the Icelandic and Norwegian leagues. The study showed that teams combining the Nordic eccentric exercise protocol and the stretching program were on average seeing 65% fewer hamstring injuries. However, when we look closely at the Nordic hamstring exercise it's clear to see that it only involves movement at one joint-the knee. We know that the hamstrings work over two joints, the hip and knee, and when we consider the mechanism of hamstring injuries then the Nordic hamstring exercise clearly doesn't replicate any of the functional activities used in football specific training.

Each player needs a specific program according to his injury risks (Table 4) which has been determined by the pre-season tests, his injury history, morphology, and his playing positions. Indeed, Mallo and Dellal (2012) have showed that the frequency of injuries was not uniformly distributed by playing positions with forwards and central defenders sustaining the greatest number of injury episodes and the highest match absence. Consequently, it is important to link the prevention program in taking in consideration the playing positions of each player in team sports.

	Strain / tear injury	Sprain	Anterior Cruciate Ligament	Groin Pain
Functional strength	X	X		X
Eccentric exercises	X			
Core stability		X	X	X
Isokinetic	X		X	
Balance/proprioception	X		X	X
Stretching	X			X
Plyometric and proprioceptive exercises on sand	X	X	X	
Training load	X	X		X

Table 4. Prevention exercises to applied for decrease the injury risk.

4. Which factors affecting injury risk?

It has been identified in two studies by Heiderscheit et al (2010) and Orchard et al (2005) that clinical experience shows us that it is extremely difficult to decide at which point during rehabilitation the athlete is ready to a return to sport, and thus this is usually based on subjective evidence. These difficulties may well be the reason why there is a conspicuously high injury recurrence rate, particularly within the first few weeks of a return, as identified by Walden et al (2005). Additionally, there are a difference of risk injury according to the age (adult vs. youth soccer players) and gender (male vs. female). Indeed, it was clearly showed that female players presented between 2 and 3 times higher risks of ACL injuries than soccer male players (Vescovi and Van Heest, 2010; Walden et al, 2011). It is cause by different knee morphology with especially an impaired alignment. All these information show that different factors could affect and be at the origin of an injury

4.1. Factors impacting the injury risk

- **Warm up.** Adapted warm up is considering as a prevention strategies because it reduces the injury risk (Fields et al, 2010; Soligard et al, 2010). These studies showed that a specific intervention program based on specific "The11" FIFA warm up focusing on core stability, eccentric training of thigh muscles, proprioceptive training, dynamic stabilization and plyometrics with straight leg alignment induce lower knee injuries in comparison to a control group. This is contrasted by Junge et al (2002) who did not find that "the11" had a preventive effect on youth soccer players, probably due to the fact that youth players are growing and they don't have a control of a large pattern. Olsen et al (2004) confirmed that specific warm up and cool down, adapted training shoes analyzed, prophylactic taping (especially in players formers sprain and ankle instability), reduce the injury risk.

- **Congested period.**Dellal et al (2013) and Dupont et al (2010) have shown that a congested period could affect and increase the injury risk. Consequently, when a team plays 6 or 7 matches in about 20 days for example, a global preventive plan has to be settled including the training load monitoring, the use of post-efforts recovery method (alternating cold and hot water immersion for example)

- **Change of temperature and external conditions.** To the best of our knowledge, no study has ever attempted to show if the brutal change of external temperature has any effect on the injury occurrence. However, it is suggested that several fast change of temperature from heat to cold induce a greater risk of injury, especially hamstring strain (personal unpublished observations). Moreover, the external conditions could modify the type of grass pitch and therefore, the run and the footstep will be altered too. When the pitch is firm, hard or soft, it affects the players' muscle contraction pattern at ground contact and thus could increase the risk of injury. For example, when the pitch is "heavy" the fatigue appears more quickly, especially at the hamstrings but to the best of our knowledge, no study has ever investigated this.

- **Equipment modification and playing surface.** Specific running shoes adapted to the players' anatomy (if the players is under pronation, supination, genu varus and rear foot with varus) could possibly be a preventive injury risk factor to be a determinant factor (Fields et al, 2010), but this has not been widely investigated. However, it is essential for the staff to pay a special attention that each player having the adequate equipment for playing football, running, to perform strength exercise training (belt), or stretching (carpet). The playing surface has a essential roles (Ekstrand et al, 2006), but as it was showed, this is the change of playing surface which induce an increase of the injury risk.

- **Fatigue and training monitoring.** The workload is the key factor to prevent injury. Periodization, and the capacity to plan and to design a schedule with the appropriate intensity and frequency of training is a key factor to avoid injury and in this context, it should be consider as a prevention strategy. Every coach, technical staff and fitness training have a special view of the planning design but whatsoever the method used, the final target is to manage and manipulate the players fatigue and level performance and to avoid injury. Technical staff has to determine and control precisely the training and the match performance.

- **Playing positions.** It was showed that the frequency of injuries was not uniformly distributed by playing positions with forwards and central defenders sustained the greatest number of injury episodes and the highest match absence (Mallo and Dellal, (2012) whereas it was the wide and central midfielders who have the lowest number of injuries during two consecutive season in Spanish professional soccer players. Complementarily, Woods et al (2004) revealed that defenders sustained 15% more hamstring strains than forwards.

However, Debedo et al (2004) demonstrated the opposite results with forwards sustained 10% more hamstring strains than defenders. Whatever, the prevention program has to be plan according to the playing position, the region, the country and the championship.

- **Injury history and re-injury.** As it was previously described, the injury history is a determinant factor to design the prevention training for players (Hagglund et al, 2006). The different adaptation resulting from previous injuries will direct the manner to manage the prevention program and to be careful for one or more specific players. Previous injuries, which are not well treated, could be the origin of a re-injury (in the same scarb area). In this context, it is very important to take the time in order to the organism recover totally its physiological and biomechanical components. The rehabilitation work, the prevention exercises and the re-training needs to pay a special attention after players took part in the collective training. The high risk of re-injury concerns the hamstring strain, and indirectly, after an ACL, there are a possibility of compensation and of re-injury on the same knee, and the contro-lateral knee, or muscle (hamstring, quadriceps, gastrocnemius).

- **Nutrition and dehydration.** A bad management of the food and the fluid intake could increase the risk of injury according to the period of the season and external conditions. Appropriate nutrition, regular and adapted hydration is the basic behavior to have.

- **The period of the season.** The risk of injury differs according to the period of the season. To illustrate it, the highest incidence of sprains was achieved during pre-season and the beginning of the competition period. The risk to sustain a muscular strain peaked at the beginning and in the final weeks of the competition period and was related ($r=0.72$; $P<0.05$) to mean heart rate during training. (Mallo and Dellal, 2012). Concerning the in-season, recent research has shown that performing an injury prevention program twice weekly for the entirety of the entire season (58 prevention sessions) can lead to significantly less muscle injuries. The findings from this study identified a multi component injury prevention training program may be appropriate for reducing the number of muscle injuries during a season but may not be adequate to reduce all other injuries. A recent study by Mendiguchia and Brughelli (2012) has attempted to provide a return-to-sport algorithm. In general, the pre-season requires a greater proprioception (ankle and knee), eccentrics, core stability and stretching program whereas the in-season needs to increase the attention to prevent the sprain with each player participating in a specific preventive training. However, sometimes it is no chance due to player-to-player contact, because it could reach 32% of the injury causes.

4.2. Prevention in young soccer players

The injury risk and the type of injury are age dependent. Soligard et al (2010) suggested that most earlier the prevention program is started, greater will be the effect. Literature showed that youth soccer players have between 61-82% of overall injuries located at the lower extremity especially at the ankle (28%) and knee (19%) (Emery and Meeuwisse, 2010; Junge et al, 2002). The incidence of injuries decreases with a specific strength program (resistance training) in youth soccer players during in-season and off-season (Lehnhard et al, 1996). Emery and

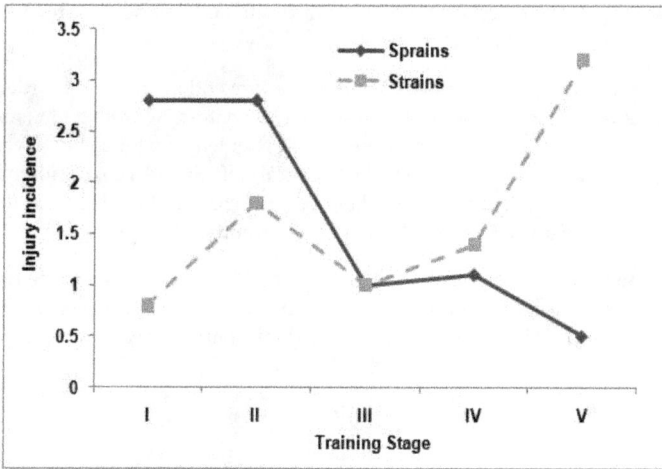

Figure 6. Ligament sprains and muscle strains incidence (per 1000 hours) during each training stage during two consecutive seasons (from Mallo and Dellal, 2012)

Meeuwisse (2010) added that most studies showed a high effect of an intervention until 88% reduction in injuries. Specifically, they showed that prevention strategies including hamstring eccentric exercise, neuromuscular training, warm up, balance board exercise, and core stability induced lower risks for acute injuries, lower extremity injuries, ankle sprain and knee sprains than no intervention strategy in youth soccer players (U13-U18). In this context, injury prevention strategies should be applied very early in youth soccer players' categories.

5. Conclusion

This particular book chapter has tried to provide an analysis of the main injury prevention strategies commonly used in soccer with the primary aim being to decrease the injury rates during both soccer training and matches. The combination of different prevention methods (functional strength, eccentric strength, isokinetic ratio, core stability, balance, proprioception, stretching, flexibility, stability, work on sand) have not been discussed due to the fact that each of them as a separate method has been reported to reduce the risk of injury.

However, the key point running throughout the chapter is the necessity to individualize prevention programs according to the athlete or players injury history, morphology, gender, age, testing data (e.g. medical and fitness tests) and their playing position. As suggested, pre-season training allows a foundation to be provided through general and sport specific training (i.e. specific musculature, joints, tendons) whereas the competitive period needs individual preventive exercises (i.e. aimed at hamstring/quads). Moreover, the prevention exercises need adjustment according to the collective training in positioned the exercises before, during or after the training (or before and after games).

Additionally, recovery strategies have constituted a prevention strategy in order to reduce injury risk because they decrease the soreness. In, this context, hydrotherapy (after training and matches), a good nutrition and hydration with supplements for some players (during, before or after the training and matches). The technical staff should also considered the warm up, the number of match played (congested period), the change of temperature, the type and change of playing surface, and adapted shoes as a preventive strategies.

Finally, all these prevention strategies will be efficient if they are include in the training, and considering the individual characteristics of all players as a unique person. However a complementary question is when the players could take part in the collective training after a specific injury.

Author details

Alexandre Dellal[1,2,3], Karim Chamari[4] and Adam Owen[3,5]

1 FIFA Medical Excellence Centre, Santy Orthopedicae Clinical, Sport Science and Research Department, Lyon, France

2 OGC Nice, Fitness Training Department, Nice, France

3 Centre de recherche et d'Innovation sur le Sport (CRIS), Université de Lyon 1, Lyon, France

4 Research and Education Centre, Aspetar, Qatar Orthopaedic and Sports Medicine Hospital, Doha, Qatar

5 Glasgow Rangers Sport Science Department (soccer), Glasgow, Scotland

References

[1] Aagaard P, Simonsen EB, Trolle M, Bangsbo J, Klausen K. Isokinetic hamstring/quadriceps strength ratio: influence from joint angular velocity, gravity correction and contraction mode. Acta Physiol Scand 1995, 154: 421-427.

[2] Alonso JM, Tscholl PM, Engebretsen L et al. Occurrence of injuries and illness during the 2009 IAAF World Athletics Championships. Br J Sports Med 2010, 44: 1100-5.

[3] Andersen JC. Stretching before and after exercise: effect on muscle soreness and injury risk. J Ath Training 2005, 40(3): 218-220.

[4] Arnason A, Sigurdsson SB, Gudmundsson A, Holme I, Engebretsen L, Bahr R. Physical fitness, injuries, and team performance in soccer. Med Sci Sports Exerc 2004a, 36: 278–285.

[5] Arnason A, Sigurdsson SB, Gudmundsson A, Holme I, Engebretsen L, Bahr R. Risk factors for injuries in football. Am J Sports Med 2004b, 32: 5S–16S.

[6] Arnasson A, Andersen TE, Holme et al. Prevention of hamstring strains in elite soccer: an intervention study. Scand J Med Sci Sports 2008, 18: 40-8.

[7] Arnasson A, Andersen TE, Home I, Engebresten I, Bahr R. Prevention of hamstring strains in elite soccer: an intervention study. Scand J Med Sci Sports 2008, 18: 40-48.

[8] Askling C, Karlsson J, Thorstensson, A. Hamstring injury occurrence in elite soccer players after preseason strength training with eccentric overload. Scand J Med Sci Sports 2003, 13(4): 244-250.

[9] Behm DG, Chaouachi A "A review of the acute effects of static and dynamic stretching on performance". Eur J Appl Physiol 2011, 111: 2633-2651.

[10] Bennell K, Wajswelner H, Lew P, Schall-Riaucour A, Leslie S, Plant D, Cirone J. Isokinetic strength testing does not predict hamstring injury in Australian Rules Footballers. Br J Sports Med 1998, 32: 309-314.

[11] Borghuis AJ, Lemmink KA, Hof AL. Core muscle response times and postural reactions in soccer players and non-players. Med Sci Sports Exerc 2011, 43(1): 108-14.

[12] Brooks JH, Fuller CW, Kemp SP et al. Incidence, risk and prevention of hamstring muscle injuries in professional rugby union. Am J Sports Med 2006, 34: 1297-306.

[13] Brughelli M, Cronin J. Altering the length-tension relationship with eccentric exercise. Implications for performance and injury. Sports Med 2007, 37(9): 807-826.

[14] Caraffa A, Cerulli G, Projetti M et al. Prevention of anterior cruciate ligament injuries in soccer: a prospective controlled study of proprioceptive training. Knee Surg Sports Traumatol Arthrosc 1996, 4: 19-21.

[15] Carling C, Le Gall F, Dupont G. Are physical performance and injury risk in a professional soccer team in match play affected over a prolonged period of fixture congestion. Int J Sports Med 2012, 33(1): 36-42.

[16] Cerilli G, Benoit DL, Caraffa A, Ponteggia F. Proprioceptive training and prevention of anterior cruciate ligament injuries in soccer. J Orthop Sports Phys Ther 2001, 31(11): 655-60 .

[17] Chamari K, Haddad M, Wong del P, Dellal A, Chaouachi A. Injury rates in professional soccer players during Ramadan. J Sports Sci 2012, 30 Suppl 1:S93-S102.

[18] Chaouachi A, Chamari K, Wong P, Castagna C, Chaouachi M, Moussa-Chamari I, Behm DG. Stretch and sprint training reduces stretch-induced sprint performance deficits in 13- to 15-year-old youth. Eur J Appl Physiol 2008, 104: 515-522.

[19] Chimera NJ, Swanik KA, Swanik CB et al. Effects of plyometric training on muscle-activation strategies and performance in female athletes. J Athl Train 2004, 39:24-31.

[20] Cometti G, Maffiuletti NA, Pousson M, Chatard JC, Mafulli N. Isokinetic strength and Anaerobic power of Elite, Subelite, and Amateur French Soccer players. Int J Sports Med 2001, 22: 45-51.

[21] Croisier JL, Ganteaume S, Binet J, Genty M, Ferret JM. Strength imbalances and prevention of hamstring injury in professional soccer players: a prospective study. Am J Sports Med 2008, 36(8): 1469-1475.

[22] Croisier JL. Factors associated with recurrent hamstring injuries. Sports Med 2004, 34(10): 681-695.

[23] Dauty M, Potiron-Josse M, Rochcongar P. Consequences and prediction of hamstring muscle injury with concentric and eccentric isokinetic parameters in elite soccer players. Annal Readapt Med Phys 2003, 46: 601-606.

[24] Dedebo B, White J, George KP. A survey of flexibility training protocols and hamstrings strains in professional football club in England: Br J Sports Med 2004, 38: 388-94.

[25] Dellal, A, Chamari, C, Wong, DP, Ahmaidi, S, Keller, D, Barros, MLR, Bisciotti, GN, and Carling, C. Comparison of physical and technical performance in European professional soccer match-play: the FA Premier League and La LIGA. Eur J Sport Sci 2011, 11(2): 51-59.

[26] Dellal A, Lago-Penas C, Rey E et al. The effects of a congested fixture period on physical performance, technical activity and injury rate during matches in a professional soccer team. Br J Sports Med 2013, 25.

[27] DiStefano LJ, Padua DA, Blackburn JT, Garrett WE, Guskiewicz KM, & Marshall SW. Integrated injury prevention program improves balance and vertical jump height in children. J Strength Cond Res 2010, 24(2): 332-42.

[28] Dupont G, Nedelec M, McCall A, et al. Effect of 2 soccer matches in a week on physical performance and injury rate. Am J Sports Med 2010, 38(9): 1752-1758.

[29] Ebben WP, Leigh DH, Long N, Clewien R, Davies JA. Electromyographical analysis of hamstring resistance training exercises. In: Proceeding of the XXIV International Symposium of the Society of Biomechanics in Sports. Salzburg (Austria): University of Salzburg, 2006, 236 – 239.

[30] Ekstrand J, Gillquist J, Moller M, Oberg B, & Liljedahl S. Incidence of soccer injuries and their relation to training and team success. Am J Sports Med 1983, 11(2): 63-67.

[31] Ekstrand J, Hagglund M & Walden M. Injury incidence and injury patterns in professional football: the UEFA injury study. Br J Sports Med 2011, 45: 553-558.

[32] Ekstrand J, Gillquist J. Prevention of sports injuries in football players. Int J Sports Med 1984, 5: 140-4.

[33] Emery CA, Meeuwisse WH. The effectiveness of a neuromuscular prevention strategy to reduce injuries in youth soccer: a cluster-randomized controlled trial. Br J Sports Med 2010, 44: 555-562.

[34] Engebretsen AH, Myklebust G, Holme I, Engebretsen L, & Bahr R. Prevention of injuries among male soccer players: a prospective, randomized intervention study targeting players with previous injuries or reduced function. Am J Sports Med 2008, 36(6): 1052-1060.

[35] Fields KB, Sykes JC, Walker KM, Jackson JC. Prevention of running injuries. Curr Sports Med Rep 2010, 9(3): 176-182.

[36] Fousekis K, Tsepis E, Vagenas G. Multivariate isokinetic strength asymmetries of the knee and ankle in professional soccer players. J Sports Med Phys Fitness 2010, 50(4): 465-74.

[37] Fousekis K, Tsepis E, Poulmedis P, Athanasopoulos S, Vagenas G. Intrinsic risk factors of non-contact quadriceps and hamstring strains in soccer: a prospective study of 100 professional players. Br J Sports Med 2011, 45:709-714.

[38] Gabett TJ Reductions in pre-season training loads reduce training injury rates in rugby league players. Br J Sports Med 2004, 38: 743-749.

[39] Goodstein B. Sports performance and injury prevention in professional soccer. NSCA' performance training journal. 2000, 10(3): 8-10.

[40] Greig M, Siegler JC. Soccer-specific fatigue and eccentric hamstrings muscle strength. J Ath Train 2009, 44:180–184.

[41] Hagglund M, Walden, M, Ekstrand J. UEFA Injury Study, an audit of European Championships 2006 – 2008. Br J Sports Med 2005, 43:483-489.

[42] Hagglund M, Walden M, Ekstrand J. Previous injury as a risk factor for injury in elite football: a prospective study over two consecutive season. Br J Sports Med 2006, 40:767-72.

[43] Hartig DE, Henderson JM. Increasing Hamstring flexibility decreases lower extremity overuse injuries in military basic trainees. Am J Sports Med 1999, 27(2): 173-176.

[44] Hawkins RD, & Fuller CW. An examination of the frequency and severity of injuries and incidents at three levels of professional football. Br J Sports Med 1998, 32(4): 326-32.

[45] Hawkins RD, & Fuller CW. Risk assessment in professional football: an examination of accidents and incidents in the 1994 World Cup finals. Br J Sports Med 1996, 30(2): 165-70.

[46] Hawkins RD, Fuller CW. A prospective epidemiological study of injuries in four English professional football clubs. Br J Sports Med 1999, 33: 196–203.

[47] Hawkins RD, Hulse MA, Wilkinson C, Hodson A, Gibson M. The association football medical research programme: an audit of injuries in professional football. Br J Sports Med 2001, 35(1): 43-7.

[48] Heidt RS, Sweeterman LM, Carlonas RL et al. Avoidance of soccer injuries with pre-season conditioning. Am J Sports Med 2000, 28: 659-62.

[49] Herbert RD, Gabriel M. Effects of stretching before and after exercising on muscle soreness and risk of injury: systematic review. Br Med J 2002, 31: 325(7362): 468.

[50] Hibbs AE, Thompson KG, French D, Wrigley A, Spears I. Optimising performance by improving core stability and core strength. Sports Med 2008, 38(12): 995-1008.

[51] Høy K, Lindblad BE, Terkelsen CJ, Helleland HE, Terkelsen CJ. European soccer injuries. A prospective epidemiologic and socioeconomic study. Am J Sports Med 1992, 20(3): 318-2.

[52] Hrysomallis C. Balance ability and athletic performance. Sports Med 2011, 41(3): 221-32.

[53] Iga J, Fruer CS, Deighan M, Croix MDS, James DVB "Nordic" Hamstrings Exercise – Engagement Characteristics and Training Responses. Int J Sports Med 2012, 33: 1000–1004 .

[54] Impellizzeri FM, Bizzini M, Rampinini E, Cereda F, Maffiuletti A. Reliability of isokinetic strength imbalance ratios measured using the Cybex NORM dynamometer. Clin Physiol Funct Imaging 2008, 28: 113-119.

[55] Impellizzeri FM, Rampinini E, Castagna C, Martino F, Fiorini S, Wisloff U. Effect of plyometric training on sand versus grass on muscle soreness and jumping and sprinting ability in soccer players. Br J Sports Med 2010, 42: 42-46.

[56] Impellizzeri, FM, Rampinini, E, Coutts, AJ, Sassi, A and Marcora, SM. Use of RPE-based training load in soccer. Med Sci Sports Exerc 2004, 36(6): 1042-1047.

[57] Junge A, & Dvorak J. Soccer injuries: a review on incidence and prevention. Sports Med 2004, 34(13): 929-38.

[58] Junge A, Rösch D, Peterson L et al. Prevention of soccer injuries: a prospective intervention study in youth amateurs players. Am J Sports Med 2002, 30: 652-9.

[59] Knapik J, Bauman C, Jones B, Harris J, & Vaughan L. Pre-season strength and flexibility imbalances associated with athletic injuries in female collegiate athletes. Am J Sports Med 1991, 19(1): 76-81.

[60] Kraemer R, Knobloch K. A soccer-specific balance training program for hamstring muscle and patellar and achilles tendon injuries: an intervention study in premier league female soccer. Am J Sports Med 2009, 37(7): 1384-93.

[61] Laskowski ER, Newcomer-Aney K, Smith J. Refining rehabilitation with proprioception training: expediting return to play. Phys Sportsmed 1997, 25 (10), 1476.

[62] Lehnhard RA, Lehnhard HR, Young R, Butterfield S. Monitoring injuries on a college soccer team: the effect of strength training. J Strength Cond Res 1996, 10(2): 115-119.

[63] Lephart SM, Pincivero DM, Giraldo JL, Fu FH. The role of proprioception in the management and rehabilitation of athletic injuries. Am J Sports Med 1997, 25(1): 130-7.

[64] Malliaropoulos N, Isinkaye T, Tsitas K et al. Reinjury after acute posterior thigh muscle injuries in elite track and field athletes. Am J Sports Med 2011, 39: 304-10.

[65] Malliaropoulos N, Mendiguchia J, Pehlivanidis H, Papadopoulos S, Valle X, Malliaras P, Maffulli N. Hamstring exercises for track and field athletes: injury and exercise biomechanics, and possible implications for exercise selection and primary prevention. Br J Sports Med 2012, 46: 846-851.

[66] Mallo J, Dellal A. Injury risk in professional football players with special reference to the playing position and training periodization. J Sports Med Phys Fitness 2012, 52(6): 631-8.

[67] Miyama M, Nosaka K. Influence of surface on muscle damage and soreness induced by consecutive drop jumps. J Strength Cond Res 2004, 18: 206-11.

[68] Morgan B, Oberlander M (2001). An Examination of Injuries in Major League Soccer. Am. J. Sports Med. 29: 426-430.

[69] O'Sullivan K, McAuliffe S, DeBurca N. The effects of eccentric training on leg lower limb flexibility: a systematic review. Br J Sports Med 2012, 46: 838-845.

[70] Olsen L, Scanlan 1, MacKay M, Babul S, Reid D, Clark M, Raina P. Strategies for prevention of soccer related injuries: a systematic review. Br J Sports Med 2004, 38: 89-94.

[71] Owen AL, Wong DP, Paul D, & Dellal A. Physical and technical comparisons between small, medium and large-sided training games within elite professional soccer. Eur J Sport Sci 2013a, in press.

[72] Owen AL, Wond DP, Dellal A, Paul DJ, Orhant E, Collie S. Effect of an injury prevention program on muscle injuries in elite professional soccer. J Strength Cond Res 2013b, 21.

[73] Owen AL, Wong DP, McKenna M, and Dellal A. Heart rate responses and technical comparison between small- vs. large-sided games in elite professional soccer. J Strength Cond Res 2011, 25(8): 2104-10.

[74] Padua DA, Di Stefano LJ, Marshall SW, Beutler AI, Motte SJ & Di Stefano MJ. Retention of movement pattern changes after a lower extremity injury prevention program is affected by program duration. Am J Sports Med 2012, 40(2): 300-6.

[75] Parry L, and Drust B. Is injury the major cause of elite soccer players being unavailable to train and play during the competitive season? Phys Ther Sport 2006, 7(2): 58-64.

[76] Paterno MV, Myer GD, Ford KR, & Hewett TE. Neuromuscular Training Improves Single-Limb Stability in Young Female Athletes. J Orthop Sports Phys Ther 2004, 34(6): 305-316.

[77] Petersen J, Thoborg K, Nielsen NB et al. Preventive effect of eccentric training on acute hamstring injuries in men's soccer: a cluster-randomized controlled trial. Am J Sports Med 2011, 39: 2296-303.

[78] Pope RP, Herbert RD, Kirwan JD, Graham BJ. A randomized trial of preexercise stretching for prevention of lower-limb injury. Med. Sci. Sports Exerc 2000, 32(2): 271-277.

[79] Proske U, Morgan DL. Muscle damage from eccentric exercise: mechanism, mechanical signs, adaptation and clinical applications. J Physiol 2001, 537: 333-345.

[80] Rey E, Lago-Peñas C, Lago-Ballesteros J, Casais L, Dellal A. The effects of a congested fixture period on the activity of elite soccer players. Biol Sport 2010, 27: 181-185.

[81] Rochcongar P. Isokinetic thigh muscle strength in spots: a review. Annal Rehab Med Phys 2004, 47: 274-281.

[82] Saliba L, Hrysomallis C. Isokinetic strength related to jumping but not kicking performance of Australian Footballers. J Sci Med Sport 2001, 4(3): 336-347.

[83] Schache AG, Wrigley TV, Baker R et al. Biomechanical response to hamstring muscle strain injury. Gait Posture 2009, 29: 332-8.

[84] Shehab R, Mirabelli M, Gorenflo D, Fetters M. Pre-exercise stretching and sports related injuries: knowledge, attitudes and practices. Clin J Sports Med 2006, 16(3): 228-231.

[85] Soligard T, Nilstad A, Steffen K, Myklebust G, Holme I, Dvorak J, Bahr R, Andersen TE. Compliance with a comprehensive warm up programme to prevent injuries in youth football. Br J Sports Med 2010, 44: 787-793.

[86] Souissi S, Wong DP, Dellal A et al. Improving functional performance and muscle power 4-to-6 months after anterior cruciate ligament reconstruction. J Sports Sci Med 2011, 10: 655-664.

[87] Stanton P, Purdham C. Hamstring injuries in sprinting – the role of eccentric exercise. J Orthop Sports Phys Ther 1989, 10: 343-349.

[88] Stasinopoulos D. Comparison of three preventive methods in order to reduce the incidence of ankle inversion sprains among female volleyball players. Br J Sports Med 2004, 38: 182-185.

[89] Thacker SB, Gilchrist J, Stroup DF, Kimsey CD. The impact of stretching on sports injury risk: a systematic review of the literature. Med Sci Sports Exerc 2004, 36(3): 371-378.

[90] Turl SE, George KP. Adverse neural tension: a factor in repetitive hamstring strain? J Orthop Sports Phys Ther 1998, 27(1): 16-21.

[91] Twellaar M, Verstappen FTJ, Huson A, van Mechelen W. Physical characteristics as risk factors for sports injuries: a four year prospective study. Int J Sports Med 1997, 18(1): 66-71.

[92] Van Beijsterveldt AMC, Van de Port GL, Krist MR et al. Effectiveness of an injury prevention programme for adult male amateur soccer players: a cluster-randomised controlled trial. Br J Sports Med 2013, 22: 1-6.

[93] Van Mechelen W, Hlobil H, Kemper HCG, et al. Prevention of running injuries by warm-up, cool-down, and stretching exercises. Am J Sports Med 1993, 21(5): 711-719.

[94] Verhagen E, van der Beek, A, Twisk J, Bouter L, Bahr R, and van Mechelen W. The effect of a proprioceptive balance board-training program for the prevention of ankle sprains: a prospective controlled trial. Am J Sports Med 2004, 32(6): 1385-1393.

[95] Verrall GM, Slavotinek JP, Barnes PG. The effect of sports specific training on reducing the incidence of hamstring injuries in professional Australian Rules football players. Br J Sports Med 2005, 39(6): 363-368.

[96] Vescovi JD, VanHeest JL. Effects of an anterior cruciate ligament injury prevention programme on performance in adolescent female soccer players. Scand J Med Sci Sports 2010, 20: 394-402.

[97] Walden M, Hagglund M, & Ekstrand J. UEFA Champions League study: a prospective study of injuries in professional football during the 2001-2002 season. Br J Sports Med 2005, 39: 542-546.

[98] Walden M, Hagglund M, Wermer J et al. The epidemiology of anterior cruciate ligament injury in football (soccer): a review of the literature from a gender-related perspective. Knee Surg Sports Traumatol Arthrosc 2011, 19: 3-10.

[99] Willardson. Core stability training: applications to sports conditioning programs. J Strength Cond Res 2007, 21(3): 979-985.

[100] Willson JD, Dougherty, CP, Ireland ML, and Davis IM. Core stability and its relationship to lower extremity function and injury. J Am Acad Orthop Sur 2005, 13(5): 316-325.

[101] Witvrouw E, Mahieu N, Danneels L, McNair P. Stretching and injury prevention. An obscure relationship. Sports Med 2004, 34(7): 443-449.

[102] Woods C, Hawkins RD, Maltby S, et al. The Football Association Medical Research Programme: an audit to injuries in professional football – analysis if hamstring injuries. Br J Sports Med 2004, 38: 36-41.

[103] Worrell TW. Factors associated with hamstring injuries: an approach to treatment and preventative measures. Sports Med 1994, 17(5): 338-345.

[104] Yeung SS, Suen AM, Yeung EW. A prospective cohort study of hamstring injuries in competitive sprinters: preseason muscle imbalance as a possible risk factor. Br J Sports Med 2009, 43: 589-594.

[105] Zakas A, Balaska P, Grammatikopoulou MG, Zakas N, and Vergou A. Acute effects of stretching duration on the range of motion of elderly women. J Bodyw Mov Ther 2005, 9(4): 270-276.

Chapter 11

Muscle Injuries in Professional Soccer Players During the Month of Ramadan

Karim Chamari, Alexandre Dellal and Monoem Haddad

Additional information is available at the end of the chapter

1. Introduction

The muscle injury risk is a major concern for soccer players and clubs in terms of health, safety, performance, and cost. Data in scientific literature must be made available through an effective muscle injury surveillance system, and knowledge of the factors that influence muscle injury is required. There is a need to identify the injury risks in soccer players and their respective dependent and independent variables, which are expected to differ in each specific population. Therefore epidemiological and etiological muscle injury data for international professional soccer need to be captured. The rates and characteristics of soccer muscle injuries during matches and training in top-level international tournaments such as English (Hawkins et al., 2001), Swedish (Hagglund et al., 2006), Norwegian (Andersen et al., 2004) league Championships, European Championships (Ekstrand et al., 2011) and World Cups (Dvorak et al., 2011) have been well documented; however only one study (Chamari et al., 2012) has focused on the muscle injury-rates of Muslim soccer players during the holy month of Ramadan. The first part of this chapter is dedicated to present muscle injury rates in soccer. The main aim of the present book chapter is presenting and discussing the muscle injury rate during the holy month of Ramadan its related possible causes. By providing a such analysis, it is hoped that this might help coaches and scientists to understand and choose a more efficient planning and manipulation of the player's internal training load during the Ramadan period in order to try to avoid muscles injuries.

2. Muscle injuries in soccer during traditional conditions

The first part of this chapter is dedicated to present muscle injury rates during matches and training sessions out of the month of Ramadan in English (Hawkins et al., 2001), Swedish

(Hagglund et al., 2006), Norwegian (Andersen et al., 2004) league Championships, European Championships (Ekstrand et al., 2011) and World Cups (Dvorak et al., 2011) in order to be able to further compare them with those found during the holy month of Ramadan.

Recently, Ekstrand et al., (2011) conducted a prospective cohort study in European Professional Soccer Players from 2001 to 2008. The study focused on seven consecutive seasons (July-May). In 2000, 14 teams from top European clubs (clubs participating at the highest level in Europe in the last decade) were selected by UEFA and invited to participate in the study of Ekstrand et al., (2011). Eleven teams agreed to participate and provided complete data for the 2001/2002 season. In the following seasons, 12 other teams were selected by UEFA and included in the study. Ekstrand et al., (2011) presented the results of the teams that have met the criteria for inclusion and comprehensive data sent over the full seasons. Table 1 shows these characteristics.

	All seven seasons	Seasons						
		2001/2002	2002/2003	2003/2004	2004/2005	2005/2006	2006/2007	2007/2008
Age	25.7 (4.4)	25.7 (4.4)	25.8 (4.0)	26.0 (4.3)	25.8 (4.1)	25.9 (4.5)	25.6 (4.6)	25.5 (4.6)
Training hours/ players	213 (71)	219 (66)	243 (64)	203 (67)	229 (65)	207 (75)	207 (75)	206 (68)
Exposure hours/ player	254 (85)	262 (80)	290 (74)	243 (80)	273 (79)	247 (89)	245 (90)	246 (83)
Match hours/ player	41 (23)	43 (22)	47 (23)	40 (24)	44 (24)	40 (23)	38 (24)	40 (24)
No of matches/ player	34 (17)	36 (16)	39 (16)	33 (17)	35 (16)	33 (17)	32 (17)	33 (17)
No of matches/ player	162 (53)	174 (53)	181 (45)	151 (47)	171 (46)	156 (55)	155 (56)	160 (52)
Values are mean (SD)								

Table 1. Characteristics of teams, players and exposure from 2001 to 2008 belonging from the best European clubs adapted from Ekstrand et al., (2011).

The authors reported 4483 injuries corresponding to 566 000 h of exposure (i.e, 475 000h of training and 91 000h of match-play) over the seven seasons, inducing a rate of 8.0 injuries / 1000 h. Muscle injuries were the highest type of injuries observed with 1581 injuries during the 566 000 h of exposure. A player performed an average of 34 games and had 162 training sessions each season (median values of 35 and 173, respectively). The overall average exposure during the football season was of 254 h, with 213 hours of training and 41 hours of games (median values being 269, 222 and 40, respectively). The rate of injuries during matches was higher than that of training (27.5 vs. 4.1, respectively, p <0.001). The rates of muscle injuries and others types of injuries during training and the match remained steady during the 8-years with no significant difference in-between seasons.

A player may undergo on average two injuries per season, thus a team of typically 25 players can expect about 50 injuries each season. Table 2 shows the different types of injuries according to their severity with the top European clubs in according to Ekstrand et al., (2011). During the competitive season, traumatic (or contact) injuries and hamstring strains were the more frequent observed sport accidents, while during the pre-season, overuse injuries/muscle injuries were more frequently reported injuries (35.27% of all injuries during the seven years studied, Table 2). Recurrent injuries accounted for 12% of all injuries recorded during the seven successive studied seasons, causing longer absences than non-recurrent injuries (24 vs. 18 days, respectively, p <0.0001). In the same context, Hawkins et al., (2001) have shown that recurrent injuries represented 7% of 6030 injuries reported with 91 clubs in English Professional Football during two consecutive seasons.

	Total	1-3 Days	4-7 Days	ays	"/> 28 Days
Injury type					
Fracture	160 (4)	7	9	59 (4)	85 (12)
Other bone injury	26	5	1	6	14 (2)
Disloaction/subluxation	50 (1)	5	4	24 (1)	17 (2)
Sprain/ligament injury	828 (18)	123 (13)	197 (34)	334 (20)	174 (25)
Mensiscus/catilage	124 (Rejeski et al.)	3	7	41 (2)	73 (10)
Muscle injury/Strain	1581 (35)	212 (22)	397 (34)	765 (46)	207 (30)
Tendon injury	327 (7)	95 (10)	71 (6)	101 (6)	60 (9)
Haematoma/contusion	744 (17)	306 (32)	282 (24)	141 (9)	15 (2)
Abrasion	7	3	3	1	0
Laceration	31	10 (1)	11	10	0
Contusion	34	5	14 (1)	14	1
Nerve injury	29	7	3	14	5
Synovitis/effusion	158 (4)	55 (6)	36 (3)	55 (3)	12 (2)
Overuse complaints	285 (6)	110 (11)	99 (9)	59 (4)	17 (2)
Other type	91 (2)	23 (2)	27 (2)	24 (1)	17 (2)
Total injuries	4483	971	1164	1651	697

Values within brackets show percentage of total injuries (lower line - values below 1% not shown)

Table 2. Injury pattern by severity of injuries from 2001 to 2008 (rate: injuries/1000 h of exposure) with the best European clubs adapted from Ekstrand et al., (2011)

The rate of injuries during trainings and matches-play in the study reported Ekstrand et al., (2011) are consistent with the data of Hawkins et al., (2001), who reported A total of 6030 injuries collected over two seasons (i.e., from July 1997 through to the end of May 1999) with an average of 1.3 injuries per player per season of professional football in England. Table 3 shows the nature of the injuries sustained during training and matches reported by Hawkins et al., (2001). Muscles injuries represented 46% of all the injuries. The rate of muscle injuries in trainings was high than during matches-play (p<0.001). In Table 3, Injuries classified as "other" report back and nerve related pathologies/injuries, vertebral column-disc derangements, and non-specific pain, no individual category amounting to more than 0.5% of all injuries. It is of interest to note that the players' dominant side showed a greater sustained number of injuries compared with the non-dominant side (50% vs. 37%, respectively, p<0.01), and the lower limbs (including the groin) was the site of 87% of the total injuries reported (Table 3).

In the Swedish Premier League, Hägglünd et al., (2006) prospectively recorded individual exposure and loss of time due to injury over two full consecutive seasons (2001 and 2002). They showed that the rate of injuries and training match between the seasons were similar (5.1 vs. 5.3 injuries/1000 h of training and 25.9 vs. 22.7 injuries/1000 h of match-play; respectively) but the analysis of injury severity and injury patterns showed variations between seasons. In Norway, Andersen et al., (2004) collected data and videotapes of injuries prospectively during regular league matches in 2000 (April to October). Over 174 matches, 425 injuries were recorded: 1.2 injuries per team per match or 75.5 injuries per 1000 hours played. A total of 121 acute injuries were reported from game, giving a rate of 0.3 injuries per match and team or 21.5 injuries per 1000 hours played. In an analysis of the rates and characteristics of injuries in the edition of the 2010 FIFA World Cup, Dvorak et al., (2011) reported 229 injuries, of which 140 injuries requiring rest. The remaining injuries did not prevent the players to take part to the consecutive training sessions. In this study, 32 finalist squads participated (including 736 players). 82 injuries during matches and 58 injuries during training requiring rest were observed, resulting in a rate of 40.1 injuries/1000-h during matches (95% CI 31.4 to 48.8) and 4.4 injuries/1000-h during training (95% CI 3.3 to 5.5). Table 4 shows the Location and diagnosis of match and training injuries during this study.

Contact with another player caused by foul-play based on the judgment of the team physician was the most common cause of injuries during matches (65%) and training sessions (40%). These data showed that the most common diagnoses were contusions at the thigh and ankle sprain (Dvorak et al., 2011). In the same context, Ekstrand et al., (2011) showed that 21% (n = 538) of all injuries recorded during matches of seven successive seasons with the best professional players were due to foul-play according to the referee, with the majority being due to foul play by an opponent (n=520). The most common foul-play injuries were ankle sprains (15%), knee sprains (9%) and thigh contusions (10%). In the two studied seasons, (2006/07 and 2007/08), the match timing of injury showed that foul-play injuries were evenly distributed among the two halves (74 vs. 84 for first and second half, respectively, p=0.47). In this context, receiving a tackle, receiving a "charge", and making a tackle were categorized as associated with a substantial injury risk, while goal punching, kicking the ball, shot on goal, set kick, and heading the ball were all categorized as exposing to a significant injury risk. With respect to match minute, Injury risk was highest in the first and last 15 minutes of the games. This probably reflects the intense engagements in the opening period of each game, during which the players are highly motivated and the effects of fatigue not yet clearly observable, and the possible effect of fatigue in the closing period. The injury risk was also concentrated in the areas of challenge where possession of the ball is the most hotly contested, i.e., the attack and defense areas near the goals. The injury rate during the 2010 FIFA World Cup was lower than in the previous three World Cups (Dvorak et al., 2011) as presented in Table 2. This may be a result of a connection to additional injury prevention, and a reduced fool play probably due to the more stringent arbitration (Dvorak et al., 2011). Dvorak et al., (2011) showed that training injuries differed substantially from match injuries with respect to diagnosis (Table 4) and cause, but not in severity. It was reported that training injuries were more often as a result of overuse and non-contact trauma than match injuries. In this context, it is interesting to note that 12 out of 104 training injuries were reported to be contact-injuries caused by foul-play. Out of these 12 injuries, 6 were reported from one team. In this case the rate of time-loss training injuries was similar to those reported for the European Championships {i.e., 1.3–3.9 per 1000 hours of exposure to Training} (Hagglund et al., 2006; Ekstrand et al., 2011).

No	All injuries %	No	Competition injuries %	No	Training injuries %	
Nature of injury						
Muscular strain/rupture	2225	37	1322	35	859†	42
Ligamentous sprain/rupture	1153	19	765	20	370	18
Muscular contusion	431	7	343	9	79†	4
Tissue bruising	336	6	263	7	64†	3
Fracture	253	4	186	5	61†	3
Other	238	4	123	3	95†	5
Tendinitus	237	4	107	3	10†	5
Inflammatory synovitis	192	3	114	3	73	4
Mensiscal tear	148	2	80	2	63‡	3
Hernia	120	2	56	1	40	2
Overuse	108	2	44	1	44†	2
Dislocation	81	1	50	1	28	1
Periostitis	75	1	52	1	23	1
Cut	73	1	60	2	13†	1
Chondral lesion	69	1	41	1	24	1
Capsular tear	54	1	47	1	6†	0
Paratendinitis	46	1	17	0	27†	1
Bursitis	29	1	10	0	18†	1
Blister	6	0	2	0	4	0
Skin abrasion	3	3	2	0	1	0
Not classified	153	101	96	3	44	2
Total*	6030		3780	98	2046	99
Location of injury						
Thigh	1388	23	889	24	468	22
Knee	1014	17	610	17	355	16
Ankle	1011	17	682	19	304†	14
Lower leg	753	12	452	12	272	13
Groin	596	10	226	6	340†	16
Neck/spine	352	6	176	5	159†	7
Foot	302	5	202	6	94	4
Upper limb	153	3	99	3	50	2
Hip	135	2	82	2	46	2
Abdomen	90	1	50	1	36	2
Chest	86	1	77	2	7†	0
Head	67	1	55	2	11†	1
Toe	63	1	50	1	12†	1
Other	15	0	12	0	1	0
Not specified	5	0	4	0	1	0
Total*	6030	99	3666	100	2160	100

* Percentage totals may subject to rounding errors associated with individual components

† p<0.01 Different proportions between training and competition

‡ p<0.05 Different proportions between training and competition

Table 3. Nature and location of injuries sustained during match-play and training with 91 professional soccer clubs in England during two consecutive seasons adapted from Hawkins et al., (2001).

Location and diagnostics	Match injuries		Training injuries	
	All	With absence	All	With absence
Head/neck	13	4	6	3
Contusion	1	1	1	0
Contusion	4	1	2	0
Muscle cramps (neck)	0	0	2	0
Upper extremity	12	6	4	2
Fracture	1	0	0	2
Sprain	4	3	0	0
Contusion	4	3	1	0
Laceration	0	0	1	0
Trunk	8	5	10	4
Contusion	5	2	3	0
Sprain/strain	2	2	1	1
Hip	2	1	1	1
Contusion	1	0	0	0
Groin	4	4	3	3
Muscle strain	3	3	1	1
Tendonitis	1	1	1	1
Muscle cramps	0	0	1	1
Thigh	36	25	19	13
Muscle strain/rupture	11	10	11	9
Contusion	12	6	2	1
Muscle cramps/tightness	9	7	3	2
Knee	9	6	16	9
Sprain	4	3	3	3
Tendinopathy	0	0	2	1
Contusion	3	1	4	1
Lower leg	19	12	18	9
Muscle strain/rupture	6	5	2	1
Contusion	11	5	9	2
Muscle cramps	0	0	2	2
Ankle	15	12	17	8
Sprain	6	4*	12	8*
Contusion	7	6	5	0*
Foot	7	7	10	6
Contusion	6	6	6	3

* Information was missing for at least one injury.

Table 4. Location and diagnosis of match and training muscle injuries (n=229) in 2001 in the Norway professional soccer season adapted from Dvorak et al., (2011).

Years		1998	2002	2006	2010
Injuries per match	all injuries	2.4	2.7	2.3	2
	time-loss injuries	0	1.7	1.5	1.3

Table 5. Average number of injuries per match in FIFA World Cups 1998–2010 (grey: all injuries; black: time-loss injuries) adapted from Dvorak et al., (2011).

Muscle injury risk can also be affected by the match schedule. Indeed, Dupont et al., (2011) showed that the muscle injury rate can be much higher when 2 matches are played during the week, compared to classical one-game per week schedule. The highest muscle injury was located at thigh (32 vs 15 injuries, respectively. These results confirmed that insufficient recovery between matches leads to fatigue and increases the risk of muscle injury. In the 2006 World-Cup (Germany), Dvorak et al., (2007) reported an injury rate slightly lower than the results of Dupont et al., (2011). In this tournament, the high rate of injuries may have been linked to the limited number of recovering days between 2 matches (given that most matches were played every 3 to 5 days) and the repetition of matches in a congested fixture schedule. Although some of the players studied probably had more than 4-days recovery between matches, this result highlights the higher risk of muscle injuries when the recovery between 2 matches is short. In this context, Ekstrand et al., (2004) reported that a congested soccer calendar increased the risk of muscle injury or underperformance. Results from these afore-mentioned studies confirm the high risk of injury during a congested calendar. Nevertheless, conflicting results come from Carling et al., (2012) who did not observe any difference in the injury rate between congested fixture period and outside such a period. In the same context, recently with a higher number of matches, Dellal et al., (Accepted 2012) showed that muscle injuries during the congested periods of fixture (3 different congested fixture periods, 6 matches in 21 days during each one of the congested periods) was not different to those reported in matches outside these periods (55.8% of total injuries from 14.4 injuries/1000h during congested period vs 55.6% from 15.6 injuries/1000h during non-congested period). Rahnama et al., (2002) assessed the exposure of English Premier League players to injury risk during the "1999–2000 season" by rating the injury potential of playing actions during competition with respect to the type of playing action, period of the game, zone of the pitch, and playing either at home or away games. Muscle injury rate was no different in away matches than at home games (Rahnama et al., 2002). From the 3836 injuries for which the timing of injury was known, Hawkins et al., (2001) found that a greater than the average frequency of injuries was observed during the final 15 minutes of the first half and the final 30 minutes of the second ($p<0.01$). Table 6 shows the distribution of the competitive match injuries with respect to timing of occurrence. Despite the increase in injury rate observed towards the later stages of the first half (i.e. the last 15 min of play, which was similar with the same trend for the second half), overall, there remained a greater number of injuries recorded in the second half compared to the first (57% v 43%, respectively, $p<0.01$). This may be the result of fatigue of the muscles and other body organs as well as muscle glycogen stores near to depletion (Reilly, 1997) and players becoming hypo-hydrated (Saltin, 1973).

Time (minutes)	Injuries (%)
0 – 15	8
>15 – 30	14.5
>30 – 45	22.5
>45 – 60	10
>60 – 75	19
>75 – 90	26
Total	100

Table 6. Timing of occurrence of injuries in matches with 91 English professional soccer clubs during two consecutive sessions adapted from Hawkins et al., (2001).

There is evidence to suggest that fatigue is associated with muscle injury. Indeed, empirical observations have shown that fatigued individuals are susceptible to muscle injury [See for review (Schlabach, 1994)]. Fatigue may not be the only cause of muscle injury, but rather a contributing factor. After reviewing the literature regarding the etiology of muscle injuries, Worrell and Perrin (1992) reported that fatigue was one of several factors that may contribute to frequency of hamstring strains (one of the common muscle injuries in soccer).

Since muscle glycogen depletion is associated with fatigue and possibly injury, it should also be treated as a potential risk factor. Muscle glycogen stores are almost entirely derived from carbohydrate intake. Both indirect and direct evidence support the notion that depleted muscle glycogen stores contribute to muscle injury. Indirectly, it is quite clear that depleted muscle glycogen stores coincide with fatigue, and fatigue in turn is associated with muscle injury as mentioned above. Although most of the evidence involves relationships rather than showing cause, many of the investigations strongly suggest a cause-and-effect relationship between low muscle glycogen stores and injury risks [See for review (Schlabach, 1994)]. Depletion up to 84-90% of intramuscular glycogen stores has been observed in soccer players at the end of a soccer match (Jacobs et al., 1982). Soccer players with low glycogen stores at the start of a match had almost no glycogen left in their working muscle and physical performance of these players decreased in the second half in comparison to those players with higher pre-game and halftime glycogen muscle levels (Jacobs et al., 1982). Because there is a limited capacity to store muscle glycogen, and because muscle glycogen is the predominant fuel in exercise of moderate to severe intensity, the nutritional focus should be on carbohydrate consumption [See for review (Schlabach, 1994)]. The absolute amount of carbohydrates in the diet may be an important factor for the recovery of muscle and liver glycogen stores after training and competition (Ivy, 2001). In this context, it is important to mention that an inadequate nutrient intake and hypohydration could affect the physical performance of the athlete and possibly contribute to sports injuries (Convertino et al., 1996). Large sweat losses, insufficient fluid intake, and consequent fluid deficits could likely impair performance and may increase the risk of hyperthermia and related problems (Bergeron et al., 2005), stressing the importance of appropriate hydration before training and matches in soccer players. In this context, as ending the day dehydrated, fasting players (as observed during Ramadan) could be exposed to higher risks of muscle injury.

Another important cause related with fatigue-associated injuries is the sleeping duration and/ or quality. Research indicates a relationship between sleep deprivation and decreased performance in adults (Taylor et al., 1997; Belenky et al., 2003). Recently, Luke et al., (2011) confirmed that fatigue-related injuries were related to sleeping less than 6 hours the night before the injury (p = 0.028) among athletes aged 6 to 18 years. In contrast, Luke et al., (2011) have reported no difference in the average amount of sleeping hours or reported sleep-deprivation between the overuse and acute injury groups of their study. However, with evidence of the obvious contributing role of fatigue in increasing muscle injury risk, planning for adequate sleep before and during training or competition events should be another notable consideration in determining a player's training schedule and setting-up an event schedule, especially if travel is involved. As sleeping schedule is acutely changed during Ramadan, this month could be a cause of higher muscle injury risks for athletes.

3. Muscle injuries in soccer during Ramadan period

Investigations describing muscle injury risk and muscle injury patterns in soccer are usually conducted over seasons of European or American Leagues (Andersen et al., 2004; Ekstrand et al., 2011; Dupont et al., 2011). To our knowledge, only one study (Chamari et al., 2012) has focused on the injury-rates of muslim soccer players during the holy month of Ramadan. In this context, to our knowledge this is the only scientific publication having studied the effect of Ramadan fasting on sports' injuries.

3.1. Ramadan characteristics

During the wholly month of Ramadan, fasting Muslims do not eat, drink, smoke, or have sexual activities daily from dawn to sunset. Since the Islamic Calendar is based on the lunar cycle, which advances 11-days compared with the seasonal year, Ramadan occurs at different times of the seasonal year over a 33-year cycle (Chaouachi et al., 2009a). This implies that Ramadan occurs at different environmental conditions between years in the same country (Leiper et al., 2003; Leiper et al., 2008). It is supposed that most Muslim soccer players fast during Ramadan, even if some exceptions are observed. Ramadan fasting is intermittent in nature, and there is no restriction to the amount of food or fluid that can be consumed after dusk and before dawn. Therefore, since the international sporting calendar is not adapted for religious observances, and Muslim soccer players continue to compete and train during Ramadan, various studies have determined whether this religious fast has any effect on athletic performance (Chaouachi et al., 2009a) and cognitive functions (Maughan et al., 2010; Water-house, 2010). These have suggested that only few aspects of physical fitness are negatively affected, and only modest decrements are observed when physical performance is considered on the basis of fitness testing (Chaouachi et al., 2009a). The evidence to date indicates that high-level athletes can maintain most of the performance measures during Ramadan if physical training, diet, and sleep are well controlled. Nevertheless, despite this, fasting athletes report higher fatigue feelings at the end of Ramadan (Chaouachi et al., 2009a; Güvenç, 2011). This could have a possible effect on performance of injury during or at the end of the month of Ramadan.

The increased perception of fatigue reported at the end of Ramadan fasting and the combination of intense training with altered carbohydrate intake, hydration-status, and sleeping pattern may place fasting Muslim athletes at greater risk of overreaching or overtraining (Chaouachi et al., 2009b; Chaouachi et al., 2009c) which could result in physical injury specifically overuse injuries (Johnson and Thiese, 1992). Most previous studies determined whether the holy month of Ramadan has any detrimental effect on performance and cognitive functions, but to our knowledge, only the study of Chamari et al., (2012) has examined the impact of the month of Ramadan and its specific socio-cultural and religious environment on the injury rates of professional elite soccer players. This pilot study presented some results on the injury rates between fasting and non-fasting players within a team before, during, and after the month of Ramadan in a professional football team during two consecutive seasons.

3.2. Muscle injury rates during Ramadan

The study of Chamari et al., (2012) presented some results on the muscle injury rate between fasting and non-fasting players within a professional soccer team during the month of Ramadan during two consecutive seasons. Ramadan occurred from 10 August to 11 September 2010 and from 1 to 30 August 2011, respectively, where the daily fast occurred from ~04 h to ~19.15 h, for a total duration of ~15h15min fasting duration. In this study, training loads (using the RPE-method), Hooper index (Hooper and Mackinnon, 1995a) {i.e., Sum of well-being subjective ratings relative to fatigue, stress, delayed onset muscle soreness (especially "heavy" legs), and sleep quality/disorders} and muscle injury were monitored in 42 professional soccer players (Age, 24 ± 4 years; height, 185 ± 8 cm; body mass, 78 ± 4 kg) a month before Ramadan, the month of Ramadan, and the month after Ramadan during each season. Injury data were considered when a player was unable to take full part in future soccer training sessions or matches owing to physical complaints (Fuller et al., 2006). Information about mechanism of injury (traumatic or muscle injury) and circumstances (training or match injury) were docu-mented. Before and after Ramadan the sessions and matches were scheduled in the afternoon (starting at 15 or 16h) and sometimes in the morning for training (for the days in which 2 training sessions were scheduled, starting at 09.30 h) while during Ramadan, training sessions and matches were performed after dusk (starting at 22h). Ambient temperature, atmospheric pressure and relative humidity were measured for each training session and are presented in Table 7.

	Year	Ambient Temperature (C°)	Atmospheric Pressure (mmHg)	Relative Humidity (%)
Before Ramadan	2010	28.83 (1.72)	1012.33 (2.25)	44.00 (5.02)
	2011	31.31 (5.38)	1011.38 (3.10)	39.15 (13.61)
Ramadan	2010	27.60 (4.04)	1014.20 (2.05)	55.80 (8.44)
	2011	24.50 (1.29)	1014.50 (2.65)	64.50 (6.56)
After Ramadan	2010	25.25 (2.06)	1014.00 (3.83)	61.50 (8.66)
	2011	28.50 (1.29)	1013.25 (3.10)	63.25 (8.54)

Values are mean (SD)

Table 7. Ambient Temperature, Atmospheric Pressure and Relative Humidity for the months of Ramadan, Before Ramadan and After Ramadan, reported by Chamari et al., (2012).

Chamari et al., (2012) have shown that muscle injuries were lower during the months prior to- and after-Ramadan with only 22.22% of total muscle injuries in both cases, while this type of injury (i.e., muscle injury) dramatically increased during Ramadan with 84.21% out of total injuries observed for the two months of Ramadan monitored. For these two periods of Ramadan (Chamari et al., 2012), the muscle injuries were distributed as follows: muscle spasms (contractures) 43.75%, tendinopathy 43.75%, and muscle strains (one tear at the hamstrings and one strain at the thigh-adductors) 12.5%. The 7 contractures were located at the hamstrings (42.86%), calf muscles (28.57%), thigh-adductors (14.29%), and knee extensors (14.29%). The tendinopathy injuries were located at the thigh-adductors (42.86%) and foot quadriceps (14.29%), with the remaining tendinopathy injuries (42.86%) located at the abdomen and pelvis. The foremost result of the study of Chamari et al., (2012) was the absence of significant difference between non-fasting and fasting players with regard to general injury rates, while the training muscle injury rates were significantly higher during Ramadan than before and after-Ramadan periods for the fasting players (Table 8).

	Before Ramadan [+]		Ramadan [+]		After Ramadan [+]	
	Fasting	Non-Fasting	Fasting	Non-Fasting	Fasting	Non-Fasting
Rate of muscle injury during matches	0 (-1.3-1.3)	0 (-1.3-1.3)	1.2 (-0.1-2.4)	0 (-1.3-1.3)	0.5 (-0.7-1.8)	0 (-1.3-1.3)
Rate of muscle injury during training	0.6 (-1.1-2.2)	0.6 (-1.1-2.2)	5.6 [b] (4.0-7.2)	3.2 (1.5-4.8)	0.5 (-1.1-2.2)	0 (-1.6-1.6)

[+] each period consisted of 4 weeks respectively in each of the two studied seasons.

[b] significantly higher than before and after-Ramadan.

Note: values in bracket are 95% confidence intervals.

Table 8. Comparisons of muscle injury rates in fasters and non-fasters for the two monitored seasons (adapted from Chamari et al., 2012).

The rates reported during the month of Ramadan (Chamari et al., 2012) were consistent with data found in Union of European Football Associations {UEFA} (Ekstrand et al., 2011), English Premier League (Hawkins et al., 2001), Swedish Premier League (Hagglund et al., 2006), Scottish league (Dupont et al., 2011), and Norwegian league (Andersen et al., 2004). Nevertheless, the muscle injury rate of the study of Chamari et al., (2012) outside the month of Ramadan is lower than what is typically reported in the literature. It has to be stressed by the authors that this muscle injury rate concerns pre-season and the start of the season and this might explain these lower rates. Indeed, pre-season is characterized by a high prevalence of endurance training and fitness training which were performed in a progressive manner. The low frequency of matches at these stages might be the cause of the low overall injury rates of the studied periods (Chamari et al., 2012). Indeed, it has been well demonstrated (as mentioned above in the present book chapter) that the match injury rates are always much higher than the training injury rates (Ekstrand et al., 2011). In this context, Koutedakis and Sharp (1998) showed that the preparation phase of the season is accompanied with fewer injuries than the competition phase. Despite a higher mean overall injury rate during the Ramadan months of the 2 studied seasons (Chamari et al., 2012), i.e. 12.3 injuries/1000-h exposure, vs 4.9 for the month's before-Ramadan and 6.7 for the month's after-Ramadan, the difference between non-fasting and fasting players being not significant, while the rate of muscle injuries during training was significantly higher during Ramadan than before- and after-Ramadan in fasting players (Table 8). Nevertheless, these groups showed differences for the Hooper's Index and perceived stress (Hooper and Mackinnon, 1995b) with fasting players having lower Hooper's Index and stress during Ramadan and after Ramadan than non-fasting players. Moreover, no difference was observed between fasting and non-fasting players for the reported quality of sleep, and quantity of delayed onset muscle soreness and fatigue during Ramadan, before, and after-Ramadan (Figure 1).

Despite the difference in Hooper Index observed, Chamari et al., (2012) showed that training load, training strain, and training duration were maintained during the 3 periods and between groups for the 2 monitored seasons (Figure 2). The technical staffs of this study (Chamari et al., 2012) had not decrease training load during Ramadan based on the key findings of Chaouachi et al., (2009a) who has suggested that elite athletes could avoid steep decrements in their physical capacities while undergoing the intermittent fast of Ramadan, when they were maintaining their usual training loads; However, although there is no study contrasting the suggestions of Chaouachi et al., (2009a), technical staffs should adapt the training load of their players based on daily observations. The suggestion of Chaouachi et al., (2009a) concerned players from elite Tunisian athletes with different characteristics of training compared to European top-level teams. Indeed, in Tunisia, there are less frequencies of matches than in European top-class teams with games played each 3-4 days almost continuously for about 10 months (about 25 to 40 games vs. 45-62 games, respectively). Another concern with Ramadan in Europe comes from the daylight duration. Indeed, fasters in Europe abstain from food and fluids for 1 to 2 hours longer than Tunisia in summer for example. In summer, with the relative heat, this could be a challenge for Muslim Fasters that are part of a European Team in which technical staffs have objectives of performance and hence, do not even think about managing the training pattern. The study of Chamari et al., (2012) reported data of players that trained

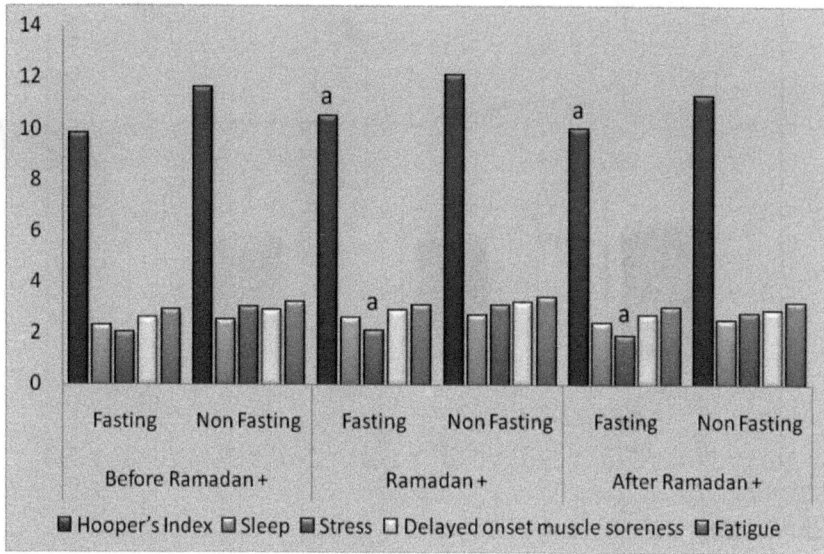

+ each period consisted of 4 weeks in each year, respectively.
a significant different from non-fasting players at p<0.05.

Figure 1. Comparisons of Hooper Index, (sleep, stress, delayed onset muscle soreness, and fatigue) {means of the 2 studied seasons} (Chamari et al., 2012).

at night during Ramadan and avoiding days including two training sessions. Consequently, their conclusions are not adaptable to such specific European Fasting players keeping training during the day (often in the morning and with some double sessions' days) and having to keep off their food and fluid intakes that are one of the pillars of recovery. Ending a high load training session at around 11h00 a.m. and having to keeping on fasting for the remaining hours until the sunset (Iftar) certainly presents a challenge, especially for the long daylight days (i.e., summer). Adding a second training session in the afternoon, is certainly not easy at all. Some recommendations in that regard have been made by Kirkendall et al., (2012) in trying to advise the technical staffs and athletes to deal with training during Ramadan. In this regard, further studies on injuries during Ramadan in different parts of the world, and through the year calendar are needed. Other specific situations should also be investigated as some players chose to fast during the week but not the day of the games. This surely presents another pattern of fasting with specific physiological adaptations and therefore injury pattern.

3.3. Possible causes of muscle injuries during Ramadan

3.3.1. Sleep disturbance and consequences

The study Chamari et al., (2012) have shown that the perceived quality of sleep was not significantly different between the months of Ramadan and the months before and after

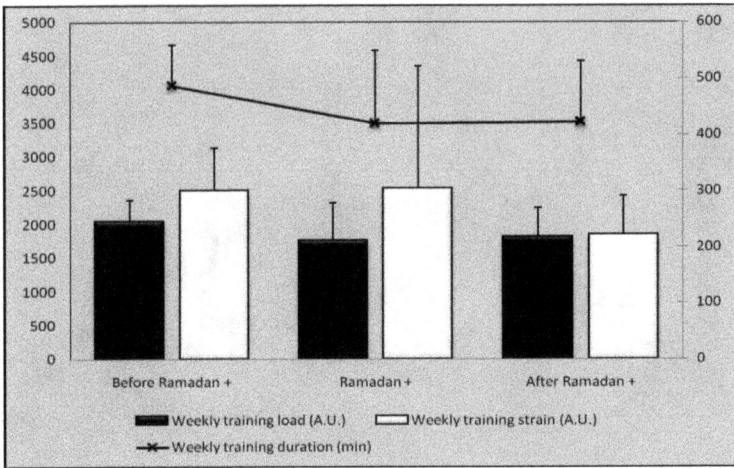

+ each period consisted of 4 weeks respectively in each season.
A.U.: arbitrary units

Figure 2. Comparisons of weekly training load, strain, and duration {mean of the 2 studied seasons} (Chamari et al., 2012).

Ramadan. Even if the reported quality of overall sleep was not altered during Ramadan, the sleeping scheduling was greatly modified with players not going to bed before 03.00-h a.m. (Chamari et al., 2012). Recently, Luke et al., (2011) showed that sleeping less than 6-h the night before the injury occurrence was associated with increased fatigue-related injuries. The results of the study of Chamari et al., (2012) show no influence of Ramadan on the perceived sleep quality of the participants. As the Hooper's index is a simple general index aiming to assess sleep quality, the absence of change does not necessary mean that sleep architecture was not altered. Even if the participants were generally satisfied about their whole 24-h sleeping quality, it may be that the time spent in the different sleeping phases was modified. In this context, it has been well established that sleeping architecture is characterized by different phases at the beginning and the end of the night (Czeisler et al., 1980; Duffy et al., 1996). The change in the sleeping and nutritional habits during Ramadan (i.e. much less night-sleep and more afternoon naps for fasters and non-fasters and major changes in eating patterns for the fasting players) may have altered the players' physiological status during Ramadan, probably leading to the observed higher over-use injury rate during the fasting month (Bogdan et al., 2001; Montelpare et al., 1992; Reilly and Waterhouse, 2007).

3.3.2. Physiological and hormonal disturbances

After sleeping architecture disturbances, an additional probable cause of higher overuse injuries could also be the end-of-Ramadan state of the fasting players. In this context, Chaoua-chi et al., (2009c) have clearly shown that elite athletes continuing to complete high training loads during Ramadan might endure higher levels of fatigue and are likely to experience a cascade of small biochemical adjustments including hormonal, immunoglobulin, and antioxidant system changes, and an elevated inflammatory response. These variations are close to what is observed in tissue traumatic processes as found in athletes in state of over-reaching or overtraining (Chaouachi et al., 2009c). Although the variations are small and may not be considered clinically relevant, they may still signal physiological stress (Chaouachi et al., 2009c). In this context, the overtraining syndrome has been referred as staleness or chronic fatigue with a mental lassitude along with some associated injuries that are observed in parallel to a significant decline in physical performance (Kenttä and Hassmén, 1998; Halson and Jeukendrup, 2004). Overtraining affects the musculoskeletal system in that sense that serum creatine kinase levels are increased and enzymatic markers of muscle tissue injury significantly elevated the day after high training loads. It is unclear whether the observed over-use injuries observed in the over-trained or over-reached athlete could be the result of excessively high training loads and/or the impaired ability to recover from training. As training load was not different between fasters and non fasters in the study of Chamari et al., (2012), it is possible that the recovery processes could be altered by Ramadan intermittent fasting.

3.3.3. Psychological alteration and general fatigue

Contradictory with many studies [see for review (Chaouachi et al., 2009a] showing that Ramadan induces additional stress on the athlete, the perceived mental stress assessed by the Hooper scale during Ramadan in the study of Chamari et al., (2012) was not different from stress measured before and after Ramadan for non-fasting players. Rather, the fasting players reported decreased stress for Ramadan and for the month after-Ramadan compared to pre-Ramadan month. It could be speculated that the religious beliefs and the well-being of living and practicing a holy month, could have led to a lower perception of stress in the latter players. The possible habituation process in the fasting players has also to be considered, as they reported that they had fasted and trained simultaneously for a mean period of seven years and thus the absence of total injury risk with respect to the non-fasting players relates to habituated fasters. Newly fasting players' data are not available from the study of Chamari et al., (2012).

3.3.4. Contextual conditions

The period of the year and changing climate has to be considered with respect to the effect of Ramadan on the incidence of sporting injuries. Indeed, the study of Chamari et al., (2012) was conducted over the 2010 and 2011 years with the months of Ramadan occurring in August/September in Tunisia where daily fasting lasted about 15h15min and the temperature was relatively high. Different fasting periods and environmental conditions have to be experimented with respect to their effects on professional soccer players' injury rates. It has also to be noted that in the latter study the training sessions occurred during the nights (22h00, i.e. about 3 hours after the "iftar" / fasting break). In that sense, the injury rates reported concern therefore "Fasting" players that were not in a fasting state, as they did break the fast about three hours earlier and were allowed to drink ad-libitum before and during the training sessions and games. Unfortunately, no data is yet available for any injury rate occurring in fasting players during training or matches.

4. Recommendations and conclusion

The only study in scientific literature (Chamari et al., 2012) on the muscle and general injury rate during the month of Ramadan was conducted in professional football players shows that many changes occurring during the Ramadan fasting may potentially affect the muscle injury risk for fasting players. In Muslim majority countries, non-fasting players may also be affected by changes in eating and sleeping habits and in the scheduling of training and match play. Preliminary data of Chamari et al., (2012), however, show the absence of the effect of the holy month of Ramadan on the general injury rates of fasting and non-fasting elite soccer players where weekly training loads were maintained during Ramadan. However, rates of non-contact injuries and rates of muscle injuries during training were higher during Ramadan than before or after Ramadan in fasting compared to the non-fasting players.

Therefore, it appears that coaches and medical staffs involved in the management of fasting players should monitor and adapt the training load according to the timing of Ramadan on the year's span (environmental conditions), and the culture and the level of the players. Pay special attention to the recovery interventions (rest, nutrition, and hydration).

Author details

Karim Chamari[1], Alexandre Dellal[2,3,4] and Monoem Haddad[5,6]

1 Research and Education Centre, Aspetar, Qatar Orthopaedic and SportsMedicine Hospital, Doha, Qatar

2 FIFA Medical Excellence Centre, Santy Orthopedicae Clinical, Sport Science and Research Department, Lyon, France

3 OGC Nice, Fitness Training Department, Nice, France

4 Centre de Recherche et d'Innovation sur le Sport (CRIS), Université de Lyon 1, Lyon, France

5 Tunisian Research Laboratory "Sport Performance Optimisation", National Center of Medicine and Science in Sports (CNMSS), Tunis, Tunisia

6 Jandouba University, ISSEP Kef, Tunisia

References

[1] Hawkins, R. D, Hulse, M. A, Wilkinson, C, Hodson, A, & Gibson, M. The association football medical research programme: an audit of injuries in professional football. British journal of sports medicine. (2001). Feb;, 35(1), 43-7.

[2] Hagglund, M, Walden, M, & Ekstrand, J. Previous injury as a risk factor for injury in elite football: a prospective study over two consecutive seasons. British journal of sports medicine. (2006). Sep;, 40(9), 767-72.

[3] Andersen, T. E, Tenga, A, Engebretsen, L, & Bahr, R. Video analysis of injuries and incidents in Norwegian professional football. British journal of sports medicine. (2004). Oct;, 38(5), 626-31.

[4] Ekstrand, J, Hagglund, M, & Walden, M. Injury incidence and injury patterns in professional football: the UEFA injury study. British journal of sports medicine. (2011). Jun;, 45(7), 553-8.

[5] Dvorak, J, Junge, A, Derman, W, & Schwellnus, M. Injuries and illnesses of football players during the 2010 FIFA World Cup. British journal of sports medicine. (2011). Jun;, 45(8), 626-30.

[6] Chamari, K, & Haddad, M. Wong del P, Dellal A, Chaouachi A. Injury rates in professional soccer players during Ramadan. Journal of sports sciences. (2012). Jul;30 Suppl 1:SS102., 93.

[7] Rejeski, W. J, Foy, C. G, Brawley, L. R, Brubaker, P. H, Focht, B. C, Norris, J. L, et al. Older adults in cardiac rehabilitation: a new strategy for enhancing physical function. Medicine and science in sports and exercise. (2002). Nov;, 34(11), 1705-13.

[8] Dupont, G, Nedelec, M, Mccall, A, Mccormack, D, Berthoin, S, & Wisloff, U. Effect of 2 soccer matches in a week on physical performance and injury rate. Am J Sports Med. (2011). Sep;, 38(9), 1752-8.

[9] Dvorak, J, Junge, A, Grimm, K, & Kirkendall, D. Medical report from the 2006 FIFA World Cup Germany. British journal of sports medicine. (2007). Sep;discussion 81., 41(9), 578-81.

[10] Ekstrand, J, Walden, M, & Hagglund, M. A congested football calendar and the well-being of players: correlation between match exposure of European footballers before the World Cup 2002 and their injuries and performances during that World Cup. British journal of sports medicine. (2004). Aug;, 38(4), 493-7.

[11] Carling, C. Le Gall F, Dupont G. Are physical performance and injury risk in a professional soccer team in match-play affected over a prolonged period of fixture congestion? International journal of sports medicine. (2012). Jan;, 33(1), 36-42.

[12] Dellal, A, Lago-peñas, C, Rey, E, Chamari, K, & Orhant, E. The effect of a congested fixture period on physical performance, technical activity and injury rate during

matches in a professional soccer team. British journal of sports medicine. Accepted (2012). In press.

[13] Rahnama, N, Reilly, T, & Lees, A. Injury risk associated with playing actions during competitive soccer. British journal of sports medicine. (2002). Oct;, 36(5), 354-9.

[14] Reilly, T. Energetics of high-intensity exercise (soccer) with particular reference to fatigue. Journal of sports sciences. (1997). Jun;, 15(3), 257-63.

[15] Saltin, B. Metabolic fundamentals in exercise. Medicine and science in sports. (1973). Fall;, 5(3), 137-46.

[16] Schlabach, G. Carbohydrate strategies for injury prevention. Journal of athletic training. (1994). , 29(3), 244-54.

[17] Worrell, T. W, & Perrin, D. H. Hamstring muscle injury: the influence of strength, flexibility, warm-up, and fatigue. J Orthop Sports Phys Ther. (1992). , 16(1), 12-8.

[18] Jacobs, I, Westlin, N, Karlsson, J, Rasmusson, M, & Houghton, B. Muscle glycogen and diet in elite soccer players. European journal of applied physiology and occupational physiology. (1982). , 48(3), 297-302.

[19] Ivy, J. L. Dietary strategies to promote glycogen synthesis after exercise. Can J Appl Physiol. (2001). Suppl:S, 236-45.

[20] Convertino, V. A, Armstrong, L. E, Coyle, E. F, Mack, G. W, Sawka, M. N, Senay, L. C, et al. American College of Sports Medicine position stand. Exercise and fluid replacement. Medicine and science in sports and exercise. (1996). Jan;28(1):i-vii.

[21] Bergeron, M. F, Mckeag, D. B, Casa, D. J, Clarkson, P. M, Dick, R. W, Eichner, E. R, et al. Youth football: heat stress and injury risk. Medicine and science in sports and exercise. (2005). Aug;, 37(8), 1421-30.

[22] Taylor, S. R, Rogers, G. G, & Driver, H. S. Effects of training volume on sleep, psychological, and selected physiological profiles of elite female swimmers. Medicine and science in sports and exercise. (1997). May;, 29(5), 688-93.

[23] Belenky, G, Wesensten, N. J, Thorne, D. R, Thomas, M. L, Sing, H. C, Redmond, D. P, et al. Patterns of performance degradation and restoration during sleep restriction and subsequent recovery: a sleep dose-response study. J Sleep Res. (2003). Mar;, 12(1), 1-12.

[24] Luke, A, Lazaro, R, Bergeron, M, Keyser, L, Benjamin, H, Brenner, J, et al. Sports-Related Injuries in Youth Athletes: Is Overscheduling a Risk Factor? Clinical journal of sport medicine. (2011). , 21(4), 307-14.

[25] Chaouachi, A, Leiper, J. B, Souissi, N, Coutts, A. J, & Chamari, K. Effects of Ramadan intermittent fasting on sports performance and training: a review. International journal of sports physiology and performance. (2009). a Dec;, 4(4), 419-34.

[26] Leiper, J. B, Molla, A. M, & Molla, A. M. Effects on health of fluid restriction during fasting in Ramadan. Eur J Clin Nutr. (2003). Dec;57 Suppl 2:S, 30-8.

[27] Leiper, J. B, Maughan, R. J, Kirkendall, D. T, Bartagi, Z, Zerguini, Y, Junge, A, et al. The F-MARC study on Ramadan and football: research design, population, and environmental conditions. Journal of sports sciences. (2008). Dec;26 Suppl 3:S, 7-13.

[28] Maughan, R. J, Fallah, J, & Coyle, E. F. The effects of fasting on metabolism and performance. British journal of sports medicine. (2010). Jun;, 44(7), 490-4.

[29] Waterhouse, J. Effects of Ramadan on physical performance: chronobiological considerations. British journal of sports medicine. (2010). Jun;, 44(7), 509-15.

[30] Güvenç, A. Effects of Ramadan Fasting on Body Composition, Aerobic Performance and Lactate, Heart Rate and Perceptual Responses in Young Soccer Journal of Human Kinetics. 2011 Tuesday, October 04, (2011). Volume 29 / September 2011):79-91., 29

[31] Chaouachi, A, Coutts, A. J, & Chamari, K. Wong del P, Chaouachi M, Chtara M, et al. Effect of Ramadan intermittent fasting on aerobic and anaerobic performance and perception of fatigue in male elite judo athletes. Journal of strength and conditioning research / National Strength & Conditioning Association. (2009). b Dec;, 23(9), 2702-9.

[32] Chaouachi, A, & Coutts, A. J. Wong del P, Roky R, Mbazaa A, Amri M, et al. Haematological, inflammatory, and immunological responses in elite judo athletes maintaining high training loads during Ramadan. Applied physiology, nutrition, and metabolism = Physiologie appliquee, nutrition et metabolisme. (2009). c Oct;, 34(5), 907-15.

[33] Johnson, M. B, & Thiese, S. M. A review of overtraining syndrome-recognizing the signs and symptoms. Journal of athletic training. (1992). , 27(4), 352-4.

[34] Hooper, S. L, & Mackinnon, L. T. Monitoring overtraining in athletes. Recommendations. Sports medicine. (1995a). , 20(5), 321-7.

[35] Fuller, C. W, Ekstrand, J, Junge, A, Andersen, T. E, Bahr, R, Dvorak, J, et al. Consensus statement on injury definitions and data collection procedures in studies of football (soccer) injuries. Scandinavian journal of medicine & science in sports. (2006). Apr;, 16(2), 83-92.

[36] Koutedakis, Y, & Sharp, N. C. Seasonal variations of injury and overtraining in elite athletes. Clin J Sport Med. (1998). Jan;, 8(1), 18-21.

[37] Hooper, S. L, & Mackinnon, L. T. Monitoring overtraining in athletes. Recommendations. Sports medicine (Auckland, NZ. (1995b). , 20(5), 321-7.

[38] Kirkendall, D. T, Chaouachi, A, Aziz, A. R, & Chamari, K. Strategies for maintaining fitness and performance during Ramadan. Journal of sports sciences. (2012). Suppl 1:S, 103-8.

[39] Czeisler, C. A, Weitzman, E, Moore-ede, M. C, Zimmerman, J. C, & Knauer, R. S. Human sleep: its duration and organization depend on its circadian phase. Science (New York, NY. (1980). Dec 12;, 210(4475), 1264-7.

[40] Duffy, J. F, Kronauer, R. E, & Czeisler, C. A. Phase-shifting human circadian rhythms: influence of sleep timing, social contact and light exposure. J Physiol. (1996). Aug 15;495 (Pt 1):289-97.

[41] Bogdan, A, Bouchareb, B, & Touitou, Y. Ramadan fasting alters endocrine and neuro-endocrine circadian patterns. Meal-time as a synchronizer in humans? Life Sci. (2001). Feb 23;, 68(14), 1607-15.

[42] Montelpare, W. J, Plyley, M. J, & Shephard, R. J. Evaluating the influence of sleep deprivation upon circadian rhythms of exercise metabolism. Can J Sport Sci. (1992). Jun;, 17(2), 94-7.

[43] Reilly, T, & Waterhouse, J. Altered sleep-wake cycles and food intake: the Ramadan model. Physiol Behav. (2007). Feb 28;90(2-3):219-28.

[44] Kenttä, G, & Hassmén, P. Overtraining and recovery. A conceptual model. Sports medicine (Auckland, NZ. (1998). Jul;, 26(1), 1-16.

[45] Halson, S. L, & Jeukendrup, A. E. Does overtraining exist? An analysis of overreaching and overtraining research. Sports medicine (Auckland, NZ. (2004). , 34(14), 967-81.

Permissions

The contributors of this book come from diverse backgrounds, making this book a truly international effort. This book will bring forth new frontiers with its revolutionizing research information and detailed analysis of the nascent developments around the world.

We would like to thank Gian Nicola Bisciotti and Cristiano Eirale, for lending their expertise to make the book truly unique. They have played a crucial role in the development of this book. Without their invaluable contribution this book wouldn't have been possible. They have made vital efforts to compile up to date information on the varied aspects of this subject to make this book a valuable addition to the collection of many professionals and students.

This book was conceptualized with the vision of imparting up-to-date information and advanced data in this field. To ensure the same, a matchless editorial board was set up. Every individual on the board went through rigorous rounds of assessment to prove their worth. After which they invested a large part of their time researching and compiling the most relevant data for our readers. Conferences and sessions were held from time to time between the editorial board and the contributing authors to present the data in the most comprehensible form. The editorial team has worked tirelessly to provide valuable and valid information to help people across the globe.

Every chapter published in this book has been scrutinized by our experts. Their significance has been extensively debated. The topics covered herein carry significant findings which will fuel the growth of the discipline. They may even be implemented as practical applications or may be referred to as a beginning point for another development. Chapters in this book were first published by InTech; hereby published with permission under the Creative Commons Attribution License or equivalent.

The editorial board has been involved in producing this book since its inception. They have spent rigorous hours researching and exploring the diverse topics which have resulted in the successful publishing of this book. They have passed on their knowledge of decades through this book. To expedite this challenging task, the publisher supported the team at every step. A small team of assistant editors was also appointed to further simplify the editing procedure and attain best results for the readers.

Our editorial team has been hand-picked from every corner of the world. Their multi-ethnicity adds dynamic inputs to the discussions which result in innovative outcomes. These outcomes are then further discussed with the researchers and contributors who give their valuable feedback and opinion regarding the same. The feedback is then collaborated with the researches and they are edited in a comprehensive manner to aid the understanding of the subject.

Apart from the editorial board, the designing team has also invested a significant amount of their time in understanding the subject and creating the most relevant covers. They scrutinized every image to scout for the most suitable representation of the subject and create an appropriate cover for the book.

The publishing team has been involved in this book since its early stages. They were actively engaged in every process, be it collecting the data, connecting with the contributors or procuring relevant information. The team has been an ardent support to the editorial, designing and production team. Their endless efforts to recruit the best for this project, has resulted in the accomplishment of this book. They are a veteran in the field of academics and their pool of knowledge is as vast as their experience in printing. Their expertise and guidance has proved useful at every step. Their uncompromising quality standards have made this book an exceptional effort. Their encouragement from time to time has been an inspiration for everyone.

The publisher and the editorial board hope that this book will prove to be a valuable piece of knowledge for researchers, students, practitioners and scholars across the globe.

List of Contributors

Giuseppe D'Antona
Department of Molecular Medicine and Interdepartmental Research Centre in Motor Activities
(CRIAMS), University of Pavia, Italy

Cristiano Eirale
Qatar Orthopaedic and Sport Medicine Hospital, FIFA Center of Excellence, Doha, Qatar
Kinemove Rehabilitation Centers, Pontremoli, Parma, La Spezia, Italy

Gian Nicola Bisciotti
Qatar Orthopaedic and Sport Medicine Hospital, FIFA Center of Excellence, Doha, Qatar

Massimo Manara
Association of Parma, Italy

Danilo Manari
FC Parma, Italy

Giulio Pasta
Pasta Associate Clinic for Imaging Diagnostics, Italy

Francisco Arroyo
Medical Director, Sport Med. FIFA Medical Clinic of Excellence Guadalajara, Mexico

Andrea Foglia, Massimo Bitocchi, Manuela Gervasi and Gianni Secchiari
Department of Physiotherapy, "Riabilita" Centre, Civitanova Marche (MC), Italy

Angelo Cacchio
Department of Life, Health & Environmental Sciences, School of Medicine, University of L'Aquila, L'Aquila, Italy

Maria Conforti
Sports Physician and Physical Therapies Physician, Bergamo, Italy
Customer Point INAIL, Milan, Italy

Cristiano Eirale and Giannicola Bisciotti
Aspetar Hospital, Doha, Qatar

Giuliano Cerulli
University of Perugia, Perugia, Italy
Nicola's Foundation ONLUS Arezzo, Italy
Let People Move Research Institute Arezzo, Perugia, Italy
International Orthopedic and Traumatologic Institute Arezzo, Italy

Enrico Sebastiani, Giacomo Placella, Matteo Maria Tei and Andrea Speziali
Residency program in Orthopedics and Traumatology, University of Perugia, Perugia, Italy

Pierluigi Antinolfi
"Santa Maria della Misericordia" Hospital, Orthopedic and Traumatology Department, Perugia, Italy

M. Giacchino
Istituto di Medicina dello Sport F.M.S.I. Torino, Italy

G. Stesina
FC Juventus, Turin, Italy

Alexandre Dellal
FIFA Medical Excellence Centre, Santy Orthopedicae Clinical, Sport Science and Research Department, Lyon, France
OGC Nice, Fitness Training Department, Nice, France
Centre de recherche et d'Innovation sur le Sport (CRIS), Université de Lyon 1, Lyon, France

Karim Chamari
Research and Education Centre, Aspetar, Qatar Orthopaedic and Sports Medicine Hospital, Doha, Qatar

Adam Owen
Glasgow Rangers Sport Science Department (soccer), Glasgow, Scotland
Centre de recherche et d'Innovation sur le Sport (CRIS), Université de Lyon 1, Lyon, France

Karim Chamari
Research and Education Centre, Aspetar, Qatar Orthopaedic and Sports Medicine Hospital, Doha, Qatar

Alexandre Dellal
FIFA Medical Excellence Centre, Santy Orthopedicae Clinical, Sport Science and Research Department, Lyon, France
OGC Nice, Fitness Training Department, Nice, France
Centre de Recherche et d'Innovation sur le Sport (CRIS), Université de Lyon 1, Lyon, France

Monoem Haddad
Tunisian Research Laboratory "Sport Performance Optimisation", National Center of Medicine and Science in Sports (CNMSS), Tunis, Tunisia
Jandouba University, ISSEP Kef, Tunisia